D1051094

POTTER'S NEW CYCLOPAEDIA

OF

BOTANICAL DRUGS AND PREPARATIONS

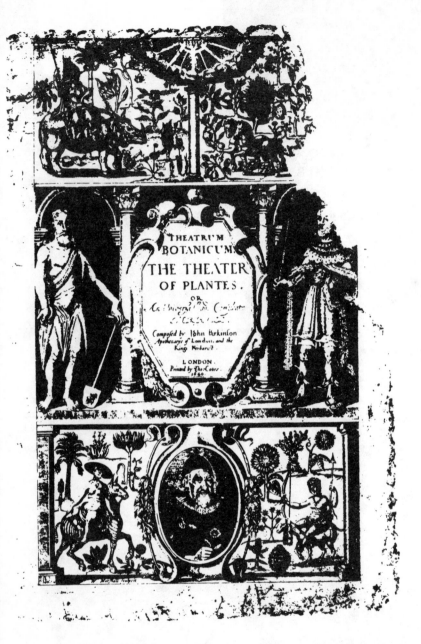

THEATRUM
BOTANICUM
THE THEATER
OF PLANTES.
OR
An Universall and Compleate
Herball.

Composed by John Parkinson
Apothecarye of London, and the
Kings Herbarist.

LONDON.
Printed by Tho. Cotes
1640

Fragment of the frontispiece to the Herball
written by John Parkinson,
King's Herbalist and printed in 1640

POTTER'S
NEW CYCLOPAEDIA
OF
BOTANICAL DRUGS
AND
PREPARATIONS

By
R. C. WREN, F.L.S.

REWRITTEN BY
ELIZABETH M. WILLIAMSON, B.Sc., Ph.D., M.R.Pharm.S., F.L.S.
AND
FRED J. EVANS,
D.Sc., B.Pharm., Ph.D., M.R.Pharm.S., F.L.S., M.N.I.M.H. (Hon.)

FOREWORD BY
T. E. WALLIS, D.Sc., F.R.I.C., F.P.S., M.I.Biol.

SAFFRON WALDEN
THE C.W. DANIEL COMPANY LIMITED

First published in 1907
and subsequently reprinted in 1915, 1923, 1932, 1939,
1950, 1956, 1968, 1970, 1971, 1973,
1980, 1982 and 1985

This completely revised edition was first published
in Great Britain in 1988 and reprinted in 1989 and 1994 by
The C. W. Daniel Company Limited
1 Church Path, Saffron Walden,
Essex, CB10 1JP, England

© Potter's (Herbal Supplies) Limited 1988

This book has been printed on 100% re-cycled
Envirowove paper

ISBN 0 85207 197 3

Designed by Jim Reader
Production in association with
Book Production Consultants, Cambridge
Typeset by Cambridge Photosetting Services
Printed and bound by Biddles, Guildford

Foreword

Many plants and parts of plants, usually in a dried condition, are still largely used in Britain as household remedies or as ingredients of orthodox medicine. It is important that reliable information should be available to enable dealers in these remedies to judge of their origin and quality. Some of them are defined and regulated by the descriptions in the *British Pharmacopoeia* and in the *British Pharmaceutical Codex*. There is, however, a very large number of materials, derived from the vegetable kingdom, which lie outside the scope of the two volumes named above. It is desirable, therefore, that some book or cyclopaedia should be compiled with the object of providing particulars by which the botanical drugs can be correctly authenticated. This kind of information is frequently needed by physicians, pharmacists and analysts, who receive inquiries relating to the identity and uses of numerous household remedies as well as those included in the pharmacopoeia and codex.

Potter's *New Cyclopaedia of Botanical Drugs and Preparations* brings together much valuable information which is scattered throughout botanical and medical literature and thus supplies a reference book which meets a need felt by both professional people and the lay public. This book has been carefully prepared and not only provides an account of characters for identification, but also gives a brief summary of the action and uses of the herbs described, together with a note of the preparations made from them.

Another direction in which difficulties frequently arise is in relation to nomenclature and this is helpfully treated in the Cyclopaedia. In addition to the accepted or scientific names, the popular names and other vernacular synonyms are included in the heading to each description and the full scientific name of the plant of origin is also given. All these names are carefully indexed and this index adds much to the value of the book and frequently enables the inquirer to ascertain the source of some obscure remedy and also to find an account of its reputed uses. The book is unique in the English language and is a valuable source of reference for all who are interested in the origin and uses of botanical drugs.

T. E. WALLIS

Preface

Potter's Cyclopaedia of botanical drugs and preparations is accepted world-wide as an authority on plant drugs and is used as a reference point for information by medical scientists, clinicians and laymen alike. To produce a new edition of this standard work was a daunting task, particularly in the present climate of renewed interest in herbal drugs, and because of the eminent status of previous editions. It is significant that this reference book has in fact been produced in eight previous editions, with a total of fourteen impressions from the date of initial publication in 1907 to the present day. Potter's Cyclopaedia therefore, with its continuing popularity as a book of reference, covers 80 years of British Herbal history and is the standard work on herbal drugs and the preparations derived from them. In this edition we have attempted to retain many of the features of the early editions. For example, where possible Biblical references and references to the herbals and philosophers of the past, introduced by R. W. Wren FLS, the son of the original author, have been retained, although in a somewhat attenuated form. We have also retained the Foreword written by Dr. T. E. Wallis, D.Sc., F.R.I.C., Ph.C, F.L.S. (Reader in Pharmacognosy, faculty of Medicine, University of London), not least because one of us now holds that appointment, but because the foreword is as pertinent today as it was in 1956. In essence we have attempted to retain the traditions of the book but at the same time to have documented recent scientific and medical research which corroborates the historical facts of earlier editions.

The first edition of the Cyclopaedia was written by Richard Cranfield Wren, F.L.S. R. C. Wren was an acknowledged authority on the cultivation, identification and preparation of herbal drugs. At that time the book was claimed to be more complete and up-to-date than any previous publication on the subject. It was obvious that Wren was concerned with the botanical authentication of the various species used in medicine and as home remedies at that time, in that he paid particular care to the documentation of the correct botanical names for the plants and included descriptions of the plants themselves. In the second edition published in 1915, R. C. Wren took his concern for authentication even further in that he collaborated with E. M. Holmes, F.L.S., curator of the Pharmaceutical Society Museum, to produce an updated version of the botanical aspects of the first edition. This collaboration was continued with the third edition when the same two authors produced a version of the Cyclopaedia in 1923 which additionally contained 200 line drawings reproduced from Benthams *Handbook of the British Flora*. These drawings, by W. H. Fitch, F.L.S. and W. S. Smith, F.L.S., were added to further assist the identification of living herbal plants growing in the countryside. Unfortunately the original line drawings are no longer capable of reproduction to modern printing standards. The fourth edition was published in 1932 and marked a development in the evolution of the Cyclopaedia in that R. W. Wren, F.L.S., M.P.S., the son of Richard Cranfield Wren, revised the book in conjunction with H. A. Potter, Ph.C.

This revision was undertaken following the death of the original author in 1930. The significant addition at that time was the inclusion of several colour plates of well known British herbal drugs. In successive editions published in 1939 and 1950 by R. W. Wren the descriptions were updated and herbal preparations were cross-referenced to official texts including the British Pharmacopoeia, the British Pharmaceutical Codex and the United States Pharmacopoeia, thereby creating a tradition of referenced authentication which has been continued in the present edition. One further revision was undertaken by Wren in 1956. For the seventh edition, and probably the edition which exhibits more of the character of that author than any other, Wren attempted to give a more philosophical background to herbal medicine and in so doing probably initiated a movement which currently has world wide support. Reference was made not only to the herbalists of antiquity such as Paracelsus, Galen, Dioscorides, Pliny and Theophrastos Eresios but also to English herbalists including John Gerard, John Hill, William Salmon, Benjamin Barton and Thomas Castle. Onto this was added a religous note in that biblical references to herbs were included. Decidedly a new feeling was created in the book. Our major problem in revising the Cyclopaedia has been to retain the philosophy of Wren and at the same time to attempt its substantiation in the light of modern scientific research. We are indebted to Mr Whittaker for revising the biblical references in this edition.

We have retained the descriptive character of the monographs because authentication of plant species, the main concern of the original author, is still a problem today. Herbal companies are required to apply ever more rigorous standards of authentication and quality control to their preparations. Such procedures require the rigid application of both botanical and chemical methods of analysis. Such protocols are available for some plant drugs from the European Pharmacopoeia and from National Pharmacopoeias around the world. Standard text books are also available for various aspects of the quality control procedure and include Jackson and Snowdon's *Powdered Vegetable Drugs*, Stahl's *Drug Analysis by Chromatography and Microscopy* and Wagner's *Thin layer Chromatographic Analysis of Plant Drugs*. Reference works available in this country include *The British Herbal Pharmacopoeia* and *Martindale, The Extra Pharmacopoeia*. Nevertheless, the descriptive passages of the Cyclopaedia are still a useful source of information. This book covers a wider range of plant species than other works, a total of 571 in all, and for some herbs provides the only readily available initial reference point. In addition the descriptions of the Cyclopaedia are of the living plants and contain notes as to habitat and time of flowering as well as listing synonyms used for the same species. The botanical names of the plants have been updated in the light of changes that continuously occur as a result of reclassification and we are grateful to the Herbarium, Kew Gardens, London for advice on this aspect of the monographs. In this edition we have given the common chemical names of the principle constituents of the herbs as far as they are known and have referenced each plant to the chemical literature. Plants contain a vast number of chemical entities, called secondary metabolites, and it is these substances which are believed to be responsible for the therapeutic activities of herbal preparations. The literature now available concerning the chemistry of plants is vast. We have made use of computer assisted literature searches in the Library of the School of Pharmacy, University of London and are grateful to Mrs. Lisgarten, the Librarian, for her assistance. The references quoted are not intended to be exhaustive in their coverage of the chemical literature of plants but represent, in our opinion, a selection of pertinent research papers. It is hoped that this information will be of assistance to analytical chemists involved in the quality control of herbal preparations and to medicinal chemists and biologists concerned with the mechanism of herbal drug actions. Such data will also be useful to herbal practitioners and to the interested laymen and may go some way towards substantiating the known therapeutic activities of plant drugs.

A further addition, introduced to this edition of the Cyclopaedia, is the regulatory status of each herb. The categories are, controlled drugs (CD), these are controlled by the misuse of drugs act, prescription only medicine (POM), a class of herbs only available on the prescription of a physician, Schedule 1 poisons as defined by the Pharmacy and Poisons Act 1933, Pharmacy medicines (P), available through a registered Pharmacist, and, general sales list (GSL) comprising drugs available for sale to the general public. Where no regulatory status is given the distribution of the herb is not controlled by British Law. Preparations of herbal drugs are referenced to the British Pharmacopoeia and to the British Pharmaceutical Codex where these are applicable. Other preparations and their dosage regemens are unchanged from previous editions, although the doses have been carefully converted to the metric system by Mr. H. Hall, M.P.S.

One essential feature of previous editions of the Cyclopaedia was the information given concerning the therapeutic usefulness of the herbs described. This information was largely drawn from tradition and represented a condensation of hundreds of years of human experience in the use of plants for the treatment of human disease. In the present edition this information has been supplemented by referencing to scientific and clinical literature, where such data is available. Some of the herbs described in *Potter's Cyclopaedia* have not as yet been the subject of recent research and further information is not available. The advent of a new Journal *Phytotherapy Research* devoted to the rapid publication of scientific and medical data relating to plant drugs bodes well for the future. Our attention to the data produced by the clinician and the biologist, in addition to purely chemical data, stems from the fact that such information is vital to the understanding of the safety and usefulness of plant drugs in medical practice. Herbs are complex mixtures of various chemicals and the whole plant or its extract represents the "drug". Individual chemical components contribute to the overall "drug" effect, known in Sino-Japanese medicine as the "Blend Effect", by virtue of complex pharmacological interactions including inhibition and synergism. In this edition of the Cyclopaedia 1381 references are made to the medical and chemical literature, many of which are concerned with the therapeutic or biological effects of plant constituents or whole plant drugs. We are grateful to Mrs. G. M. Evans for her careful reading of the manuscript and also to Mr. J. T. Hampson for not only suggesting this project to us but enabling the project to be completed on this the 175th anniversary of the foundation of Potter's Herbal Supplies Ltd.

Much has changed in the world of medicine and medical research over the 80 years of *Potter's Cyclopaedia*, but this book is still dedicated to all those with a belief in the power of herbs and plants to correct human disease conditions in a natural manner.

Fred J. Evans and
Elizabeth M. Williamson
October 1987.
The School of Pharmacy
University of London.

Contents

Introduction by H. Hall, M.P.S.
Technical Director, Potter's (Herbal Supplies) Limited

The plant kingdom has been mankind's main source of medicine since prehistoric times. So that in 1812 when Henry Potter 1st set up his business in Farringdon Street, London, as a Supplier of Herbs and Dealer in Leeches, there already existed a vast store of knowledge which had been passed down through the centuries. Much of this traditional information on the medicinal virtues of herbs has been documented in the ancient mediaeval Herbals, not only from Britain but also from the Americas, the Middle East, India and Asia.

Henry Potter 1st saw his herbal business expand in leaps and bounds. When in 1846 it passed to his nephew Henry Potter 2nd and *his* son, Henry Potter 3rd, the solid foundation for a business had been established. "Potter's" was set to become Europe's leading manufacturer of herbal remedies.

Henry Potter 3rd had one son, Henry Arthur, who had qualified as a pharmacist and, in 1896, had become a partner in the firm. In the same year his future colleague, R. C. Wren, F.L.S., who was then general manager also became a partner. The special talents which the two brought to the business, which had now become known as Potter & Clarke Limited, led to the rapid development of the company as manufacturing chemists and druggists, specialising in the extraction of crude drugs for the herbal and pharmaceutical industry, and for the well known range of Potter's proprietary herbal remedies.

R. C. Wren was particularly interested in the study of medicinal plants and, as the herbal business increased, he saw that there was an urgent need for a reference work which would serve as a complete guide for all those who used or handled botanical drugs. This was to include common and botanical titles, synonyms and therapeutic actions, with preparations and dosage. Under the title "Potter's Cyclopaedia of Botanical Drugs and Preparations as compiled by R. C. Wren", the first edition of the modern Herbal appeared in 1907.

After reorganisation in 1952, Potter's became known as Potter's (Herbal Supplies) Limited. They had then moved to their new location in Wigan, Lancashire, where the production of modern licenced herbal remedies has continued with renewed vigour. As with all other medicines, the latest and most sophisticated scientific techniques have been and continue to be used to control the manufacture and quality of a very comprehensive range of these traditional remedies. To this day, Potter's (Herbal Supplies) Limited continues its 175 year heritage by continuing to make available a full range of safe natural herbal medicines, which comply fully with all modern regulatory and legal requirements. Potter's is a government regulated licensed manufacturer of herbal medicines.

I first came to know Potter's Cyclopaedia in the third edition, published in 1923, when it really became my first textbook. Coming from a herbal background I had decided to consolidate my interest in herbal medicine within a qualification in pharmacy. This was to lead to my joining Potter's as a pharmacist in 1935 where close involvement in the herbal industry often required reference to the Cyclopaedia, then in its later editions. Now, in this the ninth edition, there is to be found a very concise and unique combination of the old with the new. The principal constituents of each herb are now given as they have been discovered in research into plant chemistry. Much of this new information on constituents is supportive of the known traditional therapeutic properties of many herbs, so, it is particularly gratifying to me to have been associated in some way with Dr. F. J. Evans and Dr. Elizabeth Williamson of London University in their re-writing of the Cyclopaedia into this modern state-of-the-art form. This new Potter's Cyclopaedia will prove invaluable to all those concerned with herbal medicine and with the scientific background to traditional herbal usage.

It is also with great satisfaction that I see that increasing numbers of medical professionals world wide are re-discovering the virtues, safety and effectiveness of time honoured herbal formulations; provided always, that the manufacturer is scientifically conscientious of proper herbal raw material identification, purity, potency and the dosage of the resulting product. Potter's sell a wide range of such products in dosage forms from the traditional herbal teas and teabags to modern capsules and tablets.

This long list of over 200 tried and tested products are especially well known for their beneficial results not only in the treatment of minor conditions but also for the treatment of more severe diseases like Arthritis, where all too often herbal medicine is the last resort, yet it is in these more difficult diseases that we often have our most outstanding results.

H. HALL, M.P.S.

Abbreviations for Weights and Measures

The following abbreviations are used in this work for the more common weights and measures—

cm	centimetre(s)
dr	drachm(s)
fl dr	fluid drachm(s)
fl oz	fluid ounce(s)
ft	foot (feet)
g	gramme(s)
gr	grain(s)
in	inch(es)
m	metres
mg	milligrammes
ml	millilitres
mm	millimetres
min	minim(s)
oz	ounce(s)
pt	pint

A

ABSCESS ROOT

Polemonium reptans L.
Fam. Polemoniaceae

Synonyms: American Greek Valerian, False Jacob's Ladder, Sweatroot.
Habitat: Native of Scandinavia.
Description: Rhizome slender, 2–5 cm long, about 3 mm diameter, with the bases of numerous stems on the upper surface, and tufts of slender, smooth, wiry, pale roots below.
Part Used: Rhizome.
Constituents: Unknown.
Medicinal Use: Diaphoretic, astringent and expectorant, it has been used in febrile and inflammatory conditions. An infusion produces copious sweating. No recent research is available.

ACACIA BARK

Acacia arabica Willd
A. decurrens Willd
Fam. Leguminosae

Synonyms: Babul Bark, Wattle Bark.
Habitat: A. *arabica* from N. Africa, *A. decurrens* from Australia.
Description: The bark appears in commerce as hard, rusty-brown pieces 3–10 mm thick, readily dividing into layers, fissured externally and striated and fibrous internally. *A. decurrens* is smoother than *A. arabica*.
Part Used: Bark.
Constituents: Condensed tannins, catechins [1], mucilage and flavonoids [2].
Medicinal Use: Seldom used medicinally although it has been used as an astringent. Joseph Miller in 1722 stated "it helps ulcers in the mouth and fastens loose teeth" [3]. Formerly used in the tanning industry.
Biblical References: Exodus 25–27, 30, 35–38; Deuteronomy 10:3; Isaiah 41:19. The references are to Shittim Wood, a variety of acacia, probably *A. arabica*, chosen for fabricating the tabernacle and its furniture due to its availability and hardness.

ACACIA GUM

Acacia senegal (L.) Willd
and other species
Fam. Leguminosae

Synonyms: Gum Acacia, Gum Arabic, Gum Senegal.
Habitat: North Africa, particularly the Sudan.
Description: The gum exudes from the tree naturally, and can be tapped from incisions made in the bark. The commercial gum appears in rounded or angular, often cracked, transparent pieces, the finest is known as Kordofan gum. Acacia gum is soluble 1:2 in water; the mucilage is usually made with hot or boiling water.

1

Constituents: The structure of the gum is not known completely, it is a high molecular weight polysaccharide containing residues of neutral sugars, e.g. galactose, arabinose and rhamnose, and acids e.g. galacturonic, glucuronic [1]. Acacia contains an oxidizing enzyme [4].

Medicinal Use: Demulcent, used for making emulsions and as an ingredient in compounds for the treatment of diarrhoea, catarrh etc. It is used more widely in the food industry as stabilizer and flavour fixative.

Preparations: Acacia and Tragacanth Powder BPC 1949; Acacia Mucilage BP; Compound Tragacanth Powder BP.

Regulatory Status: GSL.

ACONITE

Aconitum napellus L.
Fam. Ranunculaceae

Synonyms: Wolfsbane, Monkshood, Friar's Cap, Blue Rocket. There is an old story that wolves, tearing up roots of plants for food in winter, mistake this plant and die from its poison.

Habitat: It is indigenous to Central Europe, and according to Pliny is named after the Black Sea port Aconis. It is cultivated and naturalized extensively.

Description: The plant is robust, erect, with violet-blue flowers occurring in racemes, followed by capsules of angular, wrinkled seeds. The root is blackish, conical, with a 5–7 pointed star in the centre of the fracture which is white and starchy. Japanese aconite is *A. uncinatum* L. var *japonicum,* and *A. fisheri,* Indian aconite is *A. deinorhizum* and Chinese aconite *A. carmichaeli.*

Part Used: Root, occasionally leaves.

Constituents: (i) Terpenoid alkaloids, up to 1.2%, including aconitine, aconine, hypaconitine, neopelline, picraconitine, napelline, benzoylaconine, with traces of ephedrine and sparteine [1] (ii) Acids; aconitic, itaconic (iii) sugars and starch.

Medicinal Use: Sedative, anodyne, febrifuge. It is a powerful poison affecting the heart and central nervous system and therefore rarely used internally. Topically it is used for bruises, sciatica, rheumatic pain etc. It causes a tingling sensation followed by numbness. It must be borne in mind when using, that absorption through the skin may cause systemic poisoning [4]. Aconitine has a short-lived cardiotonic action followed by cardiac depression, weakening of contractility, arrhythmia and cardiac arrest. Aconine, the hydrolysed product, is very much less toxic [6]. Aconitine has a transient hypotensive activity whereas the herb, after heat treatment, has a transient pressor activity. A decoction of the herb or the total alkaloids increase coronary flow and cause vasodilation of the blood vessels in the limbs in animals [7]. Aconitine has analgesic activity, anti-inflammatory activity and local anaesthetic activity. In Chinese medicine Aconite is the principle constituent of many prescriptions for shock; and a preparation with the aconitine removed is used clinically for various forms of heart disease [7]. Recently some *Aconitum* species have been shown to have anti-tumour, antiviral, antibacterial and antipyretic activity in laboratory tests [8].

Preparations: Aconite, Belladonna and Chloroform Liniment BPC 1968; Aconite Tincture and Strong Aconite Tincture BPC 1949; Flemings Tincture of Aconite, adjusted to 0.2% w/v total alkaloid; Aconite Liniment BPC 1968.

Regulatory Status: POM.

ACORNS
Quercus robur L.
Fam. Fagaceae

Description: The fruit of the oak tree.

Constituents: Tannins, flavonoids, sugar, starch, albumin and fixed oil [2].

Medicinal Use: Astringent; an old remedy for diarrhoea, where they are powdered or grated and washed down with water. Roasted acorns have been used as a substitute for coffee although there is no mention of the taste.

ADDER'S TONGUE, AMERICAN
Erythronium americanum
Ker-Gawl
Fam. Liliaceae

Synonyms: Serpent's Tongue, Dog's Tooth Violet, Yellow Snowdrop.

Habitat: USA.

Description: Flowers; yellow, star-shaped, about 2 cm across, with 6 stamens. Leaves; two only, about 6 cm long by 2–3 cm wide, minutely wrinkled and with parallel veins. Corms spindle-shaped, up to about 2 cm long. Taste sweetish.

Part Used: Fresh leaves.

Constituents: α-methylenebutyrolactone [2]; unknown substances.

Medicinal Use: Emetic, emollient. The fresh leaves are used as a poultice for ulcers, together with an infusion taken internally. The aqueous extract has some activity against G+ve and G−ve bacteria [9].

ADDER'S TONGUE, ENGLISH
Ophioglossum vulgatum L.
Fam. Ophioglossaceae

Synonyms: Serpent's Tongue

Habitat: Moist meadows in Great Britain, it flowers in April or May.

Description: The plant has a solitary leaf, lanceolate with forked veins and bearing a stalked, linear spike of spore-cases, in double row which resembles an adder's tongue.

Part Used: Herb.

Constituents: Unknown.

Medicinal Use: Similar to that of American Adder's Tongue (qv). An ointment has been made by boiling the herb in oil or fat, for use on wounds.

ADRUE
Cyperus articulatus L.
Fam. Cyperaceae

Synonyms: Guinea Rush.

Habitat: Turkey.

Description: Blackish, top-shaped tubers, with bristly remains of former leaves, sometimes connected in twos or threes by narrow underground stems. Transverse section pale, showing a central column with darker vascular bundles. Taste bitter, odour aromatic, recalling that of lavender.

Part Used: Root.

Constituents: A sesquiterpene ketone "articulone" which is identical to cyperone [10].

Medicinal Use: Anti-emetic, a carminative and sedative in peptic disorders.

Preparations: Fluid Extract: dose 0.7–2 ml.

AGAR
Gelidium amansii Lamour and other spp of
Gelidium and *Gracilaria*
Fam. Rhodophyceae

Synonyms: Agar-Agar, Japanese Isinglass.

Habitat: The main seaweeds from which agar is prepared are indigenous to Japan, but many other countries now produce it.

Description: Agar is the dried mucilaginous extract, obtained by boiling, filtering and drying. It occurs in translucent strips or as a powder, it is colourless and tasteless and capable of absorbing up to 200 times its volume of water to form a jelly.

Part Used: Extract.

Constituents: The structure is complicated. Most agars consist of two major polygalactoses, the neutral agarose and the sulphonated poly-saccharide agaropectin, with traces of amino acids and free sugars [2].

Medicinal Use: Nutritive, bulk-laxative. Often made into an emulsion with liquid paraffin for the treatment of constipation.

Preparations: Liquid Paraffin Emulsion with Agar BPC 1949: dose 10–30 ml.

Regulatory Status: GSL.

AGARICUS
Fomes officinalis Faull.
Fam. Polyporaceae

Synonyms: White Agaric, Larch Agaric, Purging Agaric, *Boletus laricis*.

Habitat: It is a fungus growing in larch forests in Europe and Russia.

Description: Occurs in white, spongy, friable masses. The surface is brownish and the internal structure white and porous. The odour is mealy and the taste sweetish with a bitter acrid after-taste.

Part Used: Upper part (fruiting body).

Constituents: (i) Resin, including agaricin (agaric acid), (ii) Triterpene acids (iii) Polyacetylenes (unspecified) [2].

Medicinal Use: Astringent in small doses, it has been used to alleviate night sweats and diarrhoea and to dry maternal milk after weaning. Purgative in large doses, and may cause vomiting. The closely related fungus *Poria cocos* Wolf ("Hoelen") is used in Oriental medicine for many conditions; it contains the triterpenoids eburicoic acid, dehydroeburicoic acid, tumulosic and related acids, pachymic acid and polyporenic acid which are cytotoxic against hepatoma *in vitro* [11], and the polysaccharide pachyman, which although devoid of antitumour activity itself, hydrolyses to give the active pachymaran [12]. It has also been found to have a protective effect on stress-induced ulcer in mice [13]. Dose: 0.2–2 g.

AGRIMONY

Agrimonia eupatoria L.
Fam. Rosaceae

Synonyms: Cocklebur, Stickwort.

Habitat: British Isles, in hedges and fields and by ditches, flowering in July and August.

Description: The leaves, green above and silver-grey underneath, are hairy, 10 cm or longer, with 3–5 pairs of lanceolate, toothed leaflets of different sizes, and half-cordate, toothed stipules. The flowers are small and composed of five yellow petals with hairy calices, placed on long, slender spikes. The fruit is small, subconical and ribbed, with hooked bristles. Each contains two seeds. Taste astringent, slightly bitter.

Part Used: Herb.

Constituents: (i) Tannins, as condensed tannins, up to ca. 8% (ii) Coumarins (uncharacterized) (iii) Flavonoids, e.g. glucosides of luteolin, apigenin and quercetin (iv) Volatile oil (v) Polysaccharides (ca 20%) [13].

Medicinal Use: Mild astringent, diuretic, tonic, as a simple infusion. Luteolin 7-glucoside has a cholegogic action [13]. The infusion has been used clinically with some success in cutaneous porphyria [14]. Aqueous extracts inhibited *Mycobacterium tuberculosis, in vitro* [15] and ethanolic extracts have shown anti-viral effects against Colombia SK virus in mice [16]. "Agrimophol", isolated from *Agrimonia* spp., is used in Chinese Medicine.

Preparations: Liquid Extract: dose 2–4 ml.

Potter's Products: Pile Compound Herb, Rheumatic Pain Tablets, Stomach and Liver Medicinal Tea Bags, Pile Mixture No. 91.

Regulatory Status: GSL.

ALDER, BLACK, AMERICAN

Prinos verticillatus L.
Fam. Aquifoliaceae

Synonyms: Winterberry, Feverbush.
Habitat: USA and Canada.
Description: Bark: brownish-grey, in quilled thin pieces, with whitish patches surrounded by black margins on outer surface and a greenish or yellowish inner surface. Berries: resemble those of the common Holly. Taste bitter and acid.
Part Used: Bark, berries.
Constituents: Unknown.
Medicinal Use: Antiseptic, cathartic.
Preparations: Liquid Extract: dose 2–4 ml.

ALDER, ENGLISH

Alnus glutinosa Gaertn.
Fam. Betulaceae

Synonyms: Betula alnus var *glutinosa* L.
Habitat: Grows commonly in Britain in damp woods and near water, flowering in April and May.
Description: The bark usually occurs in curved or quilled thin pieces, brownish-grey externally and brownish-orange on the inner surface, the fracture is short and uneven.
Part Used: Bark, leaves.
Constituents: Bark: (i) Lignans including dimethoxyisolariciresinol [17] (ii) 10–20% Tannin (iii) Emodin (iv) Phenolic glycosides e.g. lyonoside (v) misc anulin, protanulin, phlobaphene and triterpenes [2]. Leaves: Flavonoid glycosides, resin, sugars [2].
Medicinal Use: Bark: tonic and astringent, used as a decoction as a gargle for sore throats. Leaves: rarely used for inflammations.

ALKANET

Alkanna tinctoria (L.) Tausch
Fam. Boraginaceae

Synonyms: Dyer's Bugloss, Spanish Bugloss, Anchusa, Alkanna, Orchanet.
Habitat: Indigenous to SE Europe, a common garden plant in Britain, flowering in July and August.
Description: Root up to 10 cm long, the rootbark is purplish and easily separated from the woody centre which is yellowish. The leaves are long, narrow and hairy, the flowers blue or purple and trumpet-shaped.
Part Used: Root.
Constituents: Up to 5% alkannins, which are lipophilic isohexenylnaphthazarin red pigments [18], tannin, and wax. Recently a pyrrolizidine alkaloid has been isolated from the herb [19] but it is not known whether these hepatotoxic alkaloids occur in extracts used for medicinal or food purposes.

Medicinal Use: Rarely used medicinally but has astringent properties. The alkannins have antimicrobial and wound-healing properties, they have been used clinically for indolent ulcers [18]. They are non-toxic in mice [20].

Dioscorides said that "it helps those bitten by venomous beasts, and that to chew the root and spit into the mouth of the serpent will instantly kill the reptile". Normally used in a much more mundane fashion for colouring sausages and other foodstuffs.

ALLSPICE
Pimento dioica (L.) Merr
Fam. Myrtaceae

Synonyms: Pimento, Pimenta, Jamaican Pepper, Clove pepper, *Pimenta officinalis* Lindl., *Eugenia pimenta* DC.

Habitat: Native of the West Indies, cultivated in Central America; mainly imported from Jamaica and Cuba. Flowers June–August, with berries appearing soon after.

Description: The tree is an evergreen, up to 13 m in height, bearing small white flowers. The fruits are brown, globular, about 0.75 cm in diameter with a rough surface and the remains of the calyx present as a ring of teeth at the apex. There are two kidney-shaped seeds. Odour aromatic, clove-like.

Part Used: Unripe fruit, occasionally leaves used for oil production.

Constituents: (i) Volatile oil, 3–4.5%, the major component of which is eugenol, 60–80%, with cineole, methyleugenol, α-phellandrene, caryophyllene, cadinols and many others in trace amounts [21]. The leaf oil consists mainly of eugenol (*ca* 95%) [5] (ii) Protein, lipids, vitamins A, C, B_1, B_2 and niacin, minerals.

Medicinal Use: Aromatic carminative, often used as an adjunct in the treatment of flatulence, dyspepsia and diarrhoea. Eugenol has local anaesthetic and antiseptic properties. The oil is larvicidal [22], antioxidant [23], and enhances trypsin activity [24]. It is used mainly as a condiment and spice.

Preparations: Powdered fruit, dose: 0.5–2 g. Liquid Extract, dose 2–4 ml. Pimento Oil BPC 1949, dose: 0.05 to 0.2 ml.

Regulatory Status: GSL.

ALMONDS, BITTER
ALMONDS, SWEET
Prunus amygdalus Batsch var *amara*
Prunus amygdalus Batsch var *dulcis*
Fam. Rosaceae

Synonyms: Jordan Almonds, *Prunus communis* (L.) Arc. *Amygdalus communis* L.

Habitat: The almond tree is a native of Western Asia but is extensively cultivated.

Description: The fruit is botanically a drupe, the almond is the seed and is too well known to need describing.

Part Used: Seed, oil.

Constituents: (i) Fixed oil, 35–45%, known as Almond Oil or Sweet Almond Oil, made from both varieties. It consists of triglycerides, mainly triolein and trioloelinolein, with fatty acids including palmitic, lauric, myristic and oleic. [25] (ii) Volatile oil, known as Bitter Almond Oil, distilled from Bitter Almonds only, and consisting of about 95% benzaldehyde with 2–3% amygdalin, a cyanogenetic glycoside which is removed before sale (iii) Other substances such as protein, sterols, prunasin, vitamin E and minerals [5].

Medicinal Use: Almond Oil is used largely as an emollient, alone or as an ingredient of cosmetics. It is also taken internally as a nutrient, demulcent and mild laxative. Bitter Almond Oil is used mainly as a flavouring agent, in large doses it is toxic, causing CNS depression and respiratory failure [26]. Almond flour from which the oil has been removed is used in some diabetic foods as it does not contain starch.

Preparations: Almond Oil BP, dose: 15–30 ml; Almond Mixture BPC 1934, dose; 15–30 ml; Compound Powder of Almond BPC 1934, Lotion of Bitter Almonds BPC, 1934.

Regulatory Status: GSL.

Biblical References: Genesis 43 : 11; Exodus 25 : 33–34; 37 : 19–20; Numbers 17 : 8; Ecclesiastes 12 : 5; Jeremiah 1 : 11.

ALOES

(1) Aloe barbadensis Mill
(2) Aloe ferox Mill
(3) Aloe perryi Baker
(4) other species and hybrids
Fam. Liliaceae

Synonyms: (1) Barbados Aloes, Curacao Aloes, *Aloe vera* Tourn ex L., *A. vera* (L.) Webb. (2) Cape Aloes (3) Socotrine Aloes, Zanzibar Aloes.

Habitat: (1) West Indies (2) Southern Africa (3) East Africa.

Description: Aloes is the liquid which drains from the cut leaves, evaporated to dryness. The different species can be distinguished by their appearance and by simple chemical tests: Barbados Aloes is livery or opaque and gives a crimson colour with nitric acid, Cape Aloes is translucent and gives a similar colour reaction, Socotrine Aloes is opaque but gives no colour reaction.

Constituents: (i) Anthraquinone glycosides, known as "Aloin", up to 25%; mainly barbaloin, a C-glycoside of aloe-emodin, with isobarbaloin present in Barbados Aloes only, and other minor C- and O-glycosides (ii) free aloe-emodin in small amounts (iii) chromones (iv) resins [1].

Medicinal Use: Aloes is used internally as a purgative, acting on the lower bowel, and was formerly used as an emmenagogue. It is a useful laxative but overdosage may cause gastritis, diarrhoea and nephritis [4]. The tendency to cause griping is counteracted by taking it in conjunction with anti-spasmodics such as Belladonna (q.v.) and carminatives. Aloe-emodin is reported to have anti-cancer activity *in vitro* [27]. Aloes is used as a flavouring ingredient in low concentrations and topically as an ingredient of sun creams (See also Aloe Vera), and as a paint to discourage nail biting, due to its intensely bitter taste.

Preparations: Aloes, dose: 100–300 mg; Conc. Compound Aloes Decoction BPC 1949, dose: 4–15 ml; Aloes Ext. BPC 1949, dose: 60–250 mg; Aloes and Iron Pills BPC 1949, dose: 1 or 2 pills; Aloes and Nux Vomica Pills BPC 1959, dose: 1 or 2 pills; Aloes Pills BP 1948, dose: 250–500 mg; Aloes and Nux Vomica Tablets BPC 1959, dose: 1 or 2 tablets; Aloes Tincture BPC 1949, dose: 2–8 ml.

Potter's Products: Natural Herb Tablets, Bile and Liver Tablets No. 167, Skin Eruptions Mixture, Stomach Mixture, Constipation Mixture No. 105.

Regulatory Status: GSL. Maximum dose 100 mg.

Biblical References: Numbers 24:6; Psalms 45:8; Proverbs 7:17; Song of Solomon 4:14; John 19:39. These probably refer to *Aquilaria agallocum*.

ALOE VERA

Aloe barbadensis Mill
and others; see Aloes
Fam. Liliaceae

Synonyms: Aloe Vera Gel.

Habitat: Cultivated varieties grown mainly for their reduced anthraquinone content.

Description: Aloe Vera is a mucilaginous gel obtained from the parenchyma tissue in the centre of the leaf, obtained by mechanical or chemical means. This means the product is highly variable in its properties.

Constituents: (i) Polysaccharides, mainly glucomannans [5] (ii) Anthraquinone glycosides (see Aloes) (iii) Glycoproteins [28] (iv) Others, including sterols, saponins and organic acids [5].

Medicinal Use: Topically to aid wound healing, relieve burns including sunburn, as an emollient and for colonic irrigation. Recently extracts have been shown to enhance phagocytosis in adult bronchial asthma [28]. It is an ingredient of many cosmetic preparations.

ALSTONIA BARK

Alstonia scholaris (L.) R Br.
Alstonia constricta F v Muell
Fam. Apocynaceae

Synonyms: A. scholaris = *Echites scholaris* L., Devil Tree, Dita Bark *A. constricta* = Fever Bark, Australian Quinine, Australian Febrifuge.

Habitat: A scholaris is a native of India and the Philippine Islands but is found in many areas of the tropics, *A. constricta* is native to Australia.

Description: A. scholaris occurs in irregular fragments, up to about 1 cm thick, externally rough, brownish-grey, often with darker spots. Inner surface buff coloured, fracture short and granular. *A. constricta* occurs in quilled pieces, it has a thick brown cork and is deeply fissured. The inner surface is yellowish-brown and coarsely striated, fracture fibrous. Both taste bitter.

Part Used: Bark.

Constituents: Indole alkaloids. *A. scholaris* contains akuammidine and related alkaloids, echitamine, echitenine, echitine, echitamidine, nareline, picrinine, strictamine and others, [29], scholarine, and the recently isolated scholaricine [30]. *A. constricta* contains alstonine and derivatives, alstonidine, alstoniline, reserpine, α-yohimbine, vincamajine and related alkaloids [29].

Medicinal Use: Febrifuge, spasmolytic and anti-hypertensive. The hypotensive effects of echitamine have been demonstrated [31] and reserpine is used for the same purpose. *A. scholaris* has produced a fall in temperature in human patients with fevers [32], however there is conflicting evidence as to whether it is a true anti-malarial. Echitamine has been demonstrated to be devoid of activity against a strain of *Plasmodium berghei* in one report [33] and active in another [34]. It has been used as a remedy for rheumatism, and as a tonic in the past, although this cannot be recommended. *A. constricta* is a uterine stimulant [35], this is thought to be due to the reserpine content [36], and should therefore be avoided in pregnant women.

Preparations: Powdered bark, dose: 0.1–5 g; Liquid Extract, dose: 4–40 drops (0.3–3 ml); Tincture (1 in 8), dose: 1–4 ml; Infusion, dose: 15–30 ml.

AMADOU

Fomes fomentarius (L.) Fries
Fam. Polyporaceae

Synonyms: Surgeon's Agaric, German Tinder, Oak Agaric, *Polyporus fomentarius.*

Habitat: A fungus growing upon oak and beech trees in Europe and the British Isles.

Description: A hoof-shaped, obliquely triangular, sessile fungus. The inner part is composed of short tubular fibres arranged in layers. It is prepared for use by being sliced, beaten, soaked in a solution of nitre and dried.

Constituents: Fomentaric acid, mannofucogalactan and other polysaccharides [2].

Medicinal Use: Amadou has been used for arresting haemorrhages, being applied with pressure to the affected part; and for treating ingrown toenails, by inserting between the nail and flesh.

AMARANTH

Amaranthus hypochondriacus L.
Fam. Amaranthaceae

Synonyms: Love-Lies-Bleeding, Red Cockscomb, *Amaranthus melancholicus* L.

Habitat: A common garden plant, flowering from August until the first frosts.

Description: Rounded tufts of minute flowers, hidden by tapering crimson bracts, are borne on flattened stems.

Part Used: Flowering herb.
Constituents: A magenta-red pigment consisting mainly of trisodium 3-hydroxy-4-(4-sulphonaphth-1-ylazo)-naphthalene-2,7-disulphonate, also referred to as Amaranth.
Medicinal Use: Astringent; used in menorrhagia and diarrhoea as a decoction, and internally as an application in ulcerated conditions of the mouth and throat. Amaranth is used more often as a colouring for food and medicines. Reports of teratogenicity and carcinogenicity have not been adequately substantiated and Amaranth is presumed to be safe at present [4].
Preparations: Liquid Extract, dose: 2–4 ml.

AMMONIACUM

Dorema ammoniacum Don and other spp.
Fam. Umbelliferae

Synonyms: Gum Ammoniacum.
Habitat: From the Middle East to Northern Russia.
Description: The gum-resin occurs in rounded nodules, or rarely, compacted into masses, which are opaque, whitish becoming brown with age, with a glossy fracture and an acrid taste. It forms an emulsion with water which is turned orange-red with chlorinated lime.
Part Used: Gum-resin from the flowering and fruiting stems.
Constituents: (i) Resin (60–70%), consisting mainly of amino-resinol (ii) Gum [37] (iii) Volatile oil, about 0.5%, containing ferulene as the major component, with linalyl acetate, citronellyl acetate, ferulene, doremyl alcohol and doremone [38] (iv) Free salicylic acid (v) Coumarins; not including umbelliferone which should be absent [37].
Medicinal Use: Antispasmodic, expectorant, diaphoretic. It is useful in chronic conditions of the respiratory tract, in coughs, asthma, bronchitis and catarrh.
Preparations: Powdered gum-resin; dose 0.3–1 g.
Regulatory Status: GSL.

ANGELICA

Angelica archangelica L.
Fam. Umbelliferae

Synonyms: European Angelica, *Angelica officinalis* Moench.
Habitat: Angelica is a common garden plant in Britain, and grows wild in many European countries. It flowers in June–July.
Description: The plant grows to a height of up to 2 m, with broad, pointed, serrated leaves which are larger at the base of the plant. The stalk is cylindrical and hollow, and green in colour. The flowers are small and greenish-white, arranged in large, almost spherical umbels. The fruits are whitish, plano-convex, oblong with rounded ends, about 0.5 cm long and 0.25 cm wide, winged at the margins, with three longitudinal ridges on the convex and two on the flat side. The root in commerce is 5–10 cm long, 2–5 cm in diameter, and very hard and fibrous. The fresh root when cut

11

yields a thick yellowish juice. The transverse section shows a brown bark and white inside, with numerous oil cells in the bark. American Angelica is *A. atropurpurea,* which has similar properties and a purplish root.

Part Used: Root, seeds and leaves.

Constituents: Volatile oil, obtained mainly from the root and seeds; this has a similar composition, consisting of (i) Terpenes, mainly β-phellandrene, with β-bisabolene, β-caryophyllene, α-phellandrene, α- and β-pinene, limonene, linalool, borneol, acetaldehyde, [5], menthadienes and nitro-menthadienes [39], (ii) Macrocyclic lactones including ϖ-tridecanolide, 12-methyl-ϖ-tridecanolide, ϖ-pentadecanolide [40], (iii) phthalates such as hexamethylphthalate (in a Pakistani variety) [41], (iv) Coumarins, especially furocoumarin glycosides such as marmesin, apterin and their dihydro- and hydroxyderivatives [42]; angelicin and byakangelicin derivatives [43], osthol, umbelliferone, psoralen, bergapten, imperatoren, xanthotoxol, xanthotoxin, oxypeucedanin and more, [5] (v) Miscellaneous sugars, plant acids, flavonoids and sterols [5].

Medicinal Use: Expectorant, diaphoretic, carminative and diuretic. It has been used to treat coughs and colds as well as indigestion and many other ailments. The dry extract has been shown to have anti-inflammatory activity [44], and the root oil is reported to inhibit bacterial and fungal growth [45]. Xanthotoxol has anti-nicotinic effects [46].

Many furocoumarins, notably psoralen and 8-methoxypsoralen, can cause photosensitivity (or phototoxicity), in sensitive individuals; these substances are used in the photochemotherapy of psoriasis and vitiligo. Their biological activity is due to covalent linkages formed with DNA by irradiation with long-wavelength UV light [47].

Angelica is used frequently as a flavouring; in liqueurs such as chartreuse and benedictine, in gin and vermouth; the leaves as a garnish or in salads, and the candied stalks in cakes and puddings.

In Chinese medicine, other species of Angelica are used, such as *A. sinensis,* which is very highly thought of and used widely. In a clinical trial the root of this plant was shown to be effective in improving abnormal protein metabolism in 60% of patients with chronic hepatitis or cirrhosis of the liver, and increased the erythrocyte and platelet count in many of the patients [48].

Preparations: Powdered root, dose: 0.5–2 g; Liquid Extract of Root, dose: 2–4 ml; Liquid Extract of Herb, dose: 2–4 ml, Infusion of Root, dose: a wineglassful.

Regulatory Status: GSL.

ANGOSTURA

Galipea officinalis Han.

Fam. Rutaceae

Synonyms: Cusparia Bark, *Cusparia febrifuga,* D.C., *Bonplandia trifoliata* W., *Galipea cusparia* St. Hill. Other species, including *Cusparia trifoliata* Eng. are also used, and may also be called Angostura.

Habitat: Indigenous to Venezuela, with other species growing in other parts of South America.

Description: The bark is slightly curved or quilled, in pieces about 3 mm thick, with thin laminae on the inner surface, yellowish-grey externally, outer layer sometimes soft and spongy. Transverse section dark brown. Taste, bitter; odour musty.

Part Used: Bark.

Constituents: (i) Bitter principles, known as angostura bitters 1 and 2, which are unstable glucopyranosylcyclopentane derivatives [49]. (ii) Alkaloids, including cusparine, cuspareine, galipine, galipoline, galipolidine, galipidine, quinaldine and derivatives, and others [49], [5]. (iii) Volatile oil, about 1–2%, containing galipene and cadinene [50].

Medicinal Use: Aromatic bitter, tonic, stimulant, and in large doses cathartic and emetic. It has been used as an anti-diarrhoeal and febrifuge. The alkaloids have been demonstrated to have antispasmodic properties and to affect respiration in dogs [5]. The mixer-drink "Angostura Bitters" no longer contains Angostura, but is made from Gentian and other bitters.

Preparations: Powdered bark, dose: 0.3–1 g; Liquid Extract, dose: 0.3–2 ml; Conc. Infusion of Cusparia BPC 1934, dose: 2–4 ml.

ANISEED

Pimpinella anisum L.
Fam. Umbelliferae

Synonyms: Anise, *Anisum vulgare* Gaertn. *A. officinarum* Moench.

Habitat: Originally from Egypt and Asia Minor but now widely cultivated in warmer climates.

Description: Aniseed is an annual herb reaching about 0.5 m. The fruits, sometimes called "seeds", are greyish or brownish-grey, ovate, hairy and up to 5 mm long with 10 crenate ribs, often with part of the stalk attached. Taste, sweet; odour characteristic.

Part Used: Fruit.

Constituents: (i) Volatile oil, 1–4%, consisting of mainly *trans*-anethole (70–90%), with estragole (methylchavicol), anise ketone (methoxyphenylacetone), anisic acid, β-caryophyllene, anisaldehyde, linalool [5]; the polymers of anethole, dianethole and photoanethole [51]; and in an Egyptian variety carvene, carvone, and α-zingiberene [52] (ii) Coumarins, such as bergapten, umbelliferone, scopoletin [53] (iii) Flavonoid glycosides including rutin, isovitexin and quercetin-, luteolin-, and apigeninglycosides [54] (iv) Phenylpropanoids, [51] including 1-propenyl-2-hydroxy-5-methoxy-benzene-2-(2-methyl-butyrate) recently isolated [55] (v) Miscellaneous lipids, fatty acids, sterols, proteins and carbohydrates [2].

Medicinal Use: Carminative and expectorant, in cough mixtures and lozenges, and as a flavouring and spice. Aniseed has been demonstrated to increase the mucociliary transport *in vitro* [56], thus supporting its use as an expectorant, and to significantly increase liver-regeneration in rats [57].

It has mild oestrogenic effects, thought to be due to the presence of dianethole and photoanethole, which explains the use of this plant in folk medicine to increase milk secretion, facilitate birth and increase libido [51].

Preparations: Anise Oil BP, dose: 0.05–0.2 ml, Anise Spirit BPC 1949, dose: 0.3–1.2 ml, Conc. Anise Water BPC, dose: 0.3–1 ml.

Potter's Products: Horehound and Aniseed Balsam; Lightning Cough Remedy.

Regulatory Status: GSL.

Biblical References: Matthew 23:23.

ANNATTO

Bixa orellana L.
Fam. Bixaceae

Synonyms: Annotta, Arnotta, Orellana, Orleana.

Habitat: Tropical America and cultivated elsewhere.

Description: Commercial product occurs in small circular cakes or cylindrical rolls.

Part Used: Pulp of seeds.

Constituents: Carotenoid colouring principles, mainly bixin and norbixin.

Medicinal Use: These pigments do not have any vitamin A activity despite being carotenoids, and no other documented pharmacological effects. They are used as natural colourings for foods, including fish fingers, medicines, fabrics and – reputedly – to dye maggots for fishing, to make them more tempting!

ARACHIS

Arachis hypogaea L.
Fam. Leguminosae

Synonyms: Groundnuts, Monkey Nuts, Peanuts.

Habitat: Tropical Africa, cultivated elsewhere.

Description: The lower flowers develop nuts which bury themselves in the earth to ripen. They have a well-known, characteristic appearance.

Part Used: Nuts, and oil expressed from the nuts.

Constituents: (i) Fixed oil, about 45%, consisting mainly of glycerides of oleic and linoleic acids [4] (ii) Vitamin E (iii) Vitamins B_1, B_2, and B_3; and in the skins: – (iv) Bioflavonoids, with so-called Vitamin P activity, and (v) tannins [58].

Substances of unknown structure but with demonstrable activity have also been described; there is a haemostatic principle in peanut flour which improves the condition of haemophiliacs [59, 58]; an oestrogenic factor in the oil; a goitrogenic factor in the non-liquid portion, and the skins contain a lipoxidase and protease inhibitor [33].

Medicinal Use: The oil is an ingredient of emollient creams and bath oils, and some more recent discoveries of the properties of Arachis have been described above. However its main use is as a food and cooking oil.

Preparations: Arachis Oil BP.

Regulatory Status: GSL.

ARBUTUS, TRAILING

Epigaea repens L.
Fam. Ericaceae

Synonyms: Gravel Plant, Ground Laurel, Mountain Pink, Water Pink.
Habitat: North America.
Description: Leaves broadly ovate, 2.5–4 cm long and about 2 cm broad, leathery, reticulated, with a cordate base and short pointed apex, and short hairs on undersurface.
Part Used: Herb.
Constituents: Arbutin (a hydroquinone derivative), ursolic acid, ericoline, and tannins [2].
Medicinal Use: Diuretic, astringent. Used for urinary tract conditions in the same way as Uva-Ursi and Buchu (q.v.).
Regulatory Status: GSL.

ARCHANGEL

Lamium album L.
Fam. Labiatae

Synonyms: White Deadnettle.
Habitat: A common wild plant in Britain and Europe, flowering in early spring and summer.
Description: Stem quadrangular, hairy; leaves opposite, with cordate base, acuminate apex, coarsely serrate, similar to those of the nettle (q.v.). Flowers large, white, tubular, two-lipped with two long and two short stamens. Taste, slightly bitter, odour none.
Part Used: Herb.
Constituents: (i) Tannins, mainly catechins [60] (ii) Amines, including histamine, tyramine, choline and methylamine [61] (iii) Flavonoids based on kaempferol (iv) Saponins (v) Mucilage (vi) An alkaloid, lamiine [2]. Recent scientific confirmation of these constituents is unavailable.

Other spp. of *Lamium* contain iridoid glycosides, such as lamiol, however they have not been found in *L. album* [62].
Medicinal Use: Astringent and haemostatic, particularly on the uterus, it has been used for menorrhagia and leucorrhoea. Other uses are as for nettle (q.v.).
Regulatory Status: GSL.

ARECA NUT

Areca catechu L.
Fam. Palmae

Synonyms: Betel Nut.
Habitat: Tropical India, Sri Lanka, Malaysia, Indonesia, the Philippines and parts of E. Africa.
Description: The seeds are conical or nearly spherical, about 2.5 cm in diameter, very hard, and with a deep brown testa showing fawn marbling. Taste slightly acrid, astringent, odour faint.

Part Used: Seed.

Constituents: (i) Alkaloids, mainly arecoline (0.1–0.5%), with arecaine, guvacine and others [1] (ii) Phlobaphene tannins (iii) Fixed oil.

Medicinal Use: Taenicide, used more often in veterinary medicine, to expel tapeworms. It is also astringent, and promotes the flow of saliva, and is used in Eastern countries as a masticatory. Due to the increased incidence of some types of oral cancer associated with Betel chewing [4], this habit is being discouraged. Arecoline has parasympathomimetic activity [63].

Preparations: Areca Powder BPC 1949, dose: 1–4 g; Liquid Extract, dose: 1–4 ml.

Regulatory Status: P

ARENARIA RUBRA

Spergularia rubra (L.) J & C Presl.
Fam. Caryophyllaceae

Synonyms: Sandwort, Sabline Rouge, *S. rubra* Pers., Lepigonum Rubrum, Fries., *Tissa rubra* Adans, *Buda rubra* Dum., *Arenaria purpurea* L.

Habitat: Southern France, Malta.

Description: Herb with jointed stems and flat, linear leaves about 1 cm long, with ovate, pointed stipules; flowers small, pink, in spreading panicles. Taste, saline; odour, slightly aromatic.

Part Used: Herb.

Constituents: An aromatic resin, but otherwise constituents are unknown.

Medicinal Use: Diuretic; used in Malta for diseases of the bladder.

Preparations: Liquid Extract, dose: 2–4 ml.

ARNICA

Arnica montana L.
Fam. Compositae

Synonyms: Leopard's Bane, European Arnica.

Habitat: Native to Europe, apart from Britain, cultivated in N. India.

Description: Flowerheads collected entire, the florets are yellow and the receptacle hairy.

Part Used: Flowers, occasionally the rhizome.

Constituents: (i) Sesquiterpene lactones, including the pseudoguano-lides arnifolin, the arnicolides [64], helenalin [5], and the recently isolated 6-0-isobutyryl-tetrahydrohelenalin and 2β-ethoxy-6-0-isobutyryl-2,3-dihydrohelenalin [65] (ii) Flavonoids such as eupafolin, patuletin, spinacetin and the less common laciniatin, [66] and methylated flavonoids including betuletol and hispidulin [67] (iii) Volatile oil, containing thymol and various ethers of thymol [5] (iv) Mucilage and polysaccharides [68] (v) Miscellaneous substances such as resins, bitters (arnicin), tannins, carotenes etc.

Medicinal Use: Stimulant and aid to wound-healing, particularly bruising and muscle pain. Arnica is usually applied topically rather than internally since it is toxic, as well as being irritating to mucous membranes. Recent work has shown Arnica to be an immuno-stimulant, both the sesquiterpene lactone helenalin (in high dilutions) and the polysaccharide fraction stimulate phagocytosis *in vitro* [68] when measured by Brandt's granulocyte test [69]. Sesquiterpene lactones are known to have anti-inflammatory activity, especially those with an α-methylene-γ-lactone structure, and their biological effects appear to be mediated through immunological processes [70]. Helenalin is one of the most active, which would account for the use of Arnica for pain and inflammation.

In a recent clinical trial, no effect was seen on either pain or swelling suffered by patients after the surgical removal of impacted wisdom teeth, however this was using homoeopathic dilutions of Arnica [71].

Preparations: Arnica Flower Tincture BPC 1949, Arnica Root Tincture BPC 1934, Arnica Liniment BPC 1934.

Regulatory Status: GSL, for external use only.

ARRACH
Chenopodium vulvaria L. Curt
Fam. Chenopodiaceae

Synonyms: Stinking Arrach, Goosefoot, Dog's Arrach, Goat's Arrach, *Chenopodium olidum* S. Wats.

Habitat: A British and European wild plant growing mostly on waste ground, flowering in June and July.

Description: Leaves oval, stalked, about 1 cm long, with entire margin and powdery surface. Odour strong, fishy.

Part Used: Herb.

Constituents: Trimethylamine, betaine, tannins [2].

Medicinal Use: Nervine, spasmolytic, emmenagogue, often taken as an infusion three or four times daily.

Preparations: Liquid Extract, dose: 2–4 ml.

ARROWROOT
Maranta arundinaceae L.
Fam. Marantaceae

Synonyms: Bermuda Arrowroot, Maranta.

Habitat: Tropical America and the W. Indies.

Description: Arrowroot is prepared from the rhizomes of this herbaceous plant, to form a white powder consisting of mainly starch. The grains are about 30–40 μm in diameter, with an irregular oval shape and a visible hilum near the middle.

Part Used: Starch.

Constituents: The rhizome contains about 25–27% neutral starch.

Medicinal Use: Demulcent, nutritive especially for infants and convalescence. Usually prepared by boiling in sufficient water to make a thin gruel, which may be flavoured if required.

ASAFETIDA

Ferula assa-foetida L.
Ferula rubicaulis Boiss. and other spp.
Fam. Umbelliferae

Synonyms: Gum Asafoetida, Devil's Dung.

Habitat: Native to SW Asia.

Description: The gum-resin is obtained by incising the roots, which contain a foetid juice. This solidifies to a brownish resin, sometimes with a pinkish tint, in sticky lumps with a pungent, acrid, persistent, alliaceous odour.

Part Used: Oleo-gum-resin.

Constituents: (i) Resins, about 40–60%, consisting of asaresinotannols, and their esters [37], farnesiferols, ferulic acid and other acids [5] (ii) Gum, about 25% [37] (iii) Volatile oil, about 6–17%, consisting of polysulphides such as diallyl- and allylpropyl-sulphides, 2-butylmethyl-, di-, tri-, and tetra-sulphides, propenyl sulphides [72], sulphated terpenes, pinene, cadinene and vanillin [5] (iv) Coumarins such as umbelliferone and the recently isolated sesquiterpenoid coumarin foetidin [73].

Medicinal Use: Antispasmodic, expectorant, carminative. It has been used for nervous disorders as well as for coughs, bronchitis and flatulence. Recent reports suggest it has a hypotensive effect [74], and anticoagulant effect [75], similar to that of garlic (q.v.). It is mainly used as a flavouring ingredient in low concentrations, for example in Worcester sauce, and is reputedly non-toxic [5].

Preparations: Asafetida Tincture BPC 1949, dose: 2–4 ml; Asafetida Powder (gum-resin) dose: 0.3–1 g; Aloes and Asafetida Pill BPC 1949, dose: 1 or 2 pills, Asafetida Pill BPC 1949; dose: 1 or 2 pills.

Potter's Products: Neurelax Tablets; Nerve (Neuritis) Tablets.

Regulatory Status: GSL.

ASARABACCA

Asarum europeaum L.
Fam. Aristolochiaceae

Synonyms: Hazelwort, Wild Nard, *Nardum rusticarium.*

Habitat: Grows wild in woods in Europe and the USSR, and is cultivated as a garden plant in Britain and America.

Description: A herbaceous perennial, with kidney-shaped, leathery, evergreen leaves; solitary, bell-shaped flowers, with three segments, purplish inside. The rhizome is slender, about 2 mm thick, quadrangular and tortuous, with rootlets at intervals and stem scars on the upper surface.

Part Used: Herb, rhizome.

Constituents: (i) Volatile oil, 0.7–4%; consisting of asarone up to 50%, asaraldehyde 2–3%, methyleugenol 15–20%, with bornyl acetate, terpenes and sesquiterpenes (ii) Lipids; including aliphatic alcohols such as n-dodecanol and analogues, alicyclic alcohols, higher aliphatic acids including n-hexadecylic and octodecatrienic acids [76] (iii) Miscellaneous plant acids (malic, citric etc.), flavonoids, resins, sugars and starch [2].

Medicinal Use: Emetic, purgative, stimulant in small doses. Has been used as an errhine in headache; sniffing the powder, which produces intense irritation and mucus flow, is said to relieve the headache! The root is said to have non-specific immunostimulatory activity *in vitro* [77], and a product containing the extract has been clinically shown to have anti-asthmatic activity in a trial of 90 patients [78].

In view of the fact that this plant contains asarone, the β-isomer of which is carcinogenic in animals (see Calamus), it should be used internally with caution.

Regulatory Status: GSL.

ASH

Fraxinus exelsior L.
Fam. Oleaceae

Synonyms: Common, European or Weeping Ash.
Habitat: Great Britain, Europe and N. America.
Description: The ash tree is well-known, deriving its name from the leaves and bark which are ash coloured. The bark occurs in thin, greenish-grey pieces about 2 mm thick, with longitudinal furrows and a pale brown inner surface. Taste, faintly bitter; odourless.
Part Used: Bark, leaves.
Constituents: (i) Coumarin derivatives including fraxin (approximately 0.1%), fraxetin, and fraxinol [2] (ii) Flavonoids based on aesculetin, including aescin [79], and others such as rutin and quercetin [2] (iii) Miscellaneous tannins, sugars, volatile oil and resin [2].
Medicinal Use: Laxative, anti-inflammatory, febrifuge; has been used for arthritis and rheumatism. The lipophilic fraction has been found to stimulate phagocytosis in mice inoculated with *Escherichia coli* [80]. The Ash once had a considerable reputation as a cure for snake-bite; and as a snake repellant: Pliny is reputed to have said that "if a fire and a serpent be encompassed within a circle of the boughs of an Ash Tree, it will sooner flye into the fire than into them . . ." Ash has been known to cause dermatitis [79].
Regulatory Status: GSL.
Biblical References: Isaiah 44:14, not identifiable.

ASPARAGUS

Asparagus officinalis L.
Fam. Liliaceae

Synonyms: Sparrowgrass.
Habitat: Native to Europe and Western Asia, widely cultivated.
Description: Root about 5 cm long, 1–2 cm thick, with a loose, laminate, internal structure. Rootlets long, narrow, compressed; nearly hollow with a central woody cord. Taste insipid; odourless.
Part Used: Root; young shoots as food.

Constituents: (i) Steroidal glycosides called asparagosides, at least nine of which have been isolated so far [81] (ii) Bitter glycosides, including those known as officinalisnin I and II [82], and others [5] (iii) Asparagusic acid and derivatives [83] (iv) Asparagine, arginine and tyrosine [5] (v) Flavonoids, including rutin, kaempferol and quercetin [84] (vi) Polysaccharides and inulin [85].

Medicinal Use: Diuretic, laxative, cardiac tonic and sedative. Has also been used for neuritis and rheumatism, although no clinical or pharmacological work is available to support these claims yet. Asparagusic acid has been shown to be nematocidal [5]; this and other sulphur containing compounds are hydrolysed in the body to form methylmercaptan, which appears in the urine and gives it a characteristic, peculiar smell [25].

AVENS
Geum urbanum L.
Fam. Rosaceae

Synonyms: Colewort, Herb Bennet, Geum, *Radix caryophyllata.*

Habitat: A hedgerow plant growing wild in Great Britain and Europe, flowering in May or June.

Description: A perennial, erect herb reaching 20–60 cm, with stem leaves occurring as two leaflets and one terminal, toothed lobe; insignificant small yellow flowers occurring in cymes, and distinctive fruits appearing as a brown ball of awned seeds which are covered in hooked bristles.

Part Used: Herb, root.

Constituents: (i) Phenolic glycosides such as "gein", which is eugenol vicianose, some free eugenol and sugars [86] (ii) Unconfirmed reports of the sesquiterpene lactone cnicin (see Holy Thistle), tannins and essential oil [2].

Medicinal Use: Astringent, styptic, tonic, febrifuge, stomachic. It has also been used for diarrhoea, sore throat and leucorrhoea, taken as an infusion.

Preparations: Liquid Extract (herb), dose: 1–4 ml; Liquid Extract (root), dose: 1–4 ml.

Regulatory Status: GSL.

AZEDARACH
Azadirachta indica A Juss.
Fam. Meliaceae

Synonyms: Neem, Nim, Margosa, Indian Lilac, *Melia azadirachta* L.

Habitat: Indigenous to India, now naturalized in W. Africa, particularly Nigeria, and cultivated elsewhere.

Description: A large deciduous tree. The bark is greyish-brown, externally fissured, with a buff inner surface and fibrous fracture. Taste bitter; odourless.

Part Used: Bark, leaves, seeds.

Constituents: (i) Meliacins (which are limonoids), including azadirachtin, gedunin, nimbolides A and B [87] and, in the leaves at least, a lactone nimbolide [88] (ii) Triterpenoid bitters such as nimbin, nimbidin, and nimbinin [89] (iii) Tannins, flavonoids etc. [33].

Medicinal Use: Anti-inflammatory, anti-pyretic, anthelmintic. The seed oil is used in India for the treatment of skin diseases and as a hair dressing. An extract of the leaves and bark has been found to have significant anti-inflammatory and antipyretic activity, coupled with low toxicity, in animals [90]. Nimbolide and nimbinin are antimalarial *in vitro* and in mice against *Plasmodium berghei* [91]. However there are unsubstantiated reports of renal toxicity in human patients who have treated themselves for malaria with this plant [90]. *Melia azedarach* L., also known as Persian Lilac, Bead or China Tree, is closely related and often confused in the literature [33]. Its constituents are (i) Meliacins, gedunin and derivatives, nimbolins A and B, melianins A and B, and their decomposition products fraxinellose and azedainic acid [88, 89] (ii) Protolimonoids; melianon, melianol, melianodiol and meliantol [92] (iii) Triterpenoids and steroids, including 24-methylene-cycloartanone, cycloeucalenone, cycloeucanol and others [93] (iv) Miscellaneous substances including vanillic acid and aldehyde, an alkaloid paraisine (ocaziridine), and an insect repelling substance known as meliatin [33]. It is used mainly as an anthelmintic, and for the same purposes as *Azadirachta indica*. An anti-viral factor which prevents replication of Tacaribe virus in mice [94], and an anti-neoplastic substance, also active in mice [95], have been isolated.

Preparations: Tincture, dose: 2–4 ml.

B

BAEL

Aegle marmelos Corr.
Fam. Rutaceae

Synonyms: Bel, Indian Bael, Bengal Quince.
Habitat: India.
Description: The fruits are globular or ovoid, with a hard shell, and divided internally like an orange. The flesh is reddish, with numerous seeds covered in a gummy layer. Taste mucilaginous, slightly acid.
Part Used: Unripe fruit, dried.
Constituents: (i) Coumarins, including xanthotoxol and alloimperatorin methyl ether [96] (ii) Flavonoids such as rutin and marmesin [96] (iii) Alkaloids including α-fagarine (= allocryptopine), also isolated from *Xanthoxylum* [33], O-isopentenylhalfordinol and O-methylhalfordinol [96].
Medicinal Use: Stomachic, digestive, astringent. In India, almost a specific for dysentry and diarrhoea.
Preparations: Liquid Extract, dose: 4–8 ml.

BALM

Melissa officinalis L.
Fam. Labiatae

Synonyms: Sweet Balm, Lemon Balm, Cure-all.
Habitat: A common plant in Britain, Europe, W. Asia and N. Africa, widely cultivated, flowering in Spring.
Description: A perennial herb; leaves opposite, stalked, about 3–4 cm long, ovate, wrinkled, with a coarsely serrate margin and a rounded base. Flowers small, insignificant, whitish. Taste and odour lemony.
Part Used: Herb.
Constituents: (i) Volatile oil, 0.1–0.2%, consisting mainly of citral a and b (= neral and geranial), with caryophyllene oxide, and in smaller quantities terpenes such as linalool, citronellal, β-caryophyllene, nerol, geraniol [97], traces of eugenyl acetate, β-ocimene, copaene and α-cubebene [5]. (ii) Flavonoids in low concentrations; luteolin-7-glucoside and rhamnazin [98] (iii) Polyphenolics, including protocatechuic acid, caffeic acid, rosmarinic acid and tannins [98, 99] (iv) Triterpenic acids such as ursolic and pomolic acids [100].
Medicinal Use: Carminative, sedative, diaphoretic and febrifuge. Used very widely as an ingredient of herbal teas. Hot water extracts have anti-viral properties, mainly due to the rosmarinic acid and other polyphenolics [99]. A cream containing extracts of Balm is used for the treatment of cutaneous lesions of *Herpes simplex* virus, the anti-viral activity having been confirmed *in vitro* and by clinical trial [101]. Aqueous extracts inhibit tumour cells dividing [102], and tannin-free extracts inhibit protein biosynthesis in cell-free systems of rat liver [103]. The sedative effects of

"Spirit of Melissa" have been demonstrated in the treatment of psychiatric disorders such as vegetative dystonia; significant improvement in the symptoms (restlessness, excitability, palpitations and headache) was obtained [104].

However this product contains about 75% alcohol and should therefore be used carefully [105].

The anti-hormonal effects of Balm, mainly anti-thyroid, are well-documented. Freeze-dried aqueous extracts inhibit many of the effects of exogenous and endogenous thyroid stimulating hormone (TSH) on bovine thyroid gland by interfering with the binding of TSH to plasma membranes [106] and by inhibiting the enzyme iodothyronine deiodinase *in vitro* [107]. It also inhibits the receptor binding and biological activity of immunoglobulins in the blood of patients with Graves disease [108], a condition which results in hyperthyroidism. The reputed antispasmodic effect has not been substantiated in experiments using histamine and acetylcholine as spasmogens *in vitro* [109].

Preparations: Liquid Extract, dose: 2–6 ml.
Potter's Product: Anaemia Mixture No. 103.
Regulatory Status: GSL.

BALM OF GILEAD

Populus candicans Ait
P. gileadensis Rouleau
P. tacamahacca Mill
P. balsamifera L.
P. nigra L. and others
Fam. Salicaceae

Synonyms: Poplar buds, Gileadensis, Mecca balsam, Balsam Poplar, *P. balsamifera* Du Roi is a synonym of *P. tacamahacca;* there is some confusion as to whether *P. balsamifera* L. and *P. tacamahacca* Mill. are the same species or not [5].

Habitat: *P. candicans* is a native of Arabia; *P. gileadensis* and *P. nigra* are cultivated in Europe; the others are N. American.

Description: *P. candicans* is a small tree or shrub, the others are larger trees. The buds are similar, being about 2 cm long and 0.5 cm wide, with brown scales; these are narrow, ovate, closely overlapping and polished-looking; the inner scales are sticky and resinous. Odour balsamic; taste slightly bitter.

Part Used: Leaf buds, collected in the Spring before they can open. The bark of these species is also used.

Constituents: (i) Phenolic glycosides; salicin, (salicyl alcohol glucoside), populin (benzoyl salicin) and chrysin (phloroglucin benzoate) [50]. (ii) Volatile oil, 0.5–2%, the major constituent of which is α-caryophyllene [50], with cineole, arcurcumene, bisabolene, farnesene, acetophenone and others [5]. (iii) Miscellaneous; alkanes, resins, phenolic acids [5], gallic acid, tannins [50], and other ubiquitous substances. (iv) *P. nigra* contains lignans, such as isolariciresinol mono-β-D-glucopyranoside [110].

Medicinal Use: Expectorant, stimulant, anti-pyretic and analgesic. It is a common ingredient of cough mixtures and ointments used for rheumatic and other muscular pains and for skin diseases. The phenolic glycosides such as salicin have the anti-inflammatory and anti-pyretic effects of the salicylates, and also therefore the side effects, see [4]. The volatile oil constituents have the usual antiseptic and expectorant activity [4].

Preparations: Liquid Extract, dose: 4–8 ml; Tincture, dose: 4–15 ml.

Potter's Products: Balm of Gilead Cough Mixture.

Regulatory Status: GSL.

Biblical References: Genesis 37:25; 43:11; Jeremiah 8:22; 46:11; 51:8; Ezekiel 27:17.

BALMONY

Chelone glabra L.
Fam. Scrophulariaceae

Synonyms: Bitter Herb, Snake Head, Turtle Head or Turtle Bloom.

Habitat: N. America.

Description: Leaves opposite, oblong-lanceolate, shortly stalked; flowers/fruits crowded in a short spike; seeds almost circular, winged, with a dark centre. Taste very bitter; odour slightly tea-like.

Part Used: Aerial parts collected during flowering and fruiting period.

Constituents: Very little work has been carried out on this plant. Resins and bitters only have been reported [2].

Medicinal Use: Anti-emetic, cholagogue, laxative, anti-depressant. No clinical or pharmacological work available.

Preparations: Powdered Herb, dose: 0.5–1 g; Liquid Extract, dose: 2–4 ml.

Regulatory Status: GSL.

BARBERRY

Berberis vulgaris L.
Fam. Berberidacea

Synonyms: Barbery, Berberidis, Pipperidge Bush, *Berberis dumetorum* Gouan.

Habitat: A common garden bush, native to Europe and the British Isles, naturalized in parts of N. America, flowering in April and May.

Description: A spiny, deciduous bush, reaching about 2.5 m, and bearing yellow flowers, followed by red berries, among the leaves. The stem bark is thin, externally yellowish-grey; the root bark dark brown; both with an orange-yellow inner surface. Taste very bitter.

Part Used: Bark of stem and root, root and berries.

Constituents: (i) Alkaloids of the isoquinoline type, mainly berberine, berbamine and derivatives, berberrubine (unique to *B. vulgaris*), bervulcine, columbamine, isotetrandrine, jatrorrhizine, magnoflorine, oxycanthine and vulvracine [111, 112] (ii) Miscellaneous, including chelidonic acid [37], resin, tannins etc.

Medicinal Use: Anti-pyretic, anti-haemorrhagic, anti-inflammatory and antiseptic. In the Far East, berberine-containing plants are specifically used for bacillary dysentery and diarrhoea.

Berberine has well-documented pharmacological actions; it is highly bactericidal [113], amoebicidal [114, 115] and trypanocidal [114]. The mechanism of its anti-diarrhoeal activity has been partially investigated: berberine enters into the cytosol or binds to the cell membrane and inhibits the catalytic unit of adenylate cyclase [116]. It is active *in vitro* and in animals against cholera [4]. Berberine has some anticonvulsant and uterine stimulant activity [5]; it stimulates bile secretion and has sedative and hypotensive effects in animals [117].

Berbamine is also strongly antibacterial, against some strains of *Staphylococcus aureus, Escherichia coli, Streptococcus viridans, Pseudomonas aeruginosa* and *Salmonella typhi* [118]. It has been shown to increase white blood cell and platelet counts in animals with iatrogenic leukocytopaenia [119], and has been used with some success in China to treat patients with leukopaenia due to radiotherapy and chemotherapy. Berbamine is also used there to treat essential hypotension [7].

The other alkaloids are also active: palmatine is hypotensive in a similar manner to berberine, it is a uterine stimulant [7], has anticholinesterase activity [120], and it affects the adrenal glands in animals in a complex manner which is not fully understood [7].

Jatrorrhizine has a sedative effect in animals, is hypotensive, and antifungal; isotetrandrine is antitubercular in animals and has significant anti-inflammatory action *in vitro;* oxycanthine and magnoflorine are hypotensive [7].

Many of the alkaloids are antineoplastic in a variety of *in vitro* systems [7], particularly berberine [121]. No toxicity problems have so far been observed, but it would be wise to avoid these preparations during pregnancy where the uterine-stimulant activity is obviously undesirable.

Preparations: Powdered bark, dose: 0.5–1 g; Liquid Extract, dose: 2–4 ml.
Potter's Products: Elixir of Chelidonium, Indigestion Mixture.
Regulatory Status: GSL.

BARLEY

Hordeum distichon L.
H. vulgare
Fam. Graminae

Synonyms: Pearl Barley, Perlatum, *Hordeum sativum* Pers.
Habitat: Widely cultivated throughout the world.
Part Used: Decorticated seeds, germinating seeds.
Constituents: (i) Nutrients: proteins, and prolamines such as hordein, edestin and the albumin leusosin among others, sugars, starch, fats. (ii) Vitamins of the B group (iii) Germinating radicle and leaves contain the alkaloids hordenine and gramine (iv) Leaves and husks contain hemicelluloses and glycosylflavones such as tricin and lutonarin [33] (v) An unidentified hypoglycaemic principle occurs in the seeds after fermentation [122, 123].

Medicinal Use: Nutritive and demulcent during convalescence and in cases of diarrhoea, bowel inflammation etc. Barley water is prepared from the grains; so is Malted Barley which is used to prepare Extract of Malt, used as a source of nutrients, beer and whisky.

Preparations: Malt Extract BPC, Malt Extract with Cod Liver Oil BPC, Malt Liquid Extract (BPC 1954).

Potter's Products: All the above preparations.

BASIL
Ocimum basilicum L.
Fam. Labiatae

Synonyms: Sweet or Garden Basil.

Habitat: Cultivated worldwide.

Description: An annual herb reaching about 20 cm, with an erect stem and numerous branches. The leaves are opposite, stalked, broadly ovate and pointed; usually pale green and dotted with oil glands, however purple varieties occur as ornamentals. The flowers, which appear in summer, are small and whitish, sometimes with a purple tinge, in long loose spikes. This plant should not be confused with Wild Basil, which is *Calamintha clinopodium* and has clusters of small red flowers.

Part Used: Herb.

Constituents: (i) Volatile oil, up to about 1%, the major constituents of which are linalool, up to 55%; estragole (methyl chavicol), up to 70% [5]; with, in widely varying proportions, methyl cinnamate, cineole, β-caryophyllene, α-phellandrene and derivatives, ocimene, borneol, eugenol, methyl eugenol, geraniol, anethole, cadinols, sabinene, myrcene, limonene, *p*-cymene, and camphor [124, 5]. True or "Sweet" basil oil contains little or no camphor, and is distilled in Europe and the USA, whereas African (also known as "Reunion" or "Exotic") basil oil contains more camphor and very little linalool, and is considered to be an inferior quality [5]. (ii) Miscellaneous; polyphenolic acids such as caffeic, vitamins A and C, and protein.

Medicinal Use: Aromatic, carminative, vermifuge, antibacterial, analgesic. Has been used for diseases of the kidney. Some of the vermicidal properties have been confirmed, and the antibacterial effects in acne sufferers demonstrated, in clinical trials in India [125, 126]. Basil is used more often as a flavouring in foods. The oil is reportedly non-toxic [127]; however estragole is a known hepatocarcinogen in animals [128].

BAYBERRY
Myrica cerifera L.
Fam. Myricaceae

Synonyms: Candleberry, Waxberry, Wax Myrtle.

Habitat: Native to the USA but widely cultivated in Europe and the British Isles.

Description: An evergreen shrub or small tree. The bark occurs in short quilled pieces about 2 mm thick, with a white, peeling outer layer covering a red-brown, hard inner layer. The fracture is granular; taste astringent and bitter, odour slightly aromatic.

Part Used: Bark.

Constituents: (i) Triterpenes, including taraxerol, taraxerone and myricadiol [129] (ii) Flavonoids, such as myricitrin [129] (iii) Miscellaneous tannins, phenols, resins and gums [5].

Medicinal Use: Stimulant, astringent, diaphoretic, and an ingredient of many composite remedies for a wide range of ailments, especially coughs and colds. An infusion of the bark is taken internally, and powdered bark used externally in poultices for ulcers and sores. Myricadiol has some mineralocorticoid activity, and myricitrin is bactericidal and spermatocidal [129]. The tannins and phenols extracted from the bark have been reported to exert carcinogenic activity in rats when given by injection [130] however whether this applies to oral or topical administration is not known, phenol and tannins by these routes also have reported antitumour promoting activity. The wax from the berries has been used for making candles, and it is an ingredient of Bay Rum, for the hair.

Preparations: Powdered bark, dose: 1–4 g; Liquid Extract, dose: 2–4 ml.

Potter's Products: Peerless Composition Essence, Elder Flowers and Peppermint with Composition Essence (EPC), Influenza and Feverish Colds Mixture.

Regulatory Status: GSL.

BEARSFOOT

Polymnia uvedalia L.
Fam. Compositae

Synonyms: Uvedalia, Leaf Cup, Yellow Leaf Cup.

Habitat: N. America.

Description: The root is greyish-brown, finely furrowed longitudinally, about 0.5–1 cm diameter with a tough, coarsely fibrous fracture and a thin, brittle bark. Taste; saline, faintly bitter; odour none. This is a N. American plant and must not be confused with English Bearsfoot which is *Helleborus foetidus.*

Part Used: Root.

Constituents: Unknown.

Medicinal Use: Stimulant, laxative, anodyne. Used externally as a hair tonic in the form of an ointment.

Preparations: Liquid Extract, dose: 0.5–3.5 ml.

Regulatory Status: GSL.

BEEBEERU BARK

Nectandra rodioei Hook.
Fam. Lauraceae

Synonyms: Greenheart Bark, Bibiru Bark, Bebeeru Bark.

Habitat: Guyana.

Description: Flat, heavy, hard pieces, 5–10 mm thick, grey-brown in colour with shallow depressions on the outer portions, the inner portions coarsely striated. Fracture granular.
Part Used: Bark.
Constituents: Alkaloids including bibirine, tannins [2].
Medicinal Use: Stomachic, tonic and febrifuge. Rarely used now.
Preparations: Powdered bark, dose: 1–2 g.

BELLADONNA
Atropa belladonna L.
Fam. Solanaceae

Synonyms: Deadly Nightshade, Dwale.
Habitat: Native to central and southern Europe, cultivated worldwide. Sometimes found on waste ground and in gardens in England.
Description: The herb is a perennial, reaching 1 m high. The leaves are ovate, up to 25 cm long, with an entire margin; the flowers campanulate, greenish to purplish in colour, followed by shiny black berries. All parts of the plant contain alkaloids, the leaves and root are most often used medicinally. The root in commerce is usually up to 10 cm long, 2 cm diameter, pale brown with short transverse scars and a whitish transverse section. The plant is collected when in flower.
Part Used: Herb, root.
Constituents: (i) Tropane alkaloids, up to 0.5% in both leaves and roots, consisting mainly of (−)-hyoscyamine, atropine (racemic hyoscyamine), hyoscine (1-scopolamine), belladonnine, their N-oxides, and other minor alkaloids, including cuscohygrine (in the root only) [131, 5]. (ii) Volatile pyridine and pyrrolidine bases [1]. (iii) Flavonoids such as scopoletin, scopolin, and kaempferol and quercetin derivatives [5].
Medicinal Use: Narcotic, sedative, mydriatic. The major alkaloids have anticholinergic activity, causing central nervous system stimulation followed by depression. Peripheral anticholinergic effects including the reduction of secretions and decreasing motility of the gastrointestinal tract. For these reasons Belladonna is used in stomach mixtures and powders as a sedative, in bronchial conditions as an antispasmodic, for colds and fevers to reduce nasal secretions, and externally as a liniment or plaster for rheumatic and muscular pains. Unwanted effects may include palpitations, elevated blood pressure, intense thirst and a rise in intraocular pressure. Overdosage is dangerous, causing the effects already mentioned together with dizziness, flushing, photophobia caused by mydriasis, constipation, confusion, hallucinations, delirium and death. For more details of individual alkaloids see [4].
Preparations: From leaf: Belladonna Dry Extract BP, dose: 15–60 mg; Belladonna Glycerin BPC 1959; Belladonna Tincture BP, dose: 0.5–2 ml. From root: Belladonna Liquid Extract BPC 1968; Belladonna Liniment BPC 1968; Belladonna Adhesive Plaster BP.
Regulatory Status: POM. P. at restricted strength.

BENZOIN

Styrax benzoin Dry.
S. paralleloneurus Perkins
Fam. Styraceae

Synonyms: Gum Benzoin, Gum Benjamin, Sumatra Benzoin, Palembang Benzoin.

Habitat: Sumatra and Java.

Description: Benzoin is obtained by making triangular wounds in the tree, from which the sap exudes and hardens on exposure to the air. The first exudate forms the "almonds" of benzoin, followed by greyish-brown resinous lumps; these are compressed together into a solid mass. (The greyish-brown resin alone is known as Palembang Benzoin and is considered to be of inferior quality.)

Siam benzoin is obtained from *Styrax tonkinense* (Pierre) Craib ex Hartwich, it occurs in separate "tears" coated with reddish-brown resin and has an odour of vanilla.

Part Used: Gum.

Constituents: (i) Cinnamic, benzoic and sumaresinolic acid esters, mainly coniferyl cinnamate, cinnamyl cinnamate (= styracin), coniferyl benzoate, accounting for up to 90% (ii) Free acids, benzoic acid 10–20%, cinnamic acid up to 30%, and sumaresinolic acid. (iii) Benzaldehyde (iv) Vanillin, up to about 1% [5, 4]. All are variable in proportion depending on source.

Siam benzoin contains mainly coniferyl benzoate (ca. 70%), with cinnamyl benzoate, free benzoic acid, sumaresinolic acid and vanillin [4].

Medicinal Use: Antiseptic, expectorant and astringent. Sumatra benzoin is an ingredient of Friar's Balsam which is widely used; topically on wounds and ulcers to protect and disinfect the skin and to treat mouth ulcers; as an inhalation in coughs, colds and bronchitis. Preliminary studies have shown that the lipophilic fraction of benzoin stimulates phagocytosis [80].

It is used in perfumery as an antioxidant and fixative.

Preparations: Benzoin Inhalation BP; Benzoin Tincture BPC; Compound Benzoin Tincture BP (Friar's Balsam).

Regulatory Status: GSL.

BERBERIS

Berberis aristata DC
Fam. Berberidaceae

Habitat: India.

Description: Strips of the dried stem, externally greyish-brown, internally greenish yellow, often covered with moss or lichen, and with conspicuous yellow medullary rays.

Part Used: Stem.

Constituents: Alkaloids; berberine, oxyberberine and others [2].

Medicinal Use: Used in India for intermittent fevers, in a similar manner to Golden Seal (q.v.). For actions of berberine see Barberry.

Preparations: Powder, dose: 0.5–4 g; Tincture, dose: 2–4 ml.

BETEL
Piper betle L.
Fam. Piperaceae

Synonyms: Chavica betle Miq.
Habitat: India and Malaysia, cultivated elsewhere.
Description: Leaves cordate, 6–8 cm long, about 5 cm wide, with 5–7 radiating ribs and a paler green undersurface.
Part Used: Leaf.
Constituents: Volatile oil, 0.2–1%, containing cadinene, chavicol, cineole, eugenol, caryophyllene, carvacrol and estragole [2].
Medicinal Use: Rarely used medicinally but chewed with Areca Nut (q.v.) and lime as a stimulant in some parts of the world. It increases the flow of saliva and is thought to prevent worm infestation. A dry extract of the root has been used in combination with other extracts (including Jequirity q.v.) as a long acting contraceptive in women [132], however this cannot be recommended.

BETH ROOT
Trillium erectum L.
T. pendulum Willd. and other spp.
Fam. Liliaceae

Synonyms: Birthroot, Wake Robin.
Habitat: N. America.
Description: The rhizome is dull brown, subconical, more or less compressed, 3–5 cm long and 2–3 cm diameter; often ringed with oblique lines and with numerous wrinkled rootlets on the lower surface. Taste: sweetish then acrid, odour characteristic.
Part Used: Rhizome.
Constituents: Saponin glycosides such as trillin and trillarin [37, 2]. Little work has been carried out on either *T. erectum* or *T. pendulum*. However the related species *T. kamtschaticum* Pall. and *T. tschonoskii* Maxim. which are used in Oriental medicine, have been shown to contain steroidal saponins based on 18-norspirostane; the aglycones are the pennogenins and the glycosides the trillenosides [133, 134, 135]. *T. tschonoskii* also contains about 2% diosgenin derivatives, such as dioscin and methyl protodioscin; a flavonol glycoside based on kaempferol and a sesquiterpenoid [136].
Medicinal Use: Astringent, antihaemorrhagic and expectorant. Used for menorrhagia and haematuria as an infusion, for leucorrhoea as a douche, and for varicose and other ulcers as a poultice, with Slippery Elm and a small amount of Lobelia seed (q.v.). The American Indians used to use this plant as an aid to parturition, hence the name Birthroot.
Preparations: Powdered root, dose: 0.5–1 g; Liquid Extract, dose: 4–8 ml.
Regulatory Status: GSL.

BILBERRY

Vaccinium myrtillus L.
Fam. Vacciniaceae

Synonyms: Huckleberry, Whortleberry, Hurtleberry, Blueberry.

Habitat: Grows chiefly in moorland, heaths and on acid soil in the UK, Europe and N. America and cultivated extensively. It flowers in May, the berries ripen in July.

Description: Fruits blue-black, globular, about 0.5–1 cm in diameter with the calyx ring at the apex and containing numerous small oval seeds.

Part Used: Ripe fruit.

Constituents: (i) Anthocyanosides, at least 0.3% [137] (ii) Vitamin C (iii) Plant acids such as citric and malic. Unlike other *Vaccinium* species, bilberry does not contain arbutin, or other hydroquinone derivatives [138].

Medicinal Use: Astringent, diuretic, refrigerant; used particularly for diarrhoea, as a decoction. The anthocyanosides inhibited barium induced contractions in isolated thoracic vein [139] and coronary artery smooth muscle [140] *in vitro*. These effects are thought to be mediated by stimulation of vasodilatory prostaglandin production [140]. See also Blackcurrant. Bilberries are used mainly as a food.

Preparations: Liquid Extract, dose: 2–8 ml.

BIRCH

Betula verrucosa Ehrh.
Fam. Betulaceae

Synonyms: Silver Birch, White Birch, *B. pendula* Roth., *B alba* L.

Habitat: Commonly found in woods in Britain and Europe.

Description: A fairly large tree, producing catkins of male and female flowers. The leaves are rhomboidal or oval, pointed, shiny, stalked, with a serrate margin, about 2.5–3.5 cm long and 2–3 cm broad. The young bark has a papery, layered external surface marked with linear brown lenticels; older bark is rough, blackish-brown outside with white lines showing in transverse section. Fracture short; taste astringent and bitter.

Part Used: Bark and leaves.

Constituents: Flavonoids, mainly hyperoside, with luteolin and quercetin glycosides [141]. The bark is used for the preparation of Birch Tar Oil by destructive distillation, and should not be confused with Sweet Birch Oil which is produced from *Betula lenta* L. and consists almost entirely of methyl salicylate [4].

Medicinal Use: Bitter, astringent. The leaves have been used to prepare a mouthwash. Birch Tar Oil is used in ointments for the treatment of psoriasis and eczema.

Preparations: Birch Tar Oil BPC 1949 (Oleum Rusci BPC 1949); Compound Ointment of Resorcin BPC 1949; Compound Ointment of Birch Tar 1949.

Regulatory Status: GSL, for external use only (Birch Tar Oil).

BIRTHWORT *Aristolochia clematis* L.
LONG BIRTHWORT *Aristolochia longa* L.
INDIAN BIRTHWORT *Aristolochia indica* L.
Fam. Aristolochiaceae

Habitat: A. *clematis* is European, A. *longa* from N. America, and A. *indica* from India.

Description: A. *clematis:* the root is sub-cylindrical, 2 cm or more in diameter, externally pale brown, smooth, striated or warty. Transverse fracture whitish with brown dots due to vascular bundles containing oleo-resin.

Part Used: Root.

Constituents: (i) All contain aristolochic acids and aristolactams, which are non-basic aporphinoids. A. *clematis* contains aristolochic acids I, II, III, IV and D; A. *longa* contains aristolochic acid I and aristored, and A. *indica* contains aristolochic acids I, D, D methyl ether lactam, methyl aristolochate, aristolactam, aristolactam II, aristolactam N-β-D-glucoside and aristolactam C N-β-D-glucoside [142]. A. *indica* also contains (ii) 12-secoishwaran-12-ol (iii) savinin, (iv) naphthaquinones such as aristolindoquinone (v) the alkaloid magnoflorine and (vi) *p*-coumaric acid (143].

Medicinal Use: Treatment of wounds, aromatic and stimulant. It is taken internally as well as applied topically. A. *indica* especially is also used as an abortifacient. Recent work has substantiated some of these uses.

Extracts show a pronounced enhancement of phagocytosis by leucocytes [144], granulocytes [145], and peritoneal macrophages [144, 146], due to the presence of aristolochic acids [147]; and a reduction in the rate of recurrent herpes lesions *in vivo* [147]. Aristolochic acids also appear from *in vitro* experiments to reduce some of the toxic effects of prednisolone, chloramphenicol and tetracycline [147]. Aristolochic acid in tablet form has been evaluated clinically in China for the treatment of wounds and infectious diseases; it was found to be useful for promoting wound healing in ulcers, burns and scalds, and for bronchitis, tonsillitis and nephritis as an adjuvant to antibiotic therapy.

For further information see [7], [147] and references therein. The antifertility effect of A. *indica* has been demonstrated in animals, it acts post-coitally [143]. Aristolochic acid also has an effect against adenosarcarcoma and HeLa cells in culture [147]; however it is suspected of carcinogenicity [148] and plants containing it have been withdrawn from the W. German market [147].

Preparations: Powdered root, dose: 2–4 g.

Regulatory Status: GSL.

BISTORT *Polygonum bistorta* L.
Fam. Polygonaceae

Synonyms: Snakeweed, Adderwort, English Serpentary, Dragonwort, Osterick.

Habitat: It grows in shaded places in the North of England, Europe and Asia, flowering in May and June.

Description: The rhizome is reddish-brown, about 5 cm long and 1.5 cm broad, bent twice into an S-shape (hence the synonyms). It is channelled on the upper surface and transversely striated, with root scars on the lower surface. Fracture short, showing a pinkish pith, white-grey cortex, and thick bark. Taste astringent; odourless.

Part Used: Root and rhizome.

Constituents: (i) Polyphenolic compounds such as ellagic acid [150], tannins, about 15–20% [37], mainly catechins [2] (ii) Phlobaphene, a red-brown pigment [2] (iii) Flavonoids [151] (iv) Emodin, a trace [2] (v) Miscellaneous: starch, albumin [2].

Medicinal Use: Astringent, antidiarrhoeal, anticatarrhal, antihaemorrhagic. It is used as a mouthwash and gargle, douche and ointment, as well as being taken internally as a decoction or infusion.

Preparations: Powdered rhizome, dose: 1–2 g.

Regulatory Status: GSL.

BITTER APPLE

Citrullus colocynthis Schrad.
Fam. Cucurbitaceae

Synonyms: Colocynth Pulp, Bitter Cucumber.

Habitat: Arabian Gulf, Sri Lanka, Egypt and Syria.

Description: Occurs in commerce as light, whitish balls, about 5 cm diameter, often broken. The seeds, which are oval and dark green, should be removed before use.

Part Used: Pulp of the peeled fruit.

Constituents: (i) Cucurbitacins, including cucurbitacins I and L (= elatericin B and dihydroelateracin B) which are glycosides of cucurbitacin E (= elaterin), also present (ii) Citrullol (iii) an unnamed alkaloid [152].

Medicinal Use: Cathartic, irritant, drastic purgative. It has been used for constipation and painful menstruation. It is seldom used alone because of the griping effects, and its use can no longer be recommended. Toxic effects after chronic use include hypokalaemia, oliguria and oedema, similar to acute nephritis, and symptoms resembling Crohn's disease and Addisons Disease [153]. The drug should never be taken by nursing mothers since the active constituents appear in breast milk [4]. Cucurbitacin E is highly cytotoxic [154], and extracts of Bitter Apple are carcinogenic in mice [155]. For further information on cucurbitacins see White Bryony.

Preparations: Compound Colocynth and Jalap Tablets BPC 1963, dose: 1–3 tablets; Compound Colocynth Extract BPC 1963, dose: 120–500 mg.

BITTER ROOT

Apocynum androsaemifolium L.
Fam. Apocynaceae

Synonyms: Dogsbane, Milkweed, Wild Cotton.

Habitat: Mountainous regions of Europe, flowering in June and July.

Description: The root is 3–6 mm thick, with a pale brown, transversely wrinkled and cracked bark which is about half as thick as the whitish centre. Groups of stone cells are visible in the outer bark. Taste, bitter and astringent. *Apocynum cannabinum* is often substituted, however it has a yellowish wood and no stone cells in the outer bark.

Part Used: Root.

Constituents: (i) Cardiac glycosides, including strophanthin, androsin, apocynin, cymarin, apocymarin and apobioside [2]. *A. cannabinum* contains similar compounds, particularly cymarin [4]. (ii) Essential oil containing acetovanillin [2].

Medicinal Use: Emetic, cathartic, diuretic and cardiac stimulant. For further information on these glycosides see Strophanthus. An alcoholic extract of the plant at a sub-toxic dose has been shown to damage transplanted tumours in mice [156].

The herbalist John Parkinson, in the 16th century, wrote that it was a "soveraine remedy against all poysons . . . and against the biting of a mad dogge", hence the name Dogsbane. In the light of present knowledge it would be better to give it to the mad dog than its victim.

Preparations: Powdered root, dose: 0.25–2 g; Liquid Extract, dose: 0.7–2 ml.

BITTERSWEET

Solanum dulcamara L.
Fam. Solanaceae

Synonyms: Woody Nightshade, Felonwood, Felonwort, Dulcamara.

Habitat: Found widely in hedges and on waste ground in the British Isles, Europe, Asia and N. Africa.

Description: The plant is a climber, bearing distinctive purple and yellow flowers in July, followed by oval red berries. The shoots are greenish-brown, nearly cylindrical, about 0.5 cm thick, slightly furrowed longitudinally or sometimes warty. The pith is often hollowed. The transverse section shows a green layer in the bark and a radiate ring of wood (more in older stems). Taste, bitter then sweet. Odour unpleasant when fresh; this is lost on drying. The root bark is thin and tough, blackish-grey internally, with groups of fibres of the inner bark forming pale brown wedges. Taste, astringent, slightly bitter; odourless.

Part Used: Twigs, root bark.

Constituents: (i) Steroidal alkaloids, including soladulcamaridine, soladulcidine, solanidine, solasodine, tomatidine, their hydroxy derivatives [112], and β-solamarine [157] (ii) Steroidal saponins based on tigogenin and yamogenin [158] and the solamayocinosides A-F, which are furastanol glycosides [159].

Medicinal Use: Antirheumatic, diuretic; used as a decoction and taken with milk. Bittersweet also has a long history of use as a folklore treatment for warts, tumours and skin infections. The steroidal saponins have anti-fungal activity [158] and β-solamarine is an inhibitor of Sarcoma 180 tumours in mice [157].
Preparations: Liquid Extract, dose: 2–4 ml.
Biblical References: Exodus 12 : 8 may include lettuce (wild), chicory, eryngo, horseradish and sow thistle if available.
Regulatory Status: P.

BITTERSWEET, AMERICAN

Celastrus scandens L.
Fam. Celastraceae

Synonyms: Waxwork, False Bittersweet.
Habitat: N. America.
Description: Root, bark.
Constituents: Unknown, apart from a pigment celastrol [2].
Medicinal Use: Alterative, diuretic and diaphoretic. Has been used for leucorrhoea, rheumatism and menstrual and liver disorders, but rarely used nowadays.
Preparations: Decoction, dose: 60–120 ml.

BLACKBERRY, AMERICAN

Rubus villosus Ait. and others
Fam. Rosaceae

Synonyms: Dewberry, Bramble.
Habitat: Native to the Northern United States, cultivated elsewhere.
Description: A low growing plant bearing stout prickles on the stem, the leaves are unequally divided and so distinct from the blackberry native to the UK, *R. fructicocus* L.
Part Used: Root, root bark, leaves.
Constituents: Tannins, gallic acid, villosin [5]. *R. fructicosus* leaves contain flavonoid glycosides of kaempferol and quercetin [160].
Medicinal Use: Astringent, and tonic, mainly used for diarrhoea.
Preparations: Liquid Extract, dose: 2–4 ml. Blackberry Cordial is a preparation of the root with aromatics.
Potter's Products: Spanish Tummy Mixture; Bowel Mixture. (Made with Blackberry Root Bark).
Regulatory Status: GSL.

BLACKCURRANT

Ribes nigrum L.
Fam. Saxifragaceae

Habitat: A well-known garden plant grown for its fruit.
Description: Leaves palmate, stalked, about 5 cm diameter, with three to five pointed, serrate angular lobes, and yellow glands scattered on the under surface. The fruits are shiny, purplish-black berries, about 0.5–1 cm diameter, with the calyx ring visible at the apex. Odour very characteristic.

Part Used: Leaves, fruit.

Constituents: Leaves: (i) Volatile oil, a small amount, containing mainly terpenes (ii) Tannins (iii) Vitamin C [2]. Fruit: (i) Anthocyanosides, about 0.3%, concentrated mainly in the skin, consisting mainly of glycosides of cyanidol and delphinidol [137] (ii) Vitamin C, about 120 mg per 100 g fresh weight (iii) Tannins [2].

Medicinal Use: The leaves are reputedly diuretic, hypotensive and refrigerant. They are used as an infusion for inflammatory conditions, sore throats and hoarseness. The fruits are useful in diarrhoea and as a source of Vitamin C. The anthocyanosides are reportedly bacteriostatic [161], and have vasoprotective and anti-inflammatory (so-called "Vitamin P") activity [162]. They are mildly spasmolytic, and antisecretory against cholera toxin-induced intestinal fluid secretion *in vitro* [137]. Black-currants are widely used as a food and flavouring.

Preparations: Fruit: Blackcurrant Syrup BPC.

BLACK HAW

Viburnum prunifolium L.
Fam. Caprifoliaceae

Synonyms: Stagbush, American Sloe.

Habitat: Eastern and Central USA.

Description: The young bark occurs in thin quilled pieces, with a glossy purplish-brown outer surface with scattered warts. Older bark has a greyish brown outer surface and whitish inner surface, with the thin corky layer separating away easily. Fracture short; taste astringent and bitter; odour, slightly valerianic. The root bark is reddish-brown and very bitter.

Part Used: Stem and root bark.

Constituents: (i) Coumarins, including scopoletin [163] (ii) Salicin [50] (iii) 1-Methyl-2,3-dibutyl hemimellitate [164] (iv) Miscellaneous; viburnin, plant acids, volatile oil (trace), tannin [5].

Medicinal Use: Uterine tonic, sedative, nervine antispasmodic, anti-diarrhoeal. Used particularly for preventing miscarriage in the last four or five weeks of pregnancy, although the advisability of this has not been established. It is used in dysmenorrhoea and after childbirth to check pain and bleeding. At least some of the uterine sedative effects are due to the presence of scopoletin [165], which has a number of pharmacological actions probably mediated via autonomic transmission blockade [166]. Salicin has the analgesic and other effects (including toxicity) of salicylates [4].

Preparations: Powdered bark, dose: 1–2 g; Elixir of Black Haw BPC 1949, dose: 2–8 ml, Elixir of Black Haw and Hydrastis BPC 1949, dose: 2–4 ml, Liquid Extract of Black Haw BPC 1949, dose: 4–8 ml.

Regulatory Status: GSL.

BLACK ROOT

Veronicastrum virginica (L.) Farw.
Fam. Scrophulariaceae

Synonyms: Culver's Root, Culver's Physic, Physic Root, *Leptandra virginica* (L.) Nutt., *Veronica virginica* Tourn.

Habitat: N. America.

Description: Rhizome about 0.5 cm in diameter, showing stem bases at intervals of 1–2 cm, blackish-brown, with transverse scars in rings 0.25–0.5 cm apart, chiefly on the lower surface. Rootlets wiry, brittle, with a horny fracture showing a paler core of wood and a thick brown cortex.

Part Used: Rhizome, root.

Constituents: Active constituents largely unknown, however it contains (i) Volatile oil containing esters of cinnamic acid, methoxycinnamic acid, and dimethoxycinnamic acid [37] (ii) Saponins [25] (iii) Mannitol, dextrose, tannin etc. [2].

Medicinal Use: Mild cathartic, diaphoretic, spasmolytic and cholagogue. It is used especially for chronic constipation associated with liver dysfunction.

Preparations: Powdered root bark, dose: 1–4 g; Compound Tablets of Leptandra BPC 1949 (Vegetable Laxative Tablets) dose: 1–3 tablets; Extract of Leptandra BPC 1934, dose: 30–120 mg.

Potter's Products: G.B. Tablets (No. 448); Bile and Liver Tablets (No. 167); Compound Elixir of Leptandrin; Compound Elixir of Collinsonia; Compound Elixir for Colitis; Indigestion Mixture.

Regulatory Status: GSL.

BLADDERWRACK

Fucus vesiculosus L.
Fam. Fucaceae

Synonyms: Seawrack, Kelpware, Black-tang, Bladder Fucus, Cutweed.

Habitat: A seaweed common in colder waters, such as the British coast.

Description: The fronds are flat, forked, greenish-black, about 1–2 cm broad and up to 30 cm long, with a distinct midrib and oval bladders, usually in pairs. *Fucus serratus* has no bladders and a serrate margin. Taste, mucilaginous, saline; odour, seaweed-like.

Part Used: Whole plant.

Constituents: (i) Phenolic compounds, including free phloroglucinol, its dehydropolymerization products the fucols [167], the fucophorethols which are polyhydroxyoligophenylethers [168], and high molecular weight phlorotannin derivatives [167]. (ii) Mucopolysaccharides, including algin [4], some with lectin-like properties [169] (iii) Sulphuryl-, sulphonyl- and phosphonyl-glycosyl ester diglycerides [170] (iv) Polar lipids [171] (v) Trace metals, particularly iodine, up to 0.4% [4].

Medicinal Use: Anti-obesity agent, nutritive and source of trace elements. A beneficial effect has been demonstrated on obese patients in a study carried out in Italy [172]. Bladderwrack has been shown to have antibiotic activity [167, 169]. The lectin-like mucopolysaccharides are immunomodulatory and induce lymphocyte transformation; also they have been shown to react with several *Candida* species [169]. Seaweeds are a good source of iodine, however Bladderwrack has been shown to accumulate toxic waste metals such as cadmium and strontium when grown in a polluted environment [173] and should therefore be avoided in these circumstances.

Preparations: Liquid Extract, dose: 0.5–15 ml. Solid Extract, dose: 1–2 g.

Potter's Products: Boldo Aid to Slimming Tablets; Super Kelp Tablets; Malted Kelp Tablets; Bladderwrack Tablets (No. 303); Tabritis Plus Tablets.

Regulatory Status: GSL.

BLOODROOT
Sanguinaria canadensis L.
Fam. Papaveraceae

Synonyms: Sanguinaria, Red Root, Red Indian Paint, Tetterwort.

Habitat: N. America and Canada.

Description: The rhizome is about 1 cm in diameter, 5 cm or more in length, reddish brown and longitudinally wrinkled. The fracture is short and shows a whitish transverse section with numerous red latex vessels. Rootlets are about 1 mm thick, brittle and wiry. Taste bitter and acrid; odour slight.

Part Used: Rhizome.

Constituents: Isoquinoline alkaloids, including sanguinarine (about 1%), chelerythrine, sanguidaridine, oxysanguinaridine, sanguilutine, berberine, coptisine, chelilutine, chelirubine, protopine, sanguidimerine, sanguirubine, α- and β-allocryptopine and others [174].

Medicinal Use: An ingredient of many cough preparations, since sanguinarine is an expectorant, antimicrobial, and has local anaesthetic properties. It has also been used as a tonic and to treat fevers, and externally for all kinds of skin infections and burns. Recently ointments containing blood root have been used to treat epithelial tumours and skin infections [175, 176], and a dentifrice containing the extract is reported to improve sensitive teeth [176, 177]. Both sanguinarine and chelerythrine have been shown to uncouple oxidative phosphorylation and intercalate with DNA [178], possibly helping to explain their well known anti-bacterial and anti-viral reactions.

Preparations: Powdered root, dose: 0.5–2 g; Liquid Extract, dose: 0.5–1.5 ml, Tincture, dose: 2–8 ml; Solid Extract (alc.) dose: 0.3–0.5 g.

Potter's Products: Vegetable Cough Remover.

Regulatory Status: GSL.

BLUE FLAG

Iris versicolor L.
I. caroliniana Watson
Fam. Iridaceae

Habitat: Eastern and Central North America, growing in marshy places, producing distinctive blue flowers in spring. Commonly grown in Britain as an ornamental.

Description: The rhizome is subcylindrical, about 2 cm in diameter, becoming flattened at the larger end where the cup-shaped stem scar can be seen. The outer surface is annulate, with numerous stem and root scars. Fracture short, resinous, showing a reddish-brown transverse section with a yellow endodermis and whitish vascular bundles. Taste, acrid; odour slight, aromatic.

Part Used: Rhizome.

Constituents: (i) Volatile oil, containing furfural (ii) Iridin (or irisin), a glycoside [179] (iii) Acids such as salicylic and isophthalic [37] (iv) Miscellaneous; a monocyclic C31 triterpenoid [180], gum, resin, sterols etc.

Medicinal Use: Alterative, anti-inflammatory, cathartic, diuretic, stimulant and anti-obesity agent. It is also used externally as a poultice or ointment, for skin diseases of various kinds. In one study Blue Flag has been shown to reduce food intake in rats, and it was claimed that this demonstrates anti-obesity properties [181].

Preparations: Powdered root, dose: 1 g; Liquid Extract, dose: 2–4 ml; Tincture, dose: 4–12 ml.

Potter's Products: Catarrh Mixture; Skin Eurptions Mixture; Psoriasis Mixture No. 143; Irisine; Alterative Tablet No. 34.

Regulatory Status: GSL.

BLUE MALLOW

Malva sylvestris L.
Fam. Malvaceae

Synonyms: Common Mallow, Mauls.

Habitat: A wild plant of Britain and Europe, flowering in May and June.

Description: Leaves stalked, with five to seven lobes, hairy and with prominent veins on the undersurface. Flowers mauve, with darker veins. Taste mucilaginous; odourless.

Part Used: Herb, flowers.

Constituents: (i) Sulphated flavonol glycosides; gossypin-3-sulphate, hypo-laetin-8-O-β-D-glucoside-3'-sulphate, gossypetin-8-O-β-D-glucuronide-3-sulphate [18] (ii) Mucilage [2] (iii) Flowers contain malvin, the diglucoside of malvidin, an anthocyanin, with tannins, carotene and ascorbic acid [18].

Medicinal Use: Demulcent, pectoral. The infusion is used for colds and coughs, and a poultice of the leaves applied to insect stings and bites.

Preparations: Liquid Extract, dose: 2–8 ml.

Regulatory Status: GSL.

BOLDO

Peumus boldo Mol.
Fam. Monimiaceae

Synonyms: *Boldu boldus* Lyons, *Boldea fragrans* Gay.

Habitat: Indigenous to Chile, naturalized in mountainous parts of the Mediterranean.

Description: Leaves oval, up to about 7 cm long, 3 cm broad, rather thick and brittle with an entire, slightly revolute margin and a short stalk. The upper surface is papillose, both surfaces slightly pubescent. Taste bitter, aromatic; odour camphoraceous, lemony.

Part Used: Leaves; bark for extraction of alkaloids.

Constituents: (i) Alkaloids, of the isoquinoline type, up to 0.7%, including boldine, isocorydine, N-methyllaurotetanine, norisocorydine [183], isoboldine, laurolitsine, reticuline and others [5] (ii) Volatile oil, containing mainly *p*-cymene, 1,8-cineole, ascaridole and linalool [5] (iii) Flavonoid glycosides based on isorhamnetin [184].

Medicinal Use: Cholagogue, liver stimulant and diuretic; used for the treatment of gall-stones and cystitis and as an aid to slimming. Animal studies have shown that the total alkaloidal extract has a greater choleretic activity than boldine alone [185, 186].

Preparations: Liquid Extract, dose: 0.5–2 ml.

Potter's Product: Boldo Aid to Slimming Tablets.

Regulatory Status: GSL.

BONESET

Eupatorium perfoliatum L.
Fam. Compositae

Synonyms: Feverwort, Thoroughwort.

Habitat: N. America.

Description: A perennial herb with opposite leaves, 10–15 cm long, lanceolate, tapering to a narrow point and united at the base. The margin is crenate and shiny yellow points due to the resin glands are visible on the undersurface. Taste; astringent and persistently bitter. The flowers are small and inconspicuous and occur in cymose-paniculate inflorescences.

Part Used: Herb.

Constituents: (i) Sesquiterpene lactones; eupafolin, euperfolitin, eufoliatin, eufoliatorin, euperfolide [188, 189], eucannabinolide and helenalin [48] (ii) Immunostimulatory polysaccharides, mainly 4-O-methylglucuroxylans [190] (iii) Flavonoids; quercetin, kaempferol, hyperoside, astragalin, rutin, eupatorin and others [191]. (iv) Miscellaneous; diterpenes such as dendroidinic acid, hebenolide; sterols and a small amount of volatile oil [5].

Medicinal Use: Febrifuge, expectorant, diaphoretic, tonic and laxative. Used particularly for catarrh, bronchitis and skin diseases. Both the polysaccharides and the sesquiterpene lactones are immunostimulatory in low concentrations; they enhance phagocytosis *in vitro* [190, 191]. An extract of the plant has been shown to be weakly anti-inflammatory in rats [192].

Some of the sesquiterpene lactones, and also eupatorin, are known to exhibit cytotoxic activity *in vitro* [190], and are awaiting antineoplastic *in vivo* testing.

Preparations: Powdered herb, dose: 0.5–1 g; Liquid Extract, dose: 2–4 ml; Solid Extract, dose: 0.3–0.5 g.

Potter's Products: Catarrh Compound Herb; Influenza and Feverish Cold Mixture; Pleurisy Mixture; Tonsillitis Mixture.

Regulatory Status: GSL.

BORAGE

Borago officinalis L.
Fam. Boraginceae

Synonyms: Burrage.

Habitat: Indigenous to Great Britain, Europe, and N. Africa, naturalized in N. America.

Description: A large annual. The leaves are oval, pointed, with bristles on both surfaces, about 7 cm or more in length, about 3 cm broad, and a slightly sinuous margin. The stem is robust, ridged and bristly; the flowers blue, star-shaped with the anthers forming a cone in the middle. Taste; cucumber-like, saline; odourless.

Part Used: Leaves.

Constituents: (i) Pyrrolizidine alkaloids, including lycopsamine, inter-medine and their acetyl derivatives, with amabiline and supinine [193] (ii) Choline [194]. Allantoin is reported to be absent [194].

Medicinal Use: Diuretic, demulcent, emollient, refrigerant. It is used for fevers and pulmonary disease taken as an infusion, and externally as a poultice. Although the pyrrolizidine alkaloids are present in very small amounts (2–10 ppm) in commercial samples [193], it would be advisable not to use this plant internally, especially when fresh. See Comfrey for more information on this.

Preparations: Liquid Extract, dose: 2–4 ml.

BOX

Buxus sempervirens L.
Fam. Buxaceae

Habitat: A native of Britain and Asia, cultivated here and in the USA as an ornamental.

Description: A well-known evergreen shrub or tree, with small, thick leaves and waxy yellow flowers.

Part Used: Leaves.

Constituents: Alkaloids; the mixture of which is referred to as "buxine", but which is composed of buxamine, buxaminol, buxanine, buxarine, buxatine, buxazidine B, buxazine, buxenone, buxeridine, buxetine, cyclobuxine B and D, cyclovirobuxine D, osnanine and others [195, 112].

Medicinal Use: Formerly used for "purifying the blood" and for rheumatism, but far too toxic to recommend. Symptoms of poisoning are severe abdominal pain, vomiting, convulsions and death.
Biblical References: Isaiah 41:19 and 60:13.

BOXWOOD, AMERICAN
Cornus florida L.
Fam. Cornaceae

Synonyms: American Dogwood, Flowering Cornel or Boxwood, Dog Tree.
Habitat: Eastern and Central USA.
Description: The bark occurs in slightly curved pieces, greyish and scaly, or, where the outer layer is removed, pale brown and irregularly cracked longitudinally; inner surface pinkish-brown, rough, with small raised lines. Transverse fracture shows faint medullary rays and raised groups of stone cells. Taste: astringent and bitter.
Part Used: Bark; root-bark.
Constituents: (i) Verbenalin, an iridoid glycoside (ii) Tannins, gallic and betulic acids [2].
Medicinal Use: Tonic, astringent, stimulant; used for headaches and exhaustion. Verbenalin has some parasympathomimetic activity, and is a mild laxative.
Preparations: Powdered bark, dose: 2–4 g; Liquid Extract, dose: 2–4 ml.

BROOKLIME
Veronica beccabunga L.
Fam. Scrophulariaceae

Synonyms: Water Pimpernel.
Habitat: Common in Britain and Europe in wet places.
Description: A low creeping hairless perennial, with oval stalked leaves and small (7–8 mm) blue flowers occurring in loose spikes at the base of the upper leaves.
Part Used: Herb.
Constituents: Iridoid glycosides including aucubin (ii) Miscellaneous bitters and tannins [2].
Medicinal Use: Alterative, diuretic. Culpeper said it would "provoke the urine and break away the stone and pass it away . . ." In fact aucubin has been reported to stimulate the uric acid secretion of the kidneys [196], and to have a mild laxative effect in animals [197].

BROOM
Cytisus scoparius (L.) Link.
Fam. Leguminosae

Synonyms: *Sarothamnus scoparius* (L.) Koch., *S. vulgaris* Wim., *Spartium scoparium* L. Scotch Broom, Irish Broom, Broomtops, Besom, Scoparium.

Habitat: British Isles, Europe, and naturalized in N. America, S. Africa and parts of Asia.

Description: A tall deciduous shrub with ridged stems, bearing small trefoil, lanceolate leaves and yellow, two-lipped (papilionaceous) flowers, followed by greenish-black pods, about 3 cm long and 0.5 cm broad. Taste bitter; odourless.

Part Used: Tops.

Constituents: (i) Quinolizidine alkaloids; sparteine, lupanine, 13-hydroxy-lupanine, isosparteine, ammodendrine, N-methylangustifoline, dihydrolupanine and various derivatives [198, 199]. (ii) Phenethylamines such as tyramine, hydroxytyramine, epinine and salsolidine [199] (iii) Isoflavone glycosides including genistein, 3'-O-methylorobol, 7-glucosyl-3-O-methylorobol [200], scoparin (= scoparoside) [5] and sarothamnoside [201] (iv) Other flavonoids such as quercetin, isoquercetin and spiraeoside [202, 203] (v) Essential oil, containing *cis*-3-hexen-1-ol, 1-octen-3-ol, benzylalcohol, phenol, cresols, guiacol, eugenol, isovaleric acid and benzoic acid [203] (iii) Miscellaneous: caffeic and *p*-coumaric acids [203], tannins and pigments. The seeds contain lectins (phytohaemagglutinins) [204].

Medicinal Use: Diuretic, cathartic. Sparteine has a number of pharmacological effects, including a curare-like effect on peripheral nerves which depresses respiration; it reduces the conductivity of cardiac muscle and has been used to treat tachycardia. It has an oxytocic but unpredictable effect in inducing labour [4]. The whole herb has been used to treat tumours [5].

Preparations: Liquid Extract, dose: 2–4 ml; Concentrated Decoction of Broom BPC 1949, dose: 8–15 ml; Concentrated Infusion of Broom BPC 1949, dose: 4–8 ml.

Potter's Products: Kasbah Remedy Compound Herb; Antitis Tablets; Diuretic Mixture No. 110.

Regulatory Status: GSL.

BROOMCORN

Sorghum vulgare Pers.
Fam. Graminae

Synonyms: Sorghum seeds, Darri, Durri, *Sorghum saccharatum*.

Habitat: Indigenous to N. America, grown worldwide.

Description: Seeds white, about 3 mm in diameter, rounded and slightly compressed.

Part Used: Seeds.

Constituents: Mainly protein, mucilage.

Medicinal Use: Demulcent, taken as a decoction. More often used as a food, as a cereal grain, production ranks about 5th in the world.

BRYONY, BLACK

Tamus communis L.
Fam. Dioscoreaceae

Synonyms: Blackeye Root.

Habitat: Lanes and hedgerows in Britain and Europe.

Description: A hairless perennial climber with heart-shaped leaves, bearing green, six-petalled flowers in May, followed by crimson, egg-shaped berries. The root is nearly cylindrical, 2–3 cm diameter, 6–8 cm long, with scattered, wiry, rootlets. The outside is blackish-brown, the inside whitish and yielding a slimy paste when scraped. Taste, acrid; odour slightly earthy.

Part Used: Root.

Constituents: (i) Steroidal spirostane glycosides, such as dioscin and gracillin [205] (ii) Phenanthrene derivatives, including the phenolic batatasin 1 [206], and several substituted dihydrophenanthrenes [207].

Medicinal Use: Rubifacient, diuretic. The fresh root is scraped and the pulp rubbed into the parts affected by gout, rheumatism etc. It is reputed to be a diuretic.

BRYONY, WHITE

Bryonia alba L.
B. dioica Jacq.
Fam. Cucurbitaceae

Synonyms: English Mandrake, Bryonia, Wild Vine.

Habitat: England and parts of Central and Southern Europe.

Description: Both are perennial, dioecious vines, climbing by means of tendrils (unlike Black Bryony), with large, palmate, 5-lobed leaves. The flowers are greenish-white, in small clusters, followed by red berries in the case of *B. dioica*, and black berries in *B. alba*. The root is large, up to 6 cm in diameter, and normally occurs cut transversely. The section shows concentric rings and radiating lines of medullary rays.

Part Used: Root.

Constituents: Of *B. alba:* (i) Cucurbitacins, at least 8, including cucurbitacins B, D, E, I, J, K, L and tetrahydrocucurbitacin I [208] (ii) Polyhydroxy-unsaturated fatty acids (mainly trihydroxyoctadecadienic acids [209, 210] (iii) Miscellaneous: a small amount of volatile oil, tannins etc. [37].

Medicinal Use: Cathartic, counter-irritant, hydrogogue, antirheumatic. White Bryony has been used internally in small doses for intestinal ulcers, asthma, hypertension and as an adjunct in parturition; and externally as a rubifacient for myalgia. Recent work on *B. alba* has partly substantiated these uses: the polyhydroxy acids have been shown to have prostaglandin-like activity in several biological systems such as platelet aggregation and iso-lated smooth muscle preparations [209]. They also induce hypoglycaemia under experimental conditions [210]. The cucurbitacins are cytotoxic *in vitro* and *in vivo*, with antitumour effects. The most active are cucurbitacins B, D and E [208]. An ethanolic extract of *B. dioica* has an antiviral effect *in vitro* [211]. White Bryony may precipitate menstruation. It is highly toxic, especially in large doses and should be avoided at least during pregnancy.

Preparations: Liquid Extract, dose: 0.2–2 ml.

BUCHU *Barosma betulina Bart.* et Wendl
ROUND BUCHU B. crenulata Hooker
OVAL BUCHU B. serratifolia Willd.
LONG BUCHU Fam. Rutaceae

Synonyms: Round Buchu, Oval Buchu, Long Buchu, Bucco, Diosma, *Agathosma betuline* (Berg) Pillans, *A. crenulata* (L.) Pillans, *Diosma betulina.*

Habitat: S. Africa.

Description: Small, greenish-yellow leaves with a short petiole and visible oil glands. Round or "short" buchu leaves are rhomboidal in shape, 1–2 cm long and 0.5–1.5 cm broad. The margin is serrate near the base; the apex blunt and recurved. Oval buchu leaves are oval and slightly longer, up to 3 cm long, with a blunt apex, not recurved. Long buchu leaves have a serrate margin, a truncate apex and are lanceolate in shape, up to 4 cm long. All have a large oil gland at the apex and at marginal indentations, with smaller glands scattered throughout the lamina. Taste and odour; very characteristic.

Part Used: Leaves.

Constituents: (i) Volatile oil, up to about 3% (less in long buchu), of very variable composition. The main constituents are diosphenol (= buchu camphor), up to about 12% [212]; however in long buchu there may be little or none; pulegone, (+)- and (−)-isopulegone, up to 10% and 3% each respectively, with more in long buchu; 8-mercapto-*p*-menthan-3-one (two isomers), responsible for the blackcurrant-type odour; 8-acetylthio-menthone, piperitone epoxide [212] which has been disputed [213], (+)-menthone, (−)-isomenthone, *p*-cymol, limonene, terpineol and others [5] (ii) Flavonoids; rutin, diosmin, hesperidin, quercetin and derivatives [212]. (iii) Miscellaneous; vitamins of the B group, tannin and mucilage [212].

Medicinal Use: Diuretic, diaphoretic, stimulant. The diuretic activity is due to diosphenol. Buchu is also used particularly as a urinary antiseptic, however no *in vitro* effect against urinary pathogens has yet been observed [212]. For inflammation of the bladder it is taken as an infusion.

Preparations: Concentrated Buchu Infusion BPC 1954, dose: 4–8 ml; Buchu Tincture BPC 1949, dose: 2–4 ml; Liquid Extract, dose: 2–4 ml.

Regulatory Status: GSL.

Potter's Products: Kasbah Remedy Compound Herb; Antitis Tablets; Alpine Herb Medicinal Tea Bags; Back and Kidney Tablets No. 252; Diuretic Mixture No. 110; Cystitis Mixture No. 111; Lumbago Mixture No. 117.

BUCKBEAN *Menyanthes trifoliata* L.
Fam. Menyanthaceae

Synonyms: Bogbean, Marsh Trefoil.

Habitat: Marshy ground in Britain and Europe.

Description: An aquatic or creeping perennial, with trefoil leaves and spikes of pink and white flowers, each with a five lobed petal-tube and fringed with long white hairs. Flowers April–June.

Part Used: Herb.

Constituents: (i) Iridoid glycosides; foliamenthin, dihydrofoliamenthin, menthiafolin and loganin [214, 215] (ii) Pyridine alkaloids, including gentianine [216] (iii) Coumarins, such as scopoletin [216] (iv) Phenolic acids; mainly caffeic, with protocatechuic, ferulic, sinapic, vanillic and others [217] (v) Miscellaneous; vitamin C, tannins [218], flavonoids including rutin, sterols and volatile oil [50].

Medicinal Use: Bitter tonic, deobstruent. Used also for rheumatism. Caffeic and ferulic acids have known choleretic action and it has been suggested that they may act as synergists to the iridoids [217]. It is a laxative in large doses [4].

Preparations: Liquid Extract, dose: 0.5–1.5 ml.

Potter's Products: Vinca Major Compound Mixture No. 104; Elixir for Colitis: Blood Purifying Compound Herb; Nervine Compound Herb.

Regulatory Status: GSL.

BUCKTHORN

Rhamnus catharticus L.
Fam. Rhamnaceae

Synonyms: Common Buckthorn, *Baccae spinae-cervinae.*

Habitat: Britain and parts of Europe.

Description: A deciduous shrub or small tree, often thorny, with elliptical, finely toothed leaves. The berries are globular, 8–10 mm diameter, black. The bark has a glossy reddish or greenish-brown cork.

Part Used: Berries, occasionally bark.

Constituents: (i) Anthraquinone derivatives, including emodin, aloe-emodin, chrysophanol and rhein glycosides [218], frangula-emodin, rhamnicoside [1] alaterin and physcion [219] (ii) In the bark: naphlolide glycosides of the sorigenin type [1] (iii) Flavonoid glycosides [2].

Medicinal Use: The berries are used to make Syrup of Blackthorn, which is a laxative. It is used particularly in veterinary practice. The bark may be found as an adulterant of other *Rhamnus* species (q.v.). An extract of the berries has been shown to produce tumour necrosis in mice [156].

Preparations: Buckthorn Syrup (for veterinary use), dose: 2–4 ml.

Regulatory Status: GSL.

BUCKTHORN, ALDER

Rhamus frangula L.
Fam. Rhamnaceae

Synonyms: Frangula bark, *Frangula alnus* Mill.

Habitat: Europe, Britain and the USA.

Description: A small tree, thornless, with broadly elliptical, smooth leaves. The bark occurs in thin quilled pieces, greenish-black externally, with numerous elongated whitish lenticels. There is a crimson layer just beneath the surface when abraded. Fracture fibrous; taste, sweetish then bitter; odourless.

Part Used: Bark.

Constituents: Anthraquinone derivatives, 3–7%, mainly glycosides; fran-
gulosides (= frangulin) A and B, glucofrangulosides A and B, emodin-
dianthrone, palmidin C and its monorhamnoside [1], emodin-8-O-
β-gentiobioside [220] and others, including free anthraquinones (ii)
Anthrones, anthranols and their glycosides, present in fresh bark but
readily oxidized to anthraquinones [221, 1]. These are considered to be the
emetic principles [221]. (iii) Armepavine, an alkaloid, has been reported in
the fresh (but not the dried) bark [222] (iv) Miscellaneous tannins and
flavonoids [5].

Medicinal Use: Tonic, laxative, cathartic. The dried, seasoned bark, from
one to two years old, only should be used, since fresh bark causes violent
griping pains, emesis and nausea. It is chiefly used for chronic
constipation in frequent small doses, as a decoction.

Preparations: Liquid extract dose: 2–4 ml.

Potter's Products: Lion Cleansing Herbs.

Regulatory Status: GSL.

BUGLE

Ajuga reptans L.
Fam. Labiatae

Synonyms: Common Bugle, Bugula, Middle Comfrey or Confound,
Sicklewort, Herb Carpenter.

Habitat: Europe, including the British Isles, N. Africa and parts of Asia.

Description: Leaves opposite, ovate, with a slightly toothed margin. Stems
quadrangular; flowers tubular, bluish or ash-coloured.

Part Used: Herb.

Constituents: Iridoid glycosides, including harpagide [62].

Medicinal Use: Analgesic, for bruising and other wounds, and a mild
laxative. For actions of harpagide see Devil's Claw. The old herbalist
Parkinson in 1640 recommended an ointment made "of the leaves of Bugle
two parts; of Self-heal, Sanicle and Scabious (q.v.) of each one part,
bruised and boiled in Hog's Lard or in a mixture of Sheep's Suet and Olive
Oil until the herbs are crisp and then strained forth and kept for use." This
ointment was probably effective, if rather smelly.

BUGLEWEED

Lycopus virginicus L.
Fam. Labiatae

Synonyms: Sweet Bugle, Water Bugle. Gypsywort. The closely related
L. europaeus is also called Gypsywort.

Habitat: Eastern USA. *L. europaeus* is the European species.

Description: Leaves glabrous, elliptical-lanceolate, toothed above but entire
near the base. Stem quadrangular; flowers in axillary clusters with a
purplish four-lobed corolla and only two fertile stamens. Taste bitter,
odour mint-like.

Part Used: Herb.

Constituents: (i) Phenolic acid derivatives; caffeic, rosmarinic, chlorogenic and ellagic acids. The active constituents are thought to be adducts of these formed by autoxidation [108]. (ii) *L. europaeus* contains Δ8 (9), 15-pimaric acid methyl ester [223]. Iridoids are reputed to be absent [62], however they are present in some *Lycopus* species [224].

Medicinal Use: Sedative, astringent, cough remedy. Recent work shows anti-hormonal, particularly anti-thyrotropic, activity. The freeze-dried extract of *L. virginicus* induces pituitary thyroid stimulating hormone (TSH) repletion in hypothyroid rats, and reduction of TSH levels in euthyroid rats [225]. This possibly accounts for the sedative effects. Extracts of both *L. virginicus* and *L. europaeus* also prevent bovine TSH binding to and stimulating adenyl cyclase in human thyroid membranes [108]. Bugleweed extracts have been used empirically in the treatment of Graves disease, where a thyroid-stimulating antibody is found in the blood; this antibody has been shown to bind to and be inhibited by the plant extract [108]. Antigonadotrophic activity has been demonstrated in rats; the active constituents are thought to be quinones formed from the oxidation of the phenolic acids [226].

Preparations: Liquid Extract, dose: 0.7–2 ml.

Regulatory Status: GSL.

BUGLOSS

Echium vulgare L.
Fam. Boraginaceae

Synonyms: Viper's Bugloss, Blueweed.

Habitat: A common European plant.

Description: Stems up to about 60 cm, with stiff, bulbous hairs, bearing alternate, lanceolate, bristly leaves. Flowers blue, funnel-shaped, irregularly tubular, in curved clusters. Fruit of four seed-like pyrenes, shaped like the head of a snake (hence the synonym). Taste mucilaginous; odourless.

The common Bugloss, *Anchusa arvensis* L. has smaller, wheel-shaped blue flowers and wavy, toothed leaves.

Part Used: Herb.

Constituents: Pyrrolizidine alkaloids; asperumine, echimidine, echiminine and heliosupine [227, 228]. Many species of *Echium* and *Anchusa* also contain alkannins [18] (see Alkanet).

Medicinal Use: Diuretic, demulcent, expectorant, anti-inflammatory. Normally used as an infusion, however due to the presence of these alkaloids it should not be taken internally. It would however be safe to do as Dioscorides advised: "if the leaves be held in the hand, no venomous creatures will come near the holder to sting him for that day".

BURDOCK
Arctium lappa L.
Fam. Compositae

Synonyms: Lappa, Bardane, Great or Thorny Burr, Beggar's Buttons, *Arctium majus* Bernh.

Habitat: Grows in hedges and ditches in Europe, parts of Asia, N. America; cultivated in Japan. Flowers in June and July.

Description: A large biennial with broad, blunt, cordate leaves up to about 40 cm long; flowerheads purple, globular, with hooked bracts forming burrs. The root is usually found in commerce cut or split; externally longitudinally furrowed, internally whitish or buff-coloured. The fruits are brownish-grey, wrinkled, about 6 mm long by 4 mm broad. *Arctium minus* Bernh. is also used, it is rather similar but smaller. Taste: herb, bitter; root, sweetish and mucilaginous.

Part Used: Herb, root, fruits (often called "seeds").

Constituents: (i) Lignans, including arctigenin, its glycoside arctiin, and matairesinol [229]; and in the fruits, a series of at least 8 sesqui- and dilignans known as the lappaols A, B, C etc. [230, 231] (ii) Polyacetylenes, in the root, mainly tridecadienetetraynes and tridecatrienetriynes [232], with the sulphur-containing arctic acid [5]. (iii) Sesquiterpenes, in the leaves, including arctiol, (= 8-hydroxyeudesmol), β-eudesmol, fukinone, fukinanolide and derivatives, petasitolone and eremophilene [233]. (iv) Amino acids, in the roots, such as γ-guanidino-*n*-butyric acid [234] (v) Inulin (up to 50%) in the roots (vi) Miscellaneous organic acids, fatty acids and phenolic acids; including acetic, butyric, isovaleric, lauric, myristic, caffeic and chlorogenic acids [5].

   The roots are also a rich source of dietary fibre known in Japan as "gobo" [235].

Medicinal Use: Alterative, diuretic, diaphoretic, orexigenic, anti-rheumatic, antiseptic. It is usually taken as a tea or a decoction; and for skin problems such as eczema and psoriasis in the same way or as a poultice. Burdock has also been used to treat tumours, and in fact arctigenin is a weak inhibitor of experimental tumour growth [236]. The antimicrobial properties are thought to be due to the polyacetylenes [232]. An uncharacterized desmutagenic factor of high molecular weight has been described; it reduces the effect of a number of mutagens including those which do not require metabolic activation [237]. Extracts of the fruit are reported to have hypoglycaemic activity in rats [5]. The root is eaten as a food in parts of Asia, the fibre from it has been shown to protect rats from the toxicity of various food colours [238]. There has been a report of poisoning by "Burdock Tea" [239], however it is more likely to be due to the presence of Belladonna (q.v.) than Burdock since the symptoms were atropine-like, and the leaves when dried and broken bear a superficial resemblance.

Preparations: Liquid Extract of Root, dose: 2–8 ml; Liquid Extract of Seed, dose: 0.5–2 ml.

Potter's Products: Tabritis Remedy for Arthritis; Rheumatic Pain Tablets; Skin Eruptions Mixture; Psoriasis Mixture; Compound Elixir of Trifolium; Arthritis Compound Herb Mixture; Alterative Compound; Acne Mixture No. 128.

Regulatory Status: GSL.

BURNET, GREATER

Sanguisorba officinalis L.
Fam. Rosaceae

Synonyms: Garden Burnet, Diyu (Chinese).

Habitat: Common in damp grassland in temperate regions.

Description: Leaves pinnate, with about thirteen opposite leaflets, rounded at the ends and sharply serrate. Flowerheads deep red, oblong or globose, consisting of two or three fertile flowers at the top with protruding crimson stamens and twenty or thirty barren flowers below. Taste astringent; odourless.

Part Used: Herb. In Chinese medicine the root and rhizome are used, often roasted, and then stir-fried.

Constituents: Tannins and related compounds; sanguisorbic acid dilactone (a phenolic acid), sanguiins H1, H2, and H3 (ellagitannins) [240], methyl glucoside gallates [241], galloyl catechins and procyanidins [242], galloyl hamameloses (in the root) [243], a trimeric hydrolysable tannin sanguiin H11 [244], and 3,3',4-tri-O-methylellagic acid [245]. The root contains glycosides based on ursolic acid, known as sanguisorbins A, B and E [7].

Medicinal Use: Antihaemorrhagic, astringent. Used for ulcerative colitis and diarrhoea, either internally as an infusion or tincture, or topically as a styptic or anti-haemorrhoidal. The antihaemorrhagic effect has been demonstrated in animals [245, 246], and has been shown to be due at least in part to the 3,3'4-tri-O-methylellagic acid [245]. Burnet has a therapeutic effect on burns and scalds, by reducing exudation, decreasing tissue oedema and reducing the incidence of infection. These effects were found to be due to other factors as well as the tannins [7]. It also has a mild anti-emetic action and antimicrobial activity against a variety of common pathogens [7]. Clinical studies have confirmed its usefulness in bacillary dysentery, and topically for skin diseases such as eczema and infected tinea pedis. It is also an ingredient of some Chinese compound preparations which have been tested and found to be effective for cervical erosion, uterine bleeding, and gastrointestinal haemorrhage [7]. Burnet extract is also an ingredient of a dentifrice used for the prevention and treatment of periodontal disease [247].

Regulatory Status: GSL.

BURNET SAXIFRAGE

Pimpinella saxifraga L.
Fam. Umbelliferae

Synonyms: Lesser Burnet.

Habitat: Dry grassland, particularly on lime, throughout Europe.

Description: Root spindle-shaped, brownish, up to 15 cm long, often crowned with several hollow stem bases. Fracture short, showing a thick bark dotted with resin canals and a whitish central porous woody pith. Leaves pinnate with oval serrate leaflets; flowerheads white, globular umbels. Taste, cucumber-like; odourless.

Part Used: Root, occasionally herb.

Constituents: (i) Volatile oil, about 0.4% (ii) Coumarins such as umbelliferone, bergapten, pimpinellin and isopimpinellin [2] (iii) Phenylpropanoids; the main component is epoxy-isoeugenol-(2-methylbutyrate) with pseudoisoeugenol derivatives (based on 1-(E)-propenyl-2-hydroxy-5-methoxy-benzene) [248].
Medicinal Use: Aromatic, carminative, stimulant.
Regulatory Status: GSL.

BURRA GOKEROO

Pedalium murex L.
Fam. Pedaliaceae

Synonyms: Barra Gokhru.
Habitat: India.
Part Used: Seeds.
Constituents: Unknown.
Medicinal Use: Antispasmodic, demulcent, diuretic. Has been used for incontinence, impotence and irritation of urinary organs as an infusion.

BURR MARIGOLD

Bidens tripartita L.
Fam. Compositae.

Synonyms: Water Agrimony.
Habitat: Damp places throughout Europe.
Description: Flowerheads yellow, button-like, consisting solely of disc florets; leaves lanceolate, toothed, opposite, trifid.
Part Used: Herb.
Constituents: Little information available. (i) Flavonoids, including isocoreopsin [249] (ii) Xanthophylls [249] (iii) Volatile oil, about 1.3% [250] (iv) Acetylenes [2] (v) Miscellaneous compounds including vitamins (tocopherol, ascorbic acid) sterols and tannins [250, 2].
Medicinal Use: Astringent, diaphoretic, diuretic. Used in the treatment of gout, ulcerative colitis and haematuria; and in the USSR for treating alopecia (this may be because of the effects of flavonoids on capillary blood flow, however no details are available).

BUSH TEA

Cyclopia genistoides L.
Fam. Leguminosae

Synonyms: Rooibosch, Boschori-Busch.
Habitat: S. Africa.
Description: Reddish-brown stalks 1–2.5 cm long with the aroma and taste of tea.

Constituents: Cyclopine, oxycyclopine, tannin and volatile oil [2]. Does not contain caffeine.

Medicinal Use: Used as a substitute for tea where caffeine is not advisable and for liver and kidney complaints.

BUTCHER'S BROOM
Ruscus aculeatus L.
Fam. Liliaceae

Synonyms: Kneeholm, Kneeholy, Pettigree, Sweet Broom.

Habitat: Europe, in dry woods and among rocks, often cultivated.

Description: Evergreen shrub with leaves reduced to small scales; stems flattened at the ends into oval cladodes each bearing a small whitish flower in the centre, followed by a round scarlet berry, and ending in a sharp spine.

Part Used: Herb.

Constituents: Saponin glycosides based on ruscogenin (= 1β-hydroxy-diosgenin) and others [251], similar to those found in Wild Yam (q.v.).

Medicinal Use: Anti-inflammatory, diaphoretic, aperient. Particularly used in venous insufficiency. The alcoholic extract and the ruscogenins have anti-inflammatory activity and diminish vascular permeability [1]. A hydro-alcoholic extract has recently been shown to produce α-adrenergic effects on isolated cutaneous veins causing contraction [252]. The extract may be taken internally as a decoction, or topically in the form of an ointment, or as a suppository for haemorrhoids.

BUTTERBUR
Petasites hybridus L.
Fam. Compositae

Synonyms: *P. vulgaris* Desf., *Tussilago petasites*.

Habitat: In low wet ground throughout Europe and the British Isles.

Description: A downy perennial, with very large heart-shaped leaves (up to 1 m across) and lilac-pink brush-like flowers which occur in spikes in March before the leaves appear.

Part Used: Root, herb.

Constituents: (i) Pyrrolizidine alkaloids; the major one being senecionine, with integerrrimine, senkirkine, petasitine and neopetasitine [253] (ii) Sesquiterpene lactones (eremophinolides) including petasalbin, furano-petasin, petasinolides A and B and furoeremophilone [254] (iii) Miscellaneous; volatile oil, pectin, mucilage and inulin in the root.

Medicinal Use: Tonic, stimulant, diuretic. Has been used as a remedy for asthma, fevers, colds and urinary complaints. Not recommended due to alkaloid and sesquiterpene lactone content.

Regulatory Status: GSL.

BUTTERNUT
Juglans cineraria L.
Fam. Juglandaceae

Synonyms: White Walnut, Lemon Walnut, Oilnut.
Habitat: USA.
Description: The inner bark occurs in flat or curved pieces 0.5–2 cm thick. Fracture short, having a chequered appearance due to the brown fibres alternating with the white medullary rays. Taste, bitter and slightly acrid; odour faint, rancid.
Part Used: Inner bark.
Constituents: (i) Naphthaquinones, including juglone, juglandin and juglandic acid [255, 37] (ii) Fixed and essential oil, tannins [2].
Medicinal Use: Laxative, tonic vermifuge. Butternut is used as a dermatological agent, antihaemorrhoidal and cholagogue. Juglone has antimicrobial, antineoplastic and antiparasitic activity [255]. It is a gentle purgative.
Preparations: Liquid Extract, dose: 2–4 ml; Solid Extract, dose: 0.3–0.5 g.
Regulatory Status: GSL.

BUTTON SNAKEROOT
Liatris spicata (L.) Willd.
Fam. Compositae

Synonyms: Gay-feather, Backache Root.
Habitat: USA.
Description: Rhizome 1 cm or more in diameter, somewhat tuberculate, with several cup-shaped scars. Externally brownish and slightly wrinkled; internally whitish, speckled with dark grey dots, very tough. Taste bitter; odour faintly aromatic, resembling cedar.
Part Used: Rhizome.
Constituents: (i) Sesquiterpene lactones; spicatin, euparin and desacetyl-4'-desoxyprovincalin and its epimers [256, 257] (ii) Flavonoids; quercetin-3-glucoside, the 3-rutinoside and others [257] (iii) Volatile oil, a small amount.
Medicinal Use: Has been used in kidney diseases and for menstrual disorders, often in conjunction with Unicorn Root, as an infusion. For more information on sesquiterpene lactones see Boneset and Feverfew.

C

CABBAGE TREE
Andira inermis (Sw) Kunth.
Fam. Leguminosae

Synonyms: Jamaica Cabbage Tree, Yellow Cabbage Tree, Worm Bark, *Geoffraeya inermis* Sw.

Habitat: W. Indies.

Description: The bark occurs in long flat pieces about 3 mm thick, greyish-white and fissured externally; the inner surface brownish and striated. Fracture laminated with yellow fibres. Taste; mucilaginous and bitter, odour slight but disagreeable.

Part Used: Bark.

Constituents: (i) Alkaloids: andirine, berberine and N-methyltyrosine [183] (ii) Pterocarpans including inermin [256].

Medicinal Use: Febrifuge, cathartic, vermifuge. Usually taken as an infusion.

Preparations: Liquid Extract, dose: 1–4 ml.

CACAO
Theobroma cacao L.
Fam. Sterculiaceae

Synonyms: Cocoa, Theobroma, Chocolate Tree.

Habitat: Cultivated in many tropical countries.

Description: Oval seeds, oblong compressed about 2 cm long, with a thin, papery husk. Often found broken into angular fragments. Taste and odour well-known.

Part Used: Seeds.

Constituents: (i) Xanthine derivatives and alkaloids; mainly theobromine with some caffeine; tyramine, trigonelline and others [5] (ii) Fixed oil, known as cocoa butter or theobroma oil, about 50% of the "nibs" (cotyledons) (iii) Many flavour ingredients; for full account and references see [5].

Medicinal Use: Nutritive, stimulant, diuretic. The pharmacological effects are mainly due to theobromine and caffeine, which have similar properties although theobromine is weaker than caffeine in most respects [4]. Cocoa butter is an emollient and used in cosmetic creams and as a suppository base. Cocoa is most often used as a food.

Preparations: Theobroma Oil BP.

CAJUPUT
Melaleuca leucadendron L.
Fam. Myrtaceae

Synonyms: Cajeput, White Tea Tree, Swamp Tea Tree, Paperbark Tree, *M. cajuputi* Roxb.

Habitat: S. E. Asia, Australia, cultivated elsewhere.

Description: The tree from which the oil is distilled is large with a crooked trunk. The oil is distilled from the fresh leaves and twigs and redistilled until colourless or pale yellow; it has an odour recalling that of camphor and eucalyptus.

Part Used: Oil.

Constituents: (i) Terpenoids; cineole, (usually 50–65%, but very variable) is the major component, with α-pinene, α-terpineol, nerolidol, limonene, benzaldehyde, valeraldehyde, dipentene and various sesquiterpenes [5, 4, 50] (ii) 3,5-dimethyl-4,6-di-O-methylphloroacetophenone [257].

Medicinal Use: Stimulant, antispasmodic, diaphoretic, expectorant. Used internally as an ingredient of remedies for colds, headaches, and toothaches; carminative mixtures; and externally as a rubefacient in rheumatism and muscle stiffness. The main active constituent is cineole (see Eucalyptus). It is reported to have antiseptic properties [4] and to be non-toxic [26]. It is also used as a fragrance ingredient [5].

Preparations: Cajuput Oil BPC, dose: 0.05–0.2 ml; Cajuput Spirit (from Oil), dose: 0.3–2 ml; Compound Methyl Salicylate Ointment BPC.

Regulatory Status: GSL.

CALABAR BEAN

Physostigma venenosum Balf.
Fam. Leguminosae

Synonyms: Ordeal bean, Chopnut.

Habitat: W. Africa.

Description: The plant is a woody climber, bearing papilionaceous flowers followed by pods containing two or three dark brown or blackish seeds. The seeds are kidney-shaped, up to about 3 cm long, 1.5 cm broad and 1.5 cm thick, with the hilum extending along the whole convex side. The cotyledons are whitish.

Part Used: Ripe seeds.

Constituents: Alkaloids; mainly physostigmine (eserine), with eseramine, isophysostigmine, physovenine, geneserine, calabatine, calabacine and others [1].

Medicinal Use: Rarely used medicinally except as a source of physostigmine, which is an anticholinesterase inhibitor. It is used mainly in opthalmology as a miotic and as an antidote to anticholinergics such as atropine. The beans were originally used as an ordeal poison by tribes in West Africa, for persons accused of witchcraft. They are extremely poisonous.

Regulatory Status: Schedule 1 Poison. POM.

CALAMINT

Calaminta ascendens Jord.
Fam. Labiatae

Synonyms: Common Calamint, Basil Thyme, Mountain Mint, *C. officinalis* Moench., *C. menthifolia* Host.

Habitat: Occurs on dry, often calcareous banks in Britain, Europe and N. Africa.

Description: Leaves broadly ovate, slightly serrate, stalked. Flowers pale purple; calyx with upper teeth triangular, erect, fringed with hairs, lower teeth longer, awl-shaped. Taste and odour, mint-like.

Part Used: Herb.

Constituents: Volatile oil, about 0.35%, of which the major constituent is pulegone, with other ketones and terpenes [2].

Medicinal Use: Diaphoretic, expectorant.

Regulatory Status: GSL.

CALAMUS

	Acorus calamus L.
Type I	= var *americanus*
Type II	= var *vulgaris* L. (var *calamus*)
Type III	= var *augustatus* Bess.
Type IV	= var *versus*L.
	Fam. Araceae

Synonyms: Sweet Flag, Sweet Sedge, Shuichangpu (Chinese) *Calamus aromaticus.*

Habitat: Type I is a diploid American variety, type II is a European triploid, and types III and IV are subtropical tetraploids. The plant grows on river banks and marshy places.

Description: The rhizome is pale fawn coloured, longitudinally wrinkled, with numerous oblique transverse leaf scars above, particularly near the stem, and small circular root scars underneath. Fracture short, showing a whitish, porous interior, with scattered vascular bundles visible when wetted. Taste, aromatic, pungent and bitter; odour, sweet and aromatic. The peeled rhizome is usually angular and often split.

Part Used: Rhizome.

Constituents: Volatile oil of variable composition. In types II, III and IV the major constituent is usually β-asarone (isoasarone), up to 96% [259]. In type I, β-asarone and other phenylpropanoids are absent, and the main constituents are the sesquiterpenes shyobunone, 6-epishyobunone, 2,6-diepishyobunone; together with up to 34% isoacorone, 25% acorone and acorenone and small amounts of calamendiols [259]. Other constituents of the oil are sesquiterpene hydrocarbons such as *l*-cadala-1,4,9-triene, guaiane sesquiterpene ketones [260], acoragermacrone [262], acolamone, isoacolamone, pinene, azulene, methyleugenol, methylisoeugenol, camphor, asaraldehyde and acoric acid [5].

Medicinal Use: Aromatic, spasmolytic, carminative. It is used mainly for flatulence, colic and dyspepsia and as an old remedy for ague. The rhizome (often called the root) has been used candied and in the form of an infusion since ancient times. Pharmacological studies in China have shown that extracts of Calamus have anti-arrhythmic, hypotensive, vasodilatory, anti-tussive, antibacterial and expectorant activity [7]. Toxicity studies there showed that the oil was of low toxicity in animals and adverse reactions in patients rare [7]. It has been known for some time that β-asarone is carcinogenic in animals; however recent studies have demonstrated that type I (the American variety), which does not contain β-asarone, is in fact superior in spasmolytic activity to the other types [259]. Therefore, although absolute safety has not been proven yet, it would be preferable to use this variety for internal use. Preparations containing β-asarone are banned from sale in the US.

Preparations: Powdered root, dose: 1–4 g; Liquid Extract, dose: 1–4 ml.

Regulatory Status: GSL.

Biblical References: Exodus 30:23; Song of Solomon 4:14; Ezekiel 27:19. As Sweet Cane in Isaiah 43:24 and Jeremiah 6:20.

CALOTROPIS

Calotropis procera Brown.
Fam. Asclepiadaceae

Synonyms: Mudar Bark, *Asclepias procera* Willd.

Habitat: India.

Description: The bark occurs in irregular short pieces, slightly quilled or curved, about 0.3–0.5 cm thick. Externally greyish-yellow, soft and spongy; internally yellowish-white. Fracture short; taste acrid and bitter.

Part Used: Bark.

Constituents: (i) Cardiac glycosides; cardenolides based on calotropagenin with cyclic sugars [263] (ii) Alkaloids (unspecified) have been reported in the leaves and twigs [112].

Medicinal Use: Expectorant, diuretic. Has been used in India as a remedy for dysentery, diarrhoea and other conditions, and topically for eczema.

CALUMBA

Jateorhiza palmata Miers.
Fam. Menispermaceae

Synonyms: Colombo, *Cocculus palmatus* D. C.

Habitat: E. Africa and Madagascar, cultivated in Europe.

Description: The root occurs in circular sections about 3–8 cm diameter with a depressed centre and a thick bark. Transverse section yellowish, with vascular bundles in radiating lines. Outer surface greyish-brown. Fracture short and mealy. Taste mucilaginous, very bitter; odour slight.

Part Used: Root.

Constituents: (i) Isoquinoline alkaloids, 2–3%; palmatine, jatrorrhizine and its dimer bisjatrorrhizine, columbamine (ii) Bitters including calumbin, a dilactone (iii) Dihydronaphthalenes such as chasmanthin and palmanin (iv) Volatile oil containing thymol. Tannins are absent. [1, 2, 50].

Medicinal Use: Bitter tonic, without astringency; orexigenic, carminative. Palmatine is hypotensive and a uterine stimulant; jatrorrhizine is hypotensive, sedative and antifungal [7] (see Barberry).

Preparations: Powdered root, dose: 0.5–2 g; Liquid Extract, dose: 0.5–2 ml; Concentrated Infusion of Calumba BP 1948, dose: 2–4 ml, Calumba Tincture BP 1948, dose: 2–4 ml.

Regulatory Status: GSL.

CAMPHOR

Cinnamomum camphora (L.) Nees & Eberm.
Fam. Lauraceae

Synonyms: Gum Camphor, Laurel Camphor, Camphire, *Laurus camphora* L., *Camphora officinarum* Nees.

Habitat: Central China and Japan.

Description: A colourless, crystalline, translucent mass with a characteristic odour, often imported in small square pieces. It is obtained by passing steam through the chipped wood. The distillate contains camphor which is resublimed, leaving an essential oil.

Part Used: Distillate from the wood.

Constituents: Camphor of natural origin is a dextrorotatory ketone, unlike synthetic camphor which is optically inactive. Other constituents include (i) Volatile oil, containing some camphor, safrole, borneol, heliotropin, terpineol and vanillin (ii) Lignans, of which at least 5 have been isolated including secoisosolariciresinol dimethyl ether [264] and kusunokiol [265].

Medicinal Use: Topically as a rubifacient and mild analgesic; and as an ingredient of lip balms, chilblain ointments, cold sore lotions and liniments for fibrositis and muscle stiffness. It is well known as camphorated oil. Large quantities should not be applied externally since camphor may be absorbed through the skin causing systemic toxicity. Small doses can be taken internally for colds, diarrhoea and other complaints; overdosing causes vomiting, convulsions, palpitations and can be fatal.

Ngai camphor is from *Blumea balsamifera* (Compositae) and Borneo camphor from *Dryobalanops aromatica* (Dipterocarpaceae). Both have similar uses.

Preparations: Camphor Spirit BPC 1959, dose: 0.3–2 ml; Concentrated Camphor Water BPC 1949, dose: 0.3–1 ml; Camphor Liniment BP; Camphorated Chalk BPC 1949.

Regulatory Status: GSL Restricted dose 10 mg. Maximum daily dose 30 mg.

Biblical References: Song of Solomon 1:14 and 4:13.

CANADIAN HEMP

Apocynum cannabinum L.
and other spp.
Fam. Apocynaceae

Synonyms: Black Indian Hemp, *Apocynum pubescens* Brown.

Habitat: USA and Canada.

Description: The root is about 0.5 cm or more in diameter, rarely branched, longitudinally wrinkled, sometimes fissured transversely, pale brown externally. The bark is thick, whitish, with a central, porous, radiate wood and often a small, central pith. Fracture short. Taste, bitter, disagreeable; odourless.

Part Used: Root, rhizome.

Constituents: (i) Cardiac glycosides, including strophanthin, strophanthin cymaroside, cymarol and others [2] (ii) Miscellaneous; oxyacetophenone, tannins and resin.

Medicinal Use: Diaphoretic, diuretic, emetic, expectorant. Used in the form of a decoction for cardiac dropsy. Actions similar to Strophanthus (q.v.).

Preparations: Powdered root, dose: 0.05–3 g; Liquid Extract, dose: 0.05–0.25 ml; Tincture, dose: 0.2–0.5 ml.

CANCHALAGUA
Centaurium chilensis (Willd) Druce.
Fam. Gentianaceae

Synonyms: *Erythraea chilensis* Pers.

Habitat: Pacific Coast of America.

Description: Closely resembles Centaury, but is more branched, with linear leaves and stalked flowers.

Part Used: Herb.

Constituents: Erythrocentaurin, a bitter, and tannins [2].

Medicinal Use: Bitter, tonic, stimulant. May be used as an infusion in dyspepsia and digestive complaints.

Preparations: Liquid Extract, dose: 2–4 ml.

CANELLA
Canella winterana (L.) Gaertn.
Fam. Canellaceae

Synonyms: White Cinnamon, West Indian Wild Cinnamon, *Canella alba* Murr.

Habitat: The West Indies and Florida.

Description: The bark occurs in quilled pieces, fawn coloured externally, the ash-grey cork having been removed by gentle beating; chalky white on inner surface. Transverse fracture short, with numerous bright orange-yellow resin cells visible. Taste, biting, aromatic, recalling that of cinnamon; odour, aromatic.

Part Used: Bark.

Constituents: (i) Volatile oil, about 0.75–1.25%, containing α-pinene, eugenol, caryophyllene [183] (ii) Aldehydes such as canellal, a sesquiterpene dialdehyde [1] and 3-methoxy-4,5-methylenedioxycinnamaldehyde [266] (iii) Miscellaneous; resin and mannitol, each about 8%.

Medicinal Use: Aromatic, stimulant, tonic, usually in combination. Canellal has been shown to be antimicrobial [1]. More often used as a condiment.

Preparations: Aloes and Canella Powder BPC 1934, dose: 0.2–0.6 g.

Regulatory Status: GSL.

CARAWAY
Carum carvi L.
Fam. Umbelliferae

Synonyms: Caraway Seed or Fruit, *Apium carvi* Crantz.

Habitat: Native to Europe, Asia and N. Africa, widely cultivated.

Description: The fruits are small, brown and slightly curved, about 4–8 mm long and 1–2 mm wide. They are tapered at both ends with five longitudinal ridges. Odour; characteristic.

Part Used: Fruit.

Constituents: (i) Volatile oil, consisting of carvone (40–60%) and limonene, with dihydrocarvone, carveol, dihydrocarveol, pinene, thujone, and other minor constituents [5, 1, 124] (ii) Flavonoids; mainly quercetin derivatives [267] (iii) Miscellaneous; polysaccharides, protein, fixed oil, calcium oxalate [5].

Medicinal Use: Antispasmodic, carminative, stimulant and expectorant. It is used mainly for stomach complaints in both adults and children. The antispasmodic and carminative effects have been confirmed experimentally and caraway shown to reduce gastrointestinal foam [268, 269].

Preparations: Powdered seeds, dose: 0.5–2 g; Caraway Oil, dose: 0.05–0.2 ml; Concentrated Caraway Water, dose: 0.05–0.2 ml.

Potter's Product: Acidosis Tablets.

Regulatory Status: GSL.

CARDAMON
Elettaria cardamomum (L.) Maton.
Fam. Zingiberaceae

Synonyms: Cardamom Seed.

Habitat: Malabar Coast of India, Sri Lanka, cultivated widely in the tropics.

Description: Ovoid or oblong fruit, somewhat triangular in cross-section and longitudinally finely striated. Mysore and Malabar cardamoms are usually bleached to a cream or pale buff colour, they have a smoother surface but are found less often in commerce now than the smaller, greener Alleppy or Ceylon varieties. All samples should be whole, containing seeds which are about 4 mm diameter and dark reddish-brown. Odour, highly aromatic, pleasant; taste, aromatic and pungent.

Part Used: Fruits, seeds.

Constituents: Volatile oil, about 5% but very variable. The major components are 1,8-cineole and α-terpinylacetate, with limonene, α-terpineol, sabinene and linalool [5, 50].

Medicinal Use: Carminative, stomachic, stimulant. The oil has antispasmodic activity [270] and the aqueous extract enhances the activity of trypsin *in vitro*.

Preparations: Powdered fruit, dose: 0.5–2 g; Aromatic Cardamom Tincture BP, dose: 2–4 ml; Compound Cardamom Tincture BP, dose: 2–4 ml; Liquid Extract, dose: 0.3–2 ml; Cardamom Oil BPC, dose: 0.03–0.2 ml.

Potter's Product: Acidosis Tablets.

Regulatory Status: GSL.

CAROB
Ceratonia siliqua L.
Fam. Leguminosae

Synonyms: St. John's Bread, Locust Bean.

Habitat: Native to S. E. Europe and W. Asia, cultivated elsewhere.

Description: Pods about 10–30 cm long and 3–5 cm broad, containing flattish, oval, dark brown seeds in a light brown fleshy pulp.
Part Used: Pulp.
Constituents: Nutrients: 30–70% sugars, fats, starch, protein, amino acids, gallic acid etc [5].
Medicinal Use: Antidiarrhoeal, as a decoction for catarrh and to improve the voice. Carob is used frequently as a substitute for cocoa as it contains no stimulants such as theobromine and caffeine. This plant should not be confused with the Carob Tree, *Jacaranda procera* or *J. caroba*, which is native to S. America and S. Africa, the leaves of which are reputed to be diuretic and sedative.
Preparations: Powder, for use as a food and flavouring.

CASCARA AMARGA

Picramnia antidesma Sw.
P. pentandra Sw.
P. parvifolia Engler
P. sellowi
and other spp.
Fam. Simaroubaceae

Synonyms: West Indian Snakewood *(P. antidesma)*, Bitter Bush *(P. pentandra)*.
Habitat: W. Indies and Central America.
Description: Bark usually found in small fragments about 2–3 mm thick, externally greyish, internally deep brown, inner surface nearly smooth. Fracture short, showing numerous dots due to stone cells. Taste, astringent then bitter and earthy.
Part Used: Bark.
Constituents: *P. parvifolia* contains anthraquinone derivatives based on chrysophanol, emodin, physcion and aloe-emodin [271]. *P. sellowi* contains (i) Anthraquinones based on chrysophanol, emodin and physcion (ii) Triterpenes including betulinic acid and epibetulinic acid (iii) benzoic acid [272]. *P. pentandra* contains similar triterpenes e.g. 3-epibetulinic acid [273].
Medicinal Use: Bitter tonic, alterative, laxative.
Preparations: Liquid Extract, dose 1–2 ml.

CASCARA SAGRADA

Rhamnus purshiana L.
Fam. Rhamnaceae

Synonyms: Sacred Bark, Chittem Bark, Cascara.
Habitat: Native to the Pacific Coast of N. America.
Description: Bark usually supplied in quilled or curved pieces, about 1 mm or more thick, purplish-brown, furrowed longitudinally, with transverse lenticels, and lichens and mosses visible as silver-grey or greenish patches.

The inner surface is reddish-brown, longitudinally striated and transversely wrinkled. Fracture pale to dark brown, darkening with age. Taste, bitter and nauseous; odour, leathery.

Part Used: Bark, collected in the spring and early summer and stored for at least a year before use, to eliminate constituents which cause griping.

Constituents: Up to 10% anthraquinone glycosides, consisting of the cascarosides A, B, C and D, which account for about 70% of the total [274, 275]; with other glycosides in minor concentrations, including barbaloin, frangulin, chrysaloin; glycosides based on emodin, aloe-emodin, emodin oxanthrone, and chrysophanol [1, 5], dianthrones including the heterodianthrones palmidin A, B and C (see Rhubarb) [1], and the free aglycones.

Medicinal Use: Laxative, tonic. The cascarosides act on the large intestine and stimulate peristalsis, they are more effective than the hydrolysed aloins [276]. Cascara Sagrada is used for habitual constipation, dyspepsia, digestive complaints and in the treatment of piles.

Preparations: Powdered bark, dose: 1–2.5 g; Cascara Liquid Extract BP, dose: 2–5 ml; Cascara Dry Extract BP, dose: 100–300 mg; Cascara Elixir BP, dose: 2–5 ml; Cascara tablets BP, dose: 1 or 2 tablets.

Potter's Products: Constipation Mixture No. 105; Pile Compound Herb; Pilewort Compound Tablets No. 375; Rheumatism Compound Herb.

Regulatory Status: GSL.

CASCARILLA
Croton eleuteria (L.) Sw.
Fam. Euphorbiaceae

Synonyms: Sweet Wood Bark.

Habitat: Native to the West Indies, grows also in tropical America.

Description: The bark occurs in short quilled pieces, usually with a chalky, more or less cracked, ·white surface, with black dots due to the fruit of lichens. Transverse fracture reddish-brown. Taste, aromatic, bitter; odour, aromatic, particularly when burnt, hence its use in flavouring tobacco.

Part Used: Bark.

Constituents: (i) Volatile oil, 1.5–3%, containing limonene, *p*-cymene, eugenol, β-caryophyllene, dipentene, cineole, methyl thymol, and cascarillic acid [50] (ii) Resin, about 15% [50] (iii) Miscellaneous; vanillin, betaine, cuparophenol, cascarilladiene, cascarillone [5, 50].

Medicinal Use: Stimulant, aromatic, tonic. Used in dyspepsia, flatulence and diarrhoea and as an anti-emetic, usually taken as an infusion.

Preparations: Powdered bark, dose: 1–2.5 g; Liquid Extract, dose: 2–4 ml; Tincture, dose: 2–4 ml.

Regulatory Status: GSL.

CASHEW NUT

Anacardium occidentale L.
Fam. Anacardiaceae.

Synonyms: East Indian Almond, *Cassuvium pomiferum.*

Habitat: Cultivated extensively in the Tropics.

Description: Fruit kidney-shaped, smooth, pale greyish-brown, about 2–3 cm long and 1 cm broad and thick.

Part Used: Nuts, leaves, bark.

Constituents: Leaves: (i) Flavonoids, mainly glycosides of quercetin and kaempferol (ii) Hydroxybenzoic acid [277]. Bark: A gum or balsam containing anacardic acid, anacardol, cardol and ginkgol [33]. The caustic liquid in the shell contains about 39% anacardic acid, which is a mixture of alkyl salicylic acid derivatives [33].

Medicinal Use: Leaves and bark are used as an infusion for toothache and sore gums in W. Africa, and as a febrifuge in malaria. Anacardic acid is bactericidal against *Staphylococcus aureus* [278] as well as being fungicidal, vermicidal and protozoicidal [279, 33]. Extracts of the leaves and bark are hypotensive in rats [280]. The nuts are highly regarded as a food, usually roasted.

CASSIA

Cinnamomum aromaticum Nees
Fam. Lauraceae

Synonyms: Chinese Cinnamon, False Cinnamon, *Cinnamomum cassia* Nees ex Bl., *Cassia lignea*, Rougui (Chinese).

Habitat: South East Asia, China.

Description: The bark is brown, in quilled pieces, sometimes with the remains of the outer layer present. The quills are rarely found inserted inside one another as in cinnamon (q.v.). Taste and odour, similar to cinnamon but distinct.

Part Used: Bark. Cassia Oil BPC is distilled from the leaves and twigs.

Constituents: (i) Volatile oil, consisting mainly of *trans*-cinnamaldehyde, 80–90%, with cinnamylacetate, phenylpropylacetate and numerous trace constituents including salicylaldehyde and methyleugenol [281] (ii) Diterpenes, classified into five different types, including the cinncassiols A–E and their glucosides [282, 283, 284] (iii) Tannins and polyphenols, such as (+)-catechin, (−)-epicatechin, the procyanidins B_2, B_4, B_5 and C_1, cinnamonol D_1 and D_4 (285, 286], cinnamtannins I, II, and III [286]. No hydrolysable tannins, mono- or sesquiterpenes have been isolated [284, 286].

Medicinal Use: Aromatic, stomachic, tonic, antipyretic, diaphoretic and analgesic. In Chinese medicine it is used for vascular disorders particularly. A great deal of recent research has been carried out on Cassia, showing a number of useful pharmacological actions. The volatile oil is carminative and antiseptic; cinnamaldehyde is a weak CNS stimulant at low doses and a depressant at high doses and has spasmolytic activity [7]. Cinnamaldehyde is hypotensive, hypoglycaemic and increases peripheral blood flow [287, 288], and it reduces platelet aggregability by inhibiting both the cyclooxygenase and lipoxygenase pathways of arachidonic acid metabolism [289]. It is however volatile and easily lost from the crude drug and its preparations. The therapeutic effect of the bark is not totally dependent on the cinnamaldehyde content of the bark; aqueous extracts show anti-allergic properties which have been shown to be due to anti-complement activity [290]. The cinncassiols are thought to be responsible for at least some of the anti-allergic effects [282, 283]. Cassia has shown promising results as a radiation protective agent, increasing survival times and leukocyte and platelet counts in *in vivo* experiments in China [7]. The oil is used mainly for flavouring medicines, cosmetics, toothpastes, mouthwashes and foods.

Regulatory Status: GSL.
Biblical References: Exodus 30:24; Psalm 45:8; Ezekiel 27:19.

CASSIA PODS

Cassia fistula L.
Fam. Leguminosae

Synonyms: Pudding Stick.
Habitat: Cultivated in the Tropics.
Description: The pods are up to 50 cm long, with the interior divided into compartments containing the seeds and a thin layer of black fruit pulp.
Part Used: Pulp.
Constituents: (i) Anthraquinone glycosides, sennosides A and B [183] (ii) Sugars, about 60% [2].
Medicinal Use: A pleasant fruit laxative, acting in a similar way to Senna (q.v.), but rather milder.
Preparations: Cassia Pulp BPC 1959, dose 4–8 g.
Regulatory Status: GSL.

CASTOR OIL PLANT

Ricinus communis L.
Fam. Euphorbiaceae

Synonyms: Castor Bean, Palma Christi.
Habitat: Native to India but cultivated worldwide as an ornamental.
Description: The seeds are oval, from about 1–2 cm long and 0.5–1 cm broad, slightly compressed. They are greyish-brown and often mottled with brown or black markings, with a yellowish caruncle at one end, taste, acrid; odourless.
Part Used: Oil expressed from seed.
Constituents: Fixed oil, consisting mainly of glycerides of ricinoleic, isoricinoleic acids, and to a lesser extent other acids including stearic, linoleic and dihydroxystearic. The seeds are very poisonous, but the toxic protein, ricin, is left behind in the cake after pressing. The seed also contains an alkaloid, ricinine, lectins and other substances [1].

Medicinal Use: Castor oil is used as a laxative and purgative, particularly after food or other poisoning and prior to intestinal X-ray examination. It has been used to expel worms after treatment but should not be used for this purpose since it facilitates absorption of some anthelmintics [5]. It has a folklore reputation for inducing labour. Castor oil is emollient and soothing to the skin and eye and is an ingredient of some cosmetic and ophthalmic preparations.

Preparations: Castor Oil BP, dose: 5–20 ml.

Regulatory Status: GSL.

CATECHU BLACK

Acacia catechu Willd.
Fam. Leguminosae

Synonyms: Cutch, Dark Catechu, *Catechu nigrum.*

Habitat: India and Burma.

Description: Occurs in black shining pieces or cakes, sometimes with the remains of leaf on the outside. Taste, very astringent then bitter and sweetish; odourless.

Part Used: Extract from leaves and young shoots.

Constituents: (i) Tannins; 2–20% catechin, 25–33% phlobatannins including catechutannic acid (20–50%) and others [1, 5] (ii) Flavonoids including quercetin, quercitrin, fisetin and others [1, 5] (iii) Miscellaneous; gums and resins, pigments etc.

Medicinal Use: Astringent. It is used in chronic diarrhoea, dysentery and chronic catarrh. Useful for arresting excessive mucous discharges and checking haemorrhages, and recommended as a local application for sore mouths and gums. It has also been shown to be hypotensive *in vivo* and *in vitro;* its mechansim of action is thought to be bradykinin related and due to vasodilatation [291].

Preparations: Powder, dose: 0.3–1 g.

Regulatory Status: GSL.

CATECHU PALE

Uncaria gambier Roxb.
Fam. Rubiaceae

Synonyms: Gambir, Gambier, *Terra japonica, Ourouparia gambir* Baill.

Habitat: S. E. Asia.

Description: Occurs as pale reddish to dark brownish-black cubes or lozenges, with a dull, powdery fracture. Taste similar to Black Catechu.

Part Used: Extract of leaves and shoots.

Constituents: (i) Tannins; mainly catechins, up to 35%, and catechutannic acid up to 50% (ii) Indole alkaloids including gambirine gambiridine and others [292] (iii) Flavonoids such as quercetin (iv) Pigments and gambir-fluorescin [5].

Medicinal Use: Astringent. Uses are similar to those of Black Catechu (q.v.). Gambirine is reported to be hypotensive and *d*-catechu to constrict blood vessels [5].
Preparations: Catechu Tincture, dose: 2.5–5 ml.
Regulatory Status: GSL.

CATNEP
Nepeta cataria L.
Fam. Labiatae

Synonyms: Catnip, Catmint.
Habitat: A common European herb, cultivated in Britain and the USA.
Description: Leaves stalked, cordate-ovate, pointed, with a serrate margin and a whitish, hairy undersurface. The stem is quadrangular and hairy. Flowers tubular, two-lipped, white with crimson dots, arranged in short, dense, spikes. Taste and odour mint-like but characteristic.
Part Used: Herb.
Constituents: (i) Volatile oil, up to 0.3%, containing the monoterpenes α- and β-nepetalactone, up to 42% [293], 5,9-dehydronepetalactone [294], carvacrol, citronellal, nerol, geraniol, pulegone, thymol and nepetalic acid [2, 124] (ii) Iridoids, including epideoxyloganic acid and 7-deoxyloganic acid [295] (iii) Tannins [37].
Medicinal Use: Diaphoretic, refrigerant, febrifuge, spasmolytic, anti-diarrhoeal, sedative. Used particularly for colds and colic, taken as an infusion. It has a folklore reputation as a hallucinogen [296], however this is disputed [297]. More recent studies have shown behavioural effects, although weak, in young chicks [298] and rodents [299] as well as the well-known intoxicating effect on cats [300].
Preparations: Dried herb, dose: 2–4 g.
Regulatory Status: GSL.

CAYENNE
Capsicum frutescens L.
C. annuum L.
and its varieties *C. chinense* Jacq.
C. baccata Eshbaugh
C. pendulum Ruiz et Pavon
C. minimum Roxb.
C. pubescens Willd.
Fam. Solanaceae

Synonyms: Capsicum, Chili or Chilli Pepper, Hot Pepper, Tabasco Pepper. The botanical classification is under review and any of the above names may be found. Green and Red (or Bell) Peppers and Paprika are produced by mild varieties of *C. annuum*.
Habitat: Tropical America and Africa and widely cultivated.
Description: The fruit varies in colour, size and pungency. The pods may reach 10 cm or more in length; they are conical, the colour ranging from green in the unripe fruit to yellow and red.

Part Used: Fruit.

Constituents: (i) Capsaicin, 0.1–1.5%, which is a mixture of capsaicin itself, dihydrocapsaicin, nordihydrocapsaicin, homodihydrocapsaicin and others [301] (ii) Carotenoids; capsanthin, capsorubin, carotene etc [5, 302] (iii) Steroidal saponins known as capsicidins, in the seed and root [303].

Medicinal Use: Stimulant, tonic, carminative, spasmolytic, diaphoretic, antiseptic, rubefacient and counter-irritant; this is one of the most widely used of all natural remedies. It is taken internally to improve peripheral circulation, alleviate flatulence and colic and stimulate the digestive system; as a gargle in laryngitis; and topically in the form of an ointment for muscle pain and stiffness, lumbago and unbroken chilblains. Capsicidin has antibiotic activity on some microorganisms [303]. Capsaicin has a large number of pharmacological actions, including effects on the circulatory system, smooth muscle, and heat regulation of the body. It desensitizes the sensory nerve endings to pain stimulation by depleting Substance P from the nervous system, which is the basis for its use as a local analgesic. The effects of Cayenne on the gastrointestinal system are also complex; for a full accunt of the scientific literature see [304] and references therein. Cayenne is used widely in cooking to give a hot, pungent flavour, it is non-toxic at normal doses but should be used carefully as it is very pungent.

Preparations: Cayenne or Capsicum Powder, dose: 30–120 mg; Tincture of Capsicum BPC 1973, dose: 0.3–1 ml; Strong Tincture of Capsicum BPC 1934, dose: 0.05–0.15 ml; Capsicum Oleoresin BPC, dose: 0.6–2 mg; Capsicum Ointment BPC; Compound Capsicum Ointment BPC, 1949.

Potter's Products: Composition Essence Peerless, Antispasmodic Drops, Elder Flowers and Peppermint with Composition Essence, Life Drops, Herbprin, Gout and Rheumatism Tablets No. 215, Backache and Kidney Tablets No. 252.

Regulatory Status: GSL. Oleoresin, Maximum dose, 1.2 mg. Maximum daily dose 1.8 mg.

CEDRON

Simaba cedron Planch.
Fam. Simaroubaceae

Habitat: Central America.

Description: Commercial samples of the seed usually consist of the separated cotyledons; these are flattened on one side and convex on the other, are of a greyish-yellow tint and are about 4 cm long and 1–1.5 cm wide. Taste, very bitter; odour, recalling that of coconut.

Part Used: Seeds.

Constituents: Quassinoids, including cedronine and cedronyline [305].

Medicinal Use: Febrifuge, bitter, tonic, antispasmodic. The seeds have been employed in the treatment of malaria: it is now known that these quassinoids have antimalarial and anti-inflammatory properties *in vivo* and *in vitro* [306].

Preparations: Powder, dose: 0.05–0.5 g.

CELANDINE

Chelidonium majus L.
Fam. Papaveraceae

Synonyms: Greater Celandine. (Must not be confused with Lesser Celandine, also known as Pilewort, (q.v.).

Habitat: A common garden plant in Europe, flowering in May.

Description: Leaves pinnate, green above, greyish below, 15–30 cm long and 5–8 cm wide. Leaflets opposite, deeply cut, with rounded teeth. Stems have recurved hairs and exude a saffron yellow juice when fresh and broken. The flowers are yellow, consisting of four small petals, and are followed by narrow pods containing the black shiny seeds. Taste, bitter and acrid; odour disagreeable.

Part Used: Herb.

Constituents: (i) Alkaloids, including allocryptopine, berberine, chelamine, chelerythrine, chelidonine, coptisine, magnoflorine, protopine, sanguinarine, sparteine and others [7, 112, 307] (ii) In the root: choline, histamine, tyramine, saponins, chelidoniol, chelidonic acid, carotene and vitamin C [7].

Medicinal Use: Alterative, diuretic. Has been used in the treatment of jaundice, eczema, and the fresh juice as an application for corns and warts. In Chinese medicine this herb is also highly thought of and used as an analgesic, antitussive, anti-inflammatory and detoxicant [7]. Chelidonine, α-allocryptopine and sanguinarine have *in vivo* analgesic actions [7]. Chelidonine has also been shown to relax smooth muscle spasm, including bronchospasm. An extract of the plant as well as the isolated alkaloids protopine, sanguinarine, chelerythrine and chelidonine have antibacterial activity and are antitussive [7]. Chelidonine has a number of useful actions; it produces a mild but prolonged lowering of arterial blood pressure, increases the production of urine and inhibits or delays the development of anaphylactic shock *in vivo* [7]. Clinical studies in China have concentrated mainly on its use in bronchitis and whooping cough where it is considered to be effective, however statistics were not given. Side effects were shown to be mild and infrequent and include dry mouth and dizziness; no changes in liver or kidney functions and ECG were detected [7].

Preparations: Liquid Extract, dose: 2–4 ml.

Potter's Products: Elixir of Chelidonium.

Regulatory Status: Maximum daily dose, 6 g.

CELERY

Apium graveolens L.
Fam. Umbelliferae

Synonyms: Smallage, Qincai (Chinese).

Habitat: Cultivated widely. The wild variety grows in marshy places and has an unpleasant odour.

Description: Celery is a well-known plant needing no description. The seeds are very small, abut 1 mm long, plano-convex, brown, with five paler, longitudinal ribs. Taste and odour of celery.

Part Used: Seeds. Stems of *A. graveolens* var dulce (Mill) Pers. are used as a vegetable.

Constituents: (i) Volatile oil, about 2%, containing *d*-limonene, ca. 60%, with α-selinene, santalol, α- and β-eudesmol, dihydrocarvone and others [5] (ii) Phthalides; mainly 3-*n*-butylphthalide, ligustilide, sedanolide, and sedanenolide, [308, 309, 310] (iii) Coumarins; bergapten, isoimperatorin, isopimpinellin, osthenol, apiumoside and celeroside [311, 312] (iv) Flavonoids; apiin and apigenin [313] (v) Fixed oil, fatty acids [5].

Medicinal Use: Antiinflammatory, antirheumatic, hypotensive, carminative, diuretic, tonic, reputed aphrodisiac. Some of these actions have been substantiated by experimentation; the aqueous extract has been shown to reduce adjuvant-induced arthritis in rats [314] and to be hypotensive in patients as well as animals [5, 7]. The phthalides are sedative in mice [308] and exhibit antiepileptic activity in rats and mice [310]. The volatile oil has antifungal activity [7]. Clinical studies in China have confirmed the usefulness of the tincture in cases of hypertension of various types; the drop in blood pressure is accompanied by an increased urine output and an amelioration of subjective symptoms such as an improvement in sleep patterns [7].

Preparations: Powdered seeds, dose: 1–4 g; Liquid Extract, dose: 0.3–1.5 ml; Essential oil, dose: 0.05–0.1 ml.

Potter's Products: Celery Tablets No. 218, Rheumatism Compound Herb.

Regulatory Status: GSL.

CENTAURY

Centaurium erythraea Rafn.
Fam. Gentianaceae

Synonyms: Century, Feverwort.

Habitat: Native to Europe, including the British Isles, Western Asia, North Africa and naturalized in N. America.

Description: Stem up to 30 cm high, bearing opposite, lanceolate-ovate leaves having 3–5 longitudinal ribs, hairless, and entire at margins. Flowers pink, with twisted anthers. Taste, bitter; odour, slight.

Part Used: Herb.

Constituents: (i) Secoiridoids. These glycosides are the so-called "bitter principles" and include sweroside, its *m*-hydroxybenzoyl esters centapicrin and desacetylcentapicrin, the related glucosides decentapicrin A, B and C, gentiopicroside (= gentiopicrin), and swertiamarin [315, 316] (ii) Alkaloids; gentianine, gentianidine, gentioflavine [5] (iii) Xanthone derivatives such as 1,8-dihydroxy-3,5,6,7-tetramethoxyxanthone [317] (iv) Phenolic acids including protocatechuic, *m*- and *p*-hydroxbenzoic, vanillic, syringic, *p*-coumaric, ferulic and caffeic [5] (v) Triterpenes; β-sitosterol, campesterol, brassicsterol, stigmasterol [318], α- and β-amyrin, erythrodiol and others [5].

Medicinal Use: Aromatic, bitter, stomachic, tonic. Centaury is widely used in disorders of the upper digestive tract, in dyspepsia, for liver and gallbladder complaints and to stimulate the appetite in a similar manner to gentian (q.v.). It has some antipyretic activity which is thought to be due to the phenolic acids [319]. For details of the pharmacology of gentianin, gentianidine, gentiopicroside and swertiamarin, see Gentian.

Preparations: Liquid Extract, dose: 2–4 ml.
Potter's Products: Stomach and Liver Medicinal Tea Bags.
Regulatory Status: GSL.

CHAMOMILE

Chamaemelum nobile L.
Fam. Compositae

Synonyms: English Chamomile, Roman Chamomile, Double Chamomile, *Anthemis nobilis* L.

Habitat: Cultivated mainly in Europe.

Description: Flowers mainly double, consisting of ligulate florets only, with a conical, solid receptacle, covered with lanceolate, membranous scales (palae). Leaves pinnately divided into short and hairy leaflets. Taste, aromatic and very bitter; odour characteristic. Wild chamomiles, with only an outer row of ligulate florets, are known as Scotch chamomiles.

Part Used: Flowers, herb.

Constituents: (i) Volatile oil, up to 1.75%, consisting mainly of esters of tiglic and angelic acids, with chamazulene, pinocarvone, 1,8-cineole [5], α-pinene, isobutyrate esters, cyclododecane, pinene-3-one [320] and others (ii) Sesquiterpene lactones of the germacranolide type, including nobilin, 1,10-epoxynobilin and 3-dihydronobilin (321] (iii) Flavonoids such as luteolin and apigenin and their 7-glucosides (322] (iv) Coumarins including scopoletin and its glucoside (323) (v) Phenolic acids; *trans*-caffeic and ferulic acids and their glucosides [323].

Medicinal Use: Stomachic, antiemetic, antispasmodic and mild sedative, when taken internally. As a lotion it is used as a soothing and analgesic application in toothache, earache, and neuralgia, and as a cream or ointment for wounds, sore nipples and nappy rash. The sesquiterpene lactones have anti-tumour activity *in vitro* [321]. Chamomile is an ingredient of shampoos and hair rinses for blonde hair.

Preparations: Liquid Extract, dose: 2–4 ml; Chamomile Oil BPC 1949, dose: 0.03–2 ml; Extract of Chamomile, dose: 0.1–0.5 g.
Potter's Products: Tonic and Nervine Essence, Nervine Mixture No. 90.
Regulatory Status: GSL.

CHAMOMILE, GERMAN

Matricaria recutita L.
Fam. Compositae

Synonyms: Single Chamomile, Hungarian Chamomile, Pin Heads, *M. chamomilla* L., *Chamomilla recutita*. The botanical classification is again being revised and any of the above names may be found in the literature.

Habitat: Native to Europe, N. W. Asia; naturalized in N. America and extensively cultivated.

Description: The flowerheads are much smaller than the preceding, and have only one row of ligulate florets which are usually bent backwards when dried. The receptacle is conical and hollow, and has no membranous bracts. Taste, bitter and aromatic; odour similar to the former but weaker.

Part Used: Flowers.

Constituents: (i) Volatile oil, up to about 2%, containing α-bisabolol up to 50% [324], azulenes including chamazulene, guiazulene and matricine, α-bisabolol oxides A and B, α-bisabolone oxide A, farnesene and others [325, 5] (ii) Flavonoids including apigenin and luteolin, and their glycosides and acetylglucosides, patuletin and quercetin [326, 327] (iii) Spiroethers, such as *cis*- and *trans*-en-yn-dicycloether [328] (iv) Coumarins; e.g. umbelliferon and herniarin [5] (v) Polysaccharides; xyloglucurans [147].

Medicinal Use: Sedative, carminative, antispasmodic, analgesic, antiinflammatory and antiseptic. It is often used as a tea, sometimes in the form of tea-bags, for insomnia; for gout, sciatica, indigestion and diarrhoea, and topically in the same way as Chamomile (q.v.). It has a particular place in the treatment of childrens ailments, for colic, teething pains and infantile convulsions. Recent work has substantiated many of the claims made for German Chamomile. Matricine and (−)-α-bisabolol have significant antiinflammatory and analgesic activity; chamazulene, guiazulene and the oxides of α-bisabolol considerably less as measured by a number of *in vivo* and *in vitro* systems [329, 330]. Natural (−)-α-bisabolol has been shown to be more effective than synthetic racemic bisabolol in healing burns; it also decreases the temperature of skin exposed to UV light [331]. Bisabolol also has an ulceroprotective effect; it prevents the formation of ulcers induced by indomethacin and alcohol and also reduces the healing time [332]. The total extract of German Chamomile has an *in vitro* antispasmodic effect which is due to a number of constituents: (−)-α-bisabolol has a spasmolytic effect comparable with that of papaverine; the oxides are about half as potent [333]. The spiroethers, particularly the *cis*-isomer which is about ten times as potent as papaverine [328], and the flavonoids, especially apigenin, which is about three times as potent [333], are also spasmolytic. The flavonoids also inhibit Croton-oil induced oedema of mouse ear [327]. Chamazulene and α-bisabolol have antimicrobial properties, umbelliferone is fungistatic [5] and an extract demonstrates inhibition of poliovirus replication *in vitro* [334]. German Chamomile is considered non-toxic and tests done on α-bisabolol at least have shown no problems and no teratogenicity [335]. The polysaccharides are immunostimulating; they activate macrophages and B lymphocytes [147], thus demonstrating a scientific basis for the use of chamomile in wound healing.

Preparations: Powdered flowers, dose 2–8 g; Liquid Extract, dose: 0.5–4 ml.

Regulatory Status: GSL.

CHAULMOOGRA

Hydnocarpus kurzii (King) Warb.
H. anthelmintica
H. wightiana Blume
and other spp.
Fam. Flacourtaceae

Synonyms: Hydnocarpus, *Taraktogenos kurzii* = *H. kurzii*. Species of *Chaulmoogra* have been used, however the botanical origin is not always apparent.

Habitat: Indian subcontinent, Malaysia.

Description: Seeds greyish, about 2–3 cm long and 1.5 cm diameter, irregularly angular with rounded ends. Kernel oily, enclosing two thin, heart-shaped, three-veined cotyledons and a straight radicle. Taste, acrid; odour, disagreeable.

Part Used: Seeds, oil expressed from the seeds.

Constituents: Fixed oil, constituting about 55–60% of the kernel, containing cyclopentenic acids including hydnocarpic, dihydrohydnocarpic, gorlic, chaulmoogric, dihydrochaulmoogric, taraktogenic, isogaleic and arachnic acids and their esters [2, 336].

Medicinal Use: Antileprotic, dermatic, febrifuge, sedative, The oil is used particularly for skin diseases, such as eczema and psoriasis, as an ointment, and in the form of injections for leprosy [337]. Internally it is taken as an emulsion. The seeds may be taken powdered in the form of pills.

Preparations: Oil, dose: 0.3–1 ml.

CHEKEN

Eugenia chequen Mol.
Fam. Myrtaceae

Synonyms: *Myrtus cheken* Spreng.

Habitat: Chile.

Description: Leaves leathery, ovate, about 1–1.5 cm long, 0.5–1 cm wide, entire margins, very shortly stalked with numerous minute, round, translucent oil cells. Taste, astringent aromatic and bitter, recalling that of bay leaves; odour slight.

Part Used: Leaves.

Constituents: (i) Volatile oil, about 1% (ii) Bitters, including chekenone, chekenetin, chekenine (iii) Tannins [2].

Medicinal Use: Diuretic, expectorant, tonic.

Preparations: Liquid Extract, dose: 2–4 ml.

CHERRY LAUREL

Prunus laurocerasus L.
Fam. Rosaceae

Synonyms: Cherry-bay.

Habitat: Native to Russia but cultivated in many temperate countries.

Description: Leaves leathery, glossy, about 10–15 cm long by 3–5 cm wide, oblong, lanceolate, serrate with a recurved margin and pointed apex. On the undersurface there are two or three punctate glands close to the midrib near the base. Odour, when the fresh leaves are bruised, like oil of bitter almonds.

Part Used: Leaves.

Constituents: (i) Cyanogenetic glycosides, about 1.5%, mainly mandelonitrile glucosides, the *d*-isomer of which is prunasin and the *l*-isomer sambunigrin. The racemic mixture of these is referred to as prulaurasin (ii) Volatile oil, composed of benzaldehyde, benzyl alcohol and traces of hydrocyanic acid (iii) Miscellaneous; ursolic acid, tannin etc. [5].

Medicinal Use: Sedative, antitussive, stomachic. Mostly used to produce cherry-laurel water for medicinal use. The oil, with the hydrocyanic acid removed, is used as a flavouring.

Preparations: Cherry-laurel Water BPC 1949, dose: 2–8 ml.

CHERRY STALKS

Prunus avium
and other species.
Fam. Rosaceae

Description: Fruit stalks about 4 cm long and 1 mm thick, enlarged at one end. The stalks of various species were collected indiscriminately.

Medicinal Use: Not used nowadays but at one time were considered a good astringent tonic.

CHESTNUT

Castanea sativa Mill.
Fam. Fagaceae

Synonyms: Sweet Chestnut, Spanish Chestnut, *C. vulgaris* Lam., *C. vesca*, *Fagus castanea*. American Chestnut leaves are from *C. dentata* Borkh, (= *C. americana* Michx.).

Habitat: Europe.

Description: Leaves leathery, about 15–20 cm long, 6–8 cm broad, oblonglanceolate with sharply dentate margin. In American Chestnut leaves the teeth are curved forward.

Part Used: Leaves.

Constituents: (i) Tannins, (about 8 or 9% in the American species [5]) (ii) Plastoquinones [37] (iii) Miscellaneous, organic acids, mucilage etc.

Medicinal Use: Antitussive, astringent, antirheumatic. Used especially for paroxysmal coughs, catarrh and whooping cough, and for diarrhoea. The infusion can be used as a gargle in pharyngitis.

Preparations: Liquid Extract, dose: 1–4 ml.

Regulatory Status: GSL.

Biblical References: Genesis 30:37; Ezekiel 31:8 – the oriental Plane.

CHICKWEED

Stellaria media Vill.
Fam. Caryophyllaceae

Synonyms: Starweed, *Alsine media* L.

Habitat: A common weed. As Joseph Miller says "it grows everywhere in moist places and in gardens too frequently".

Description: Stem jointed, with a line of hairs down one side only, leaves ovate, about 1 cm long by 0.5 cm broad. Flowers singly in the axils of the upper leaves, petals white and narrow, equal in length to the sepals. Taste, slightly saline; odourless.

Part Used: Herb.

Constituents: (i) Saponin glycosides (ii) Coumarins and hydroxycoumarins (iii) Flavonoids (iv) Carboxylic acids (v) Triterpenoids (no details, [338]) (vi) Vitamin C, about 150–350 mg per 100 g [339].

Medicinal Use: Antipruritic, vulnerary, emollient, antirheumatic. Most often used in the form of an ointment. Culpeper writes of an ointment made by boiling "in oil of trotters or sheep's fat"; today Chickweed is still used as an ointment, though not in the same base, and as a poultice for eczema, psoriasis, ulcers, and boils. It is used internally for rheumatism, and was formerly used as a source of vitamin C.

Preparations: Liquid Extract, dose: 1–4 ml.

Regulatory Status: GSL.

CHICORY

Cichorium intybus L.
Fam. Compositae

Synonyms: Succory.

Habitat: Native to Europe and parts of Asia, naturalized in the USA and cultivated extensively.

Description: Root brownish, with tough, loose, reticulated, white layers surrounding a radiate woody column. Often crowned with remains of the stem.

Part Used: Root.

Constituents: (i) Inulin, up to 58%, in the root (ii) Sesquiterpene lactones including lactucin and lactupicrin (= intybin) (iii) Coumarins; chicoriin, esculetin, esculin, umbelliferone and scopoletin, in the herb [340] (iv) Miscellaneous; taraxesterol, sugars etc. in the root. The roasted root also contains a large number of flavour ingredients including acetophenone [341] and the β-carboline alkaloids harman and norharman [342].

Medicinal Use: Diuretic, tonic, laxative. A decoction has been used for liver complaints, gout and rheumatism. An alcoholic extract has been shown to depress heart rate and amplitude *in vitro* [343] and has antiinflammatory effects *in vitro* [344]. The roasted root is used in coffee mixtures and substitutes.

Potter's Products: Pile Mixture No. 91.

Regulatory Status: GSL.

CHINA

Smilax china L.
Fam. Liliaceae

Habitat: Native to Japan but grows elsewhere in the Far East.

Description: Tubers cylindrical, often somewhat flattened, 10–15 cm long and 2–5 cm diameter, with short, knotty branches and a rusty, shiny bark. Internally, pale fawn coloured. Taste, insipid, odourless.

Part Used: Tuber.

Constituents: Steroidal saponins, thought to be similar to those found in Sarsaparilla (q.v.) [2].

Medicinal Use: Alterative. Has been used occasionally as a substitute for Sarsaparilla.

CHIRETTA

Swertia chirata Buch.-Ham.
Fam. Gentianaceae

Synonyms: Brown Chirata, White Chirata, Chirayta, *Ophelia chirata*.

Habitat: Northern India.

Description: Stems brown or purplish, 2–4 mm thick, cylindrical below and becoming quadrangular upwards, containing a wide, yellowish pith, leaves opposite, lanceolate or ovate, entire with three to seven longitudinal ribs. Flowers small and panicled; fruit, a two-valved capsule. Taste, intensely bitter; odourless.

Green Chiretta, from *Andrographis paniculata* Ness (Fam. Acanthaceae), has an equally bitter but not an earthy taste. It contains andirographin, andrographolide etc. [2].

Part Used: Herb.

Constituents: (i) Oxygenated xanthone derivatives, including decussatin (1-hydroxy-3,7,8-trimethoxyxanthone) [345], mangiferin [1,3,6,7-tetrahydroxyxanthone C_2-β-D-glucoside) [346], swerchirin (1,8-dihydroxy-3,5-dimethoxyxanthone [347], swertianin [1,7,8-trihydroxy-3-methoxyxanthone), isobellidifolin (1,6,8-trihydroxy-4-methoxyxanthone) and others [5] (ii) Iridoids, including amarogentin (chiratin) [5] (iii) Alkaloids; gentianine, gentiocrucine, enicoflavine [348] (iv) Glycosyl flavones (unspecified) [346].

Medicinal Use: Bitter tonic, orexigenic, febrifuge, antimalarial, stomachic. Several of the constituents including amarogentin are hepatoprotective against carbon tetrachloride *in vitro* toxicity [349]. Swertianin and other xanthones are reputedly antituberculous [350] and swerchirin has *in vivo* antimalarial activity in rodents [347]. *Swertia japonica* is used in oriental medicine; it has similar types of constituents. For information see [349].

Preparations: Powder, dose, 0.5–2 g; Liquid Extract, dose: 2–4 ml, Concentrated Infusion of Chiretta BPC 1949, dose: 2–4ml.

Regulatory Status: GSL.

CICELY, SWEET

Myrrhis odorata (L.) Scop.
Fam. Umbelliferae

Synonyms: Sweet Chervil, Great Chervil.

Habitat: Southern Europe, cultivated as a garden plant elsewhere.

Description: Leaves large, tripinnate, leaflets ovate-lanceolate, usually with white splashes near the base, hairy on the veins below and on the margins. Root, whitish, 1–4 cm broad, with a radiate structure. Taste and odour, sweet and anise-like. American Sweet Cicely is from *Osmorhiza longistylis* DC.

Part Used: Root, herb.

Constituents: No information available.

Medicinal Use: Carminative, stomachic, expectorant. The dried root is used as a decoction for coughs and flatulence, and the herb as an infusion for anaemia and as a tonic.

Cicely Root and Angelica were used to "prevent" infection in the time of the plague.

CINCHONA

Cinchona succirubra Pav ex Klotsch
C. calisaya Wedd.
C. ledgeriana Moens ex Trim.
and their hybrids and varieties
Fam. Rubiaceae

Synonyms: Peruvian Bark, Jesuit's Bark, Red Cinchona (cinchona rubra) is *C. succirubra* (= *C. pubescens* Vahl). Yellow Cinchona (cinchona flava) is *C. calisaya* and *C. ledgeriana*.

Habitat: Native to mountainous regions of tropical America, cultivated in S. E. Asia and parts of Africa.

Description: The bark occurs in quills or flat pieces up to 30 cm long, and 3–6 mm thick. The external surface is brownish-grey, usually fissured with an exfoliating cork, and lichens and mosses may be seen as greyish-white or greenish patches. Inner surface yellowish to reddish-brown. Fracture fibrous. Taste, bitter and astringent; odour slight.

Part Used: Bark of stem and root.

Constituents: (i) Quinoline alkaloids, up to 16% but usually less, consisting mainly of quinine, quinidine, cinchonine and cinchonidine. Other alkaloids include epi- and hydro- derivatives of these, quinamine and many others [1, 4, 5] (ii) Glycosides such as quinovin [5] (iii) Miscellaneous; tannins, including the phlobatannin cinchotannic acid, quinic acid, resin, wax etc. [1].

Medicinal Use: Antimalarial, febrifuge, tonic, orexigenic, spasmolytic and astringent. The bark is used for the extraction of the alkaloids quinine and quinidine. Quinine is the most potent of the alkaloids as an antimalarial; it is becoming important again in the treatment of those types of malaria which are resistant to the newer synthetic drugs. Both quinine and particularly quinidine act as cardiac depressants, quinidine is used clinically for this purpose. Quinine salts are used in the prevention of leg cramps and are an ingredient of many analgesic and cold and flu remedies. Chronic overdosage can result in the condition known as cinchonism, which is characterized by headache, abdominal pain, rashes and visual disturbances. Cinchona and quinine should not be taken in large doses during pregnancy except in malarial patients.

Preparations: Powdered Bark, dose: 0.3–1 g; Cinchona Liquid Extract BPC 1954, dose: 0.3–1 ml; Cinchona Extract BPC 1954, dose: 0.3–1 ml; Cinchona Tincture BPC 1949, dose: 2–4 ml.

Potter's Products: Herbprin Tablets.

Regulatory Status: GSL. Maximum dose 50 mg.

CINERARIA MARITIMA

Senecio cineraria DC
Fam. Compositae

Synonyms: Dusty Miller, *S. maritimus* L.

Habitat: Native to the W. Indies but introduced into Britain, the USA and elsewhere as a garden plant.

Description: Leaves 15–20 cm long and about 5–6 cm wide, pinnate, each segment three-lobed, white with a dense white covering of hairs beneath. Flowerheads yellow, about 1 cm across.

Part Used: Juice of the plant.

Constituents: Pyrrolizidine alkaloids including jacobine, jacodine and senecionine [112].

Medicinal Use: The sterilized juice of the plant has been employed for the treatment of capsular and lenticular cataract of the eye, and was applied to the eye by means of a medicine dropper.

CINNAMON

Cinnamomum verum J S Presl.
and its varieties var *verum* (= var *vulgare*
and var *subcordata*
Fam. Lauraceae

Synonyms: Ceylon Cinnamon, *C. zeylanicum* Garc. ex Blume.

Habitat: Native to Sri Lanka but cultivated elsewhere.

Description: Pale brown, thin quills, several rolled inside one another. Quills usually 0.5–1 cm wide, not exceeding 1 mm in thickness. Taste, sweet pungent and aromatic; odour, characteristic.

Varieties: Saigon cinnamon, from *C. laureirii* Nees., appears as thin greyish brown quills and Batavian or Padang cinnamon is from *C. burmanii* (Nees.) Bl.

Cassia, or Chinese Cinnamon, is from *C. aromaticum*. NB: "Oil of Cinnamon NF", (USA) is obtained from Cassia (q.v.).

Part Used: Inner (peeled) bark; oil distilled from bark and leaves.

Constituents: (i) Essential oil, up to about 4% in the bark, consisting of cinnamaldehyde, (ca. 60–75%), cinnamyl acetate, cinnamyl alcohol, cuminaldehyde, eugenol and methyleugenol, in variable amounts, and many other constituents. The leaf oil has a much greater proportion of eugenol, around 80% [1, 4, 5] (ii) Tannins, consisting of polymeric tetrahydroxyflavandiols [351], probably similar to those found in Cassia (q.v.) (iii) Cinnzelanin and cinnzelanol [352] (iv) Coumarin [351].

Medicinal Use: Aromatic, astringent, stimulant, carminative. Cinnamon has been used for thousands of years to treat nausea and vomiting, diarrhoea, rheumatism, colds, hypertension, female complaints and many other disorders, with justification. Cinnamaldehyde is hypotensive, spasmolytic and increases peripheral blood flow; and it inhibits cyclooxygenase and lipoxygenase enzymes of arachidonic acid metabolism [287, 288, 289]. Cinnamon bark oil and extracts exhibit antifungal antibacterial and antiviral activities [5, and refs. therein] and enhance trypsin activity [24]. The leaf oil is antiseptic and anaesthetic, due to the eugenol content. It is not interchangeable with the bark oil and is usually used as a source of eugenol and as a fragrance ingredient in cosmetics. Cinnamon bark and oil are used widely as a flavouring in manufactured and home-cooked foods as well as in mouthwashes, cosmetics, tonics and other pharmaceuticals.

Preparations: Powdered Bark, dose: 0.3–1.2 g; Cinnamon Oil BP, dose: 0.05–0.2 ml; Cinnamon Tincture BPC 1949, dose: 2–4 ml; Spirit of Cinnamon BPC 1949, dose: 0.3–1.2 ml; Concentrated Cinnamon Water BP.

Regulatory Status: GSL.

Biblical References: Biblical References: Exodus 30:23; Proverbs 7:17; Sons of Solomon 4:14; Revelation 18:13.

CLARY

Salvia sclarea L.
Fam. Labiatae

Synonyms: Clary Sage, Clary Wort, Clarry, Cleareye, Muscatel Sage.

Habitat: Native to Southern Europe, cultivated worldwide.

Description: Leaves large, heart-shaped, pointed, wrinkled, covered with velvety hairs. Flowers, appearing in June-August, blue or white, with large membranous bracts longer than the calyx. Taste, warm and aromatic, slightly bitter; odour, aromatic, recalling that of Tolu.

Part Used: Herb, and at one time the seeds.

Constituents: (i) Volatile oil, about 0.1%, consisting mainly of linalyl acetate; with linalool, β-pinene, β-myrcene, phellandrene and others [5 and refs. therein] (ii) Diterpene alcohols manool and sclareol [353].

Medicinal Use: Antispasmodic, balsamic. Usually used in digestive disorders and for kidney diseases. The oil has been reported to be anticonvulsant in animals and to potentiate the effects of some hypnotics [354]. The mucilage of the seeds as well as a decoction of the herb has been used in ophthalmic preparations.

CLIVERS
Galium aparine L.
Fam. Rubiaceae

Synonyms: Cleavers, Goosegrass, Hayriffe, Erriffe, Burweed, Goosebill.

Habitat: A common wild plant. Culpeper says "It is also an inhabitant in gardens that it ramps upon and is ready to choak what ever grows near it", a statement that is still true today.

Description: Leaves lanceolate, about 1–2 cm long and 0.5 cm broad, in whorls of six, with backward pointing bristly hairs at the margins. Stem quadrangular. Flowers small, insignificant, dull white; fruits nearly globular, about 3 mm diameter, covered with hooked bristles. Taste, slightly saline; odourless.

Part Used: Herb.

Constituents: (i) Iridoids, including asperuloside and deacetylasperulosidic acid [355] (ii) Polyphenolic acids, such as caffeic, *p*-coumaric, gallic and *p*-hydroxybenzoic acids [356] (iii) Anthraqinone derivatives, including alizarin and derivatives, xanthopurpurin and its esters, galiosin and simple anthraquinones. These are in the roots and have been shown to be absent from the herb [356]. (iv) *n*-Alkanes, mainly C_{29} alkanes (v) Flavonoids, such as luteolin [357] (vi) Miscellaneous; tannins [358], coumarins (unspecified) [2].

Medicinal Use: Diuretic, aperient, tonic, alterative, mild astringent. It is used particularly for enlarged lymph glands and in cystitis and psoriasis. Asperuloside in common with other iridoids is a mild laxative in animals [197]. Extracts of Clivers lower arterial blood pressure in dogs without slowing the heart rate or showing any toxic effects [359]. Asperuloside can be chemically converted to prostanoid intermediates and may find an important use here [360].

Preparations: Liquid Extract, dose: 2–4 ml.

Potter's Products: Alpine Herb Medicinal Tea Bags; Kasbah Remedy Compound Herb; Sciargo Medicinal Tea Bags; Stomach and Liver Medicinal Tea Bags; Liver and Bile Medicinal Tea Bags; Tabritis Remedy for Arthritis; Antitis Tablets; Cystitis Mixture No 111; Lumbago Mixture No. 117.

Regulatory Status: GSL.

CLOVES
Syzygium aromaticum (L.) Merr. et Perry
Fam. Myrtaceae

Synonyms: *Eugenia caryophyllus* Spreng., *E. caryophyllata* Thunb. *E. aromatica* (L.) Baill.

Habitat: Native to the Molucca Islands, Indonesia; introduced into Tanzania, Madagascar, Penang, Brazil and other tropical parts.

Description: The cloves, or flowerbuds, are brown, about 1–1.5 cm long, the lower portion consisting of the calyx tube enclosing in its upper half the ovary filled with minute ovules. There are numerous stamens and four calyx teeth, surrounded by the unopened, globular corolla of four concave, overlapping petals. Taste and odour, characteristic. On pressing with the fingernail, oil should exude.

Part Used: Unexpanded flowerbuds and the oil distilled from them.

Constituents: (i) Volatile oil, about 15–20%, consisting mainly of eugenol (usually 85–90% but variable), with acetyl eugenol, α- and β-caryophyllene, methyl salicylate, benzaldehyde [1, 4, 5], and the sesquiterpenes α-copaene, γ- and δ-cadinene and α-cubebene [361] (ii) Flavonoids; kaempferol, rhamnetin (iii) Sterols; sitosterol, campesterol and stigmasterol (iv) Miscellaneous; crategolic acid methyl ester, lipids, etc [5].

Medicinal Use: Stimulant, aromatic, carminative, antiemetic. Clove oil particularly is also used as an anodyne in toothache and constituent of various dental preparations. It also has antiseptic, antispasmodic, antihistaminic and anthelmintic properties [5, 268]. Aqueous extracts and the oil potentiate the activity of trypsin [24]. Cloves and clove oils are used in the preparation of certain types of cigarette, such as Indian "beedis" and Indonesian "kretaks", for their stimulant action, in perfumery and in cookery.

Preparations: Powder, dose: 120–300 mg; Clove Oil BP, dose: 0.05–0.2 ml; Concentrated Clove Infusion BPC 1954, dose: 2–4 ml; Concentrated Clove Water BPC 1934, dose: 0.3–1 ml.

Potter's Products: Asthma and Bronchitis Medicinal Tea Bags; Indigestion Mixture No. 147.

Regulatory Status: GSL.

CLUBMOSS

Lycopodium clavatum L.
Fam. Lycopodiaceae

Synonyms: Lycopodium Seed, Vegetable Sulphur.

Habitat: Central and Northern Europe including Northern Britain, and many other places.

Description: Stem woody, slender, elongated, with a few lateral, forked branches, and a few scattered, whitish roots below. Leaves crowded and scale-like, hair-tipped. Spore cases in spikes borne on erect forked, club-shaped branches, at right angles to the prostrate stem. Spores yellow, somewhat triangular, forming a mobile powder which floats on water without being wetted.

Part Used: Plant and spores.

Constituents: Alkaloids, about 0.1–0.2%, of which the major one is lycopodine; with clavatine, clavatoxine, nicotine and many others [2, 362, 363] (ii) Polyphenolic acids including dihydrocaffeic (iii) Flavonoids including apigenin (iv) Miscellaneous; triterpenes [2].

Medicinal Use: Sedative. It has been used for urinary disorders, in the treatment of spasmodic retention of urine, catarrhal cystitis and chronic kidney disorders, and as a gastric sedative in indigestion and gastritis. However the alkaloids can be toxic and should be used with care. Lycopodine produces uterine contractions and stimulates peristalsis in the small intestine in rodents [362].

COCA

Erythroxylum coca Lam.
E. novogranatense (Morris) Hieron
Fam. Erythroxylaceae

Synonyms: Bolivian Coca is *E. coca;* Peruvian Coca is *E. novogranatense* (= *E. truxillense* Rusby).

Habitat: Native to the S. American Andes, cultivated there and elsewhere at altitudes above 450 m.

Description: *E. coca* leaves are brownish green, oval, thin but tough, up to 5 cm long and 2.5 cm wide, with two lines on the undersurface parallel to the midrib, margins entire, apex rounded, and a faint projecting line occurring on the upper surface of the midrib. *E. novogranatense* leaves are green, oblanceolate, and very brittle, about 4 cm long and 1.5 cm broad without any projecting line on the midrib.

Part Used: Leaves.

Constituents: (i) Tropane alkaloids, up to 2.5%, mainly cocaine, with other derivatives of ecgonine; hygrine, cuscohygrine, α-truxillense and nicotine, and others [1, 5, 364, 365] (ii) Volatile oil, containing methyl salicylate, *trans*-2-hexenal, *cis*-3-hexenal, 1-hexanol, N-methylpyrrole and dihydro-benzaldehyde [366] (iii) Flavonoids such as rutin and isoquercetin (iv) Miscellaneous; vitamin A, riboflavin, minerals [5].

Medicinal Use: Central nervous system stimulant, local anaesthetic. The pharmacological effects are due almost entirely to the presence of cocaine. Cocaine is increasingly being used illicitly as a stimulant; it causes dependance with frequent use and an unpleasant withdrawal syndrome when the habit is stopped. The medical indications of cocaine are now restricted to its use as a local anaesthetic, mainly in ophthalmic surgery, apart from occasional and declining use in mixtures for terminally ill patients. Coca leaves are chewed by native workers to relieve hunger and fatigue. Coca leaf extract with the cocaine removed is used to flavour soft drinks.

Regulatory Status: CD (Misuse of Drugs Act 1973). POM.

COCCULUS INDICUS

Anamirta cocculus (L.) Wight et Arnott.
Fam. Menispermaceae

Synonyms: Fish Berries, Levant Berries, *Anamirta paniculata* Colebr.

Habitat: Indonesia.

Description: Fruits kidney-shaped, about 1 cm long, blackish, containing a horseshoe-shaped seed. Fruitshell tasteless, seed bitter and oily.

Part Used: Berries or seeds.

Constituents: (i) Picrotoxin, 0.6–5%, with menispermine, and para-menispermine [2].

Medicinal Use: Stimulant, parasiticide. Though very poisonous, it has occasionally been given internally for similar purposes to Nux Vomica (q.v.). Picrotoxin is a powerful central nervous system stimulant and was formerly used to counteract barbiturate poisoning.

Regulatory Status: POM.

COCILLANA
Guarea rusbyi Rusby
Fam. Meliaceae

Synonyms: Guapi Bark, Huapi Bark, Grape Bark, *Sycocarpus rusbyi* (Britt).
Habitat: Eastern Andes.
Description: The bark occurs as flat or curved pieces; the outer surface is fissured and grey-brown in colour with orange-brown patches where the cork has been removed. Inner surface brown and longitudinally striated. Taste, astringent, slightly nauseous; odour characteristic. It is considered likely that other species of *Guarea* ar being used, however these have not been specified [366].
Part Used: Bark.
Constituents: No recent research available. (i) Alkaloids, of unknown structure, including rusbyine (ii) Volatile oil (iii) Miscellaneous; tannins, flavonols, anthraquinones etc [366]. Other species of *Guarea* which have been investigated have yielded (i) Limonoids, such as dreagenin and methyl 6-acetoxyangolensate, in *G. cedrata* and *G. thompsonii* [367] (ii) Sesquiterpenes and glycerides, in *G. cedrata* and *G. thompsonii* [367] (iii) Pentacarbocyclic triterpenoids, including glabretal, in *G. glabra* [368] (iii) Dihydrogedunun, in *G. thompsonii,* timber [368].
Medicinal Use: Expectorant. Used widely in cough syrups in a similar way to Ipecacuanha (q.v.). No pharmacological or clinical results available. Another species, *G. guidonia,* which is used in Brazil as an antiinflammatory agent, has demonstrable *in vivo* activity [369].
Preparations: Powdered Bark, dose: 0.5–1 g; Cocillana Liquid Extract BPC, dose: 0.5–1 ml; Compound Syrup of Cocillana BPC 1949, dose: 1.5–3.5 ml.
Regulatory Status: GSL.

COFFEE
Coffea arabica L.
C. canephora Pierre ex Froehner
C. liberica
and other species and hybrids.
Fam. Rubiaceae

Synonyms: Arabian Coffee is from *C. arabica;* Robusta Coffee is from *C. canephora* (syn. *C. robusta* Linden ex De Wild.).
Habitat: Cultivated in many tropical countries.
Description: The beans are oval-concave on one side, flat on the other, with a central longitudinal groove, grey-green when fresh and brown when roasted.
Part Used: Kernel of the dried ripe seed.
Constituents: (i) Caffeine, about 0.06–0.32% when fresh, less when roasted, [5]. (ii) Miscellaneous: trigonelline, chlorogenic acid, polyamines, tannins, B vitamins, carbohydrates, oil; for a full account and references see [5].
Medicinal Use: Stimulant, diuretic, antinarcotic, antiemetic. Most of these effects are due to the caffeine content [1, 4, 5]. As a beverage coffee is well-

known. If taken in excess it results in unpleasant side effects such as tachycardia, wakefulness etc. Coffee is not used medicinally very often but caffeine is an ingredient of many analgesic preparations as it potentiates the effect of paracetamol and aspirin and produces a feeling of well-being.

Preparations: Prepared Coffee BPC 1968.

COHOSH, BLACK

Cimicifuga racemosa Nutt.
Fam. Ranunculaceae

Synonyms: Black Snakeroot, Bugbane, Rattleroot, Rattleweed, Squawroot, *Actaea racemosa* L., *Macrotys actaeoides* Rafin.

Habitat: USA and Canada.

Description: Rhizome thick, hard and knotty, with short lateral branches, cylindrical, compressed, marked with transverse leaf scars. Transverse section horny with a hard, thick, bark. Rootlets, when present, show a Maltese Cross effect in transverse section. Taste, bitter and acrid; odour, disagreeable.

Part Used: Rhizome.

Constituents: (i) Triterpene glycosides, including actein, cimigoside, cimifugine (= macrotin) and racemoside [370, 371, 372] (ii) Isoflavones such as formononetin [373] (iii) Isoferulic acid [5] (iv) Miscellaneous; volatile oil, tannin [5].

Medicinal Use: Sedative, anti-inflammatory, diuretic, antitussive, emmenagogue. Black Cohosh is used for a wide variety of ailments, such as dysmenorrhoea, whooping cough, sciatica, bronchitis and rheumatism. Pharmacological studies have shown that the methanol extract binds to oestrogen receptors *in vitro* and in rat uteri; this is thought to be due to the presence of formononetin [373]. It is also hypotensive in animals, causes peripheral vasodilation in man [374], is a central nervous system depressant and antispasmodic in mice [375] and has hypoglycaemic and antiinflammatory activity [192, 5]. Racemoside has antiulcer activity in mice [371] and isoferulic acid lowers body temperature in rats [375]. In Chinese medicine a number of other *Cimicifuga* species are used, including *C. heracleifolia* Kom., *C. dahurica* Turcz., and *C. foetida* L. These are referred to as "Shengma" and are used to treat measles, headache, gingivitis, uterine prolapse and rectal prolapse caused by chronic diarrhoea. They have been shown to have analgesic, anticonvulsant and antibacterial action in animals, and to depress heart rate and blood pressure [7].

Preparations: Powdered Root, dose: 0.3–2 g; Liquid Extract BP 1898, dose: 0.3–2 ml; Tincture BPC 1934, dose: 2–4 ml.

Potter's Products: Rheumatism Mixture No. 92, Antispasmodic Tincture.

Regulatory Status: GSL.

COHOSH BLUE   *Caulophyllum thalictroides* Mich.
                                    Fam. Berberidaceae
Synonyms: Papoose Root, Squawroot, *Leontice thalictroides* L.
Habitat: USA.
Description: Rhizome brownish grey, about 10 cm long and 0.5–1 cm thick,
    knotty with short branches; with numerous, crowded, concave stem scars
    on the upper surface, and long, paler brown, tough rootlets about 1 mm
    thick underneath. Internally whitish with narrow, woody rays. Taste,
    sweetish, then bitter and acrid; nearly odourless.
Part Used: Rhizome.
Constituents: (i) Alkaloids, including the lupin-type alkaloids caulo-
    phylline (= methylcytisine), anagyrine, baptifoline; and magnoflorine
    [376, 377] (ii) Saponins known as "caulosaponin" [376]. *C. robustum*
    Maxim., which is used in the USSR, contains the fungicidal saponin
    glycosides caulosides A–G, based on hederagenin [377, 378].
Medicinal Use: Antiinflammatory, antispasmodic, diuretic, vermifuge and
    emmenagogue. Used particularly for rheumatism, and for female com-
    plaints such as amenorrhoea and threatened miscarriage, but should be
    avoided during the first trimester of pregnancy. The North American
    Indians used the rhizome to facilitate childbirth, hence the synonyms.
    Experiments have shown that extracts stimulate phagocytosis in mice
    [379] and are antiinflammatory in the rat paw oedema test [192].
Preparations: Powdered root, dose: 0.3–2 g; Liquid Extract BPC 1934,
    dose: 0.6–2 ml.
Potter's Products: Rheumatism Mixture No. 92.
Regulatory Status: GSL.

COLCHICUM   *Colchicum autumnale* L.
                                      Fam. Liliaceae
Synonyms: Meadow Saffron, Naked Ladies.
Habitat: N. Africa and Europe, including parts of the British Isles.
Description: The plant produces a crocus-like pale purple flower in the
    autumn. The corm is usually found in transverse slices, notched on one
    side, kidney-shaped in outline and white and starchy internally. Taste,
    sweetish at first then bitter and acrid. The seeds are dull brown, nearly
    spherical, very hard, finely pitted, with a crest-like projection at the
    hilum. Taste, bitter and acrid; odourless.
Part Used: Corm, seeds.
Constituents: (i) Alkaloids, the most important of which is colchicine, with
    demecolcine, 2-demethyl colchicine, colchiceine, N-formyl-N-desacetyl
    colchicine, lumicolchicine and many others [380] (ii) Flavonoids, including
    apigenin [381] (iii) Plant acids, including chelidonic, 2-hydroxy-6-
    methoxy benzoic and salicyclic [381] (iv) Miscellaneous; sugars and
    phytosterols etc. [381].
Medicinal Use: Colchicine is used specifically for the relief of pain in acute
    gout, usually when other methods have failed. It has been used as an

ingredient of antirheumatic preparations in the same way, but as it is highly toxic it must be used with extreme caution. It is a mitotic poison which inhibits microtubule formation during cell division, and for this reason has been used in the treatment of leukaemia, but without any great success. Side effects include severe gastro-intestinal pain, nausea, diarrhoea, and with larger doses renal damage and alopecia. Colchicine may cause foetal abnormalities. The fatal dose can be as little as 7 mg [4].

Preparations: Colchicum Liquid Extract BP 1973, Colchicum Dry Extract BP 1948, dose: 10–30 mg; Colchicum Tincture BP 1973, dose: 0.5–2 ml.

Regulatory Status: POM.

COLEUS

Coleus forskohlii Briq.
Fam. Labiatae

Habitat: India.

Description: Not found in commerce yet.

Part Used: Herb.

Constituents: Labdane diterpenes, including forskolin. [382].

Medicinal Use: Coleus has only recently come into prominence. It is used as a source of forskolin rather than as a herbal remedy, however this may change shortly. Forskolin is cardiotonic, antihypertensive and vaso-dilatory [383]. It has a positive inotropic effect upon the heart, and is a potent inhibitor of platelet aggregation, due to activation of adenylate cyclase [383, 384]. It is currently undergoing clinical trials.

COLOPHONY

Pinus palustris Mill.
and other species
Fam. Pinaceae

Synonyms: Rosin.

Habitat: Worldwide.

Description: Colophony resin is the residue left after the distillation of turpentine. It varies in colour from pale yellow to brown, and appears in brittle masses. For medicinal use the paler resin is preferred.

Part Used: Resin.

Constituents: (i) Diterpene resin acids including abietic, dihydroabietic, neoabietic, palustric, pimaric and isopimaric acids and others [385] (ii) Diterpene alcohols and aldehydes (iii) Miscellaneous sterols and phenolic acids [385].

Medicinal Use: Used principally in ointments and plasters. The ointment is used for boils and ulcers. In Chinese medicine colophony from oriental *Pinus* species is used to treat rheumatism, ringworm, bronchitis and other conditions, and is taken internally as well as applied externally. Colophony has many other uses in the printing and adhesives industries.

Preparations: Colophony Ointment BPC 1959.

Potter's Preparations: Brown Marshmallow Ointment.

Regulatory Status: GSL, for external use only.

COLTSFOOT

Tussilago farfara L.
Fam. Compositae

Synonyms: Coughwort, Horsehoof, Foal's Foot, Bull's Foot.

Habitat: A common wild plant in Britain and Europe, growing in damp places. The flowers appear in early spring before the leaves.

Description: Leaves hoof-shaped, with angular teeth on the margins, about 10 cm in diameter, long-stalked, green above and coated with matted, long white hairs on the lower surface and on the upper surface when young. The flowers are bright yellow, up to 2 cm diameter, with a scaly pedicel. Taste, Mucilaginous, slightly bitter, astringent; odourless.

Part Used: Leaves, flowers.

Constituents: (i) Flavonoids; rutin, hyperoside and isoquercetin [386] (ii) Mucilage, about 8%, consisting of polysaccharides based on glucose, galactose, fructose, arabinose and xylose; and inulin [387, 388] (iii) Pyrrolizidine alkaloids, including senkirkine and tussilagine, in very small amounts (about 0.015%) [398, 390] (iv) Tannin.

Medicinal Use: Expectorant, demulcent, antitussive, anticatarrhal. Coltsfoot is used for pulmonary complaints, irritating or spasmodic coughs, whooping cough, bronchitis, laryngitis and asthma. Recent research has shown that the polysaccharides are antiinflammatory and immuno-stimulating [388, 147] as well as demulcent, and the flavonoids also have antiinflammatory and antispasmodic action [327]. A total extract and a lipophilic fraction stimulate phagocytosis in mice inoculated with *E. coli*, again showing stimulation of the immune system [80]. These experimental results help to explain the efficacy of coltsfoot. The pyrrolizidine alkaloids have caused hepatotoxicity in rats fed daily on high doses, but not on daily low dose regimes [391]. They have been shown not to cause any damage to human chromosomes *in vitro* [392].

Preparations: From leaves: Liquid Extract, dose: 2–4 ml; Solid Extract, dose: 0.3–0.6 g. From flowers: Liquid Extract BPC 1934, dose: 0.6–2 ml.

Potter's Products: Antibron Tablets, Vegetable Cough Remover.

Regulatory Status: GSL.

COLUMBO, AMERICAN

Frasera carolinensis Walt.
Fam. Gentianaceae

Synonyms: *F. walteri, F. canadensis.*

Habitat: USA and Canada.

Description: Root usually occurs in pieces 8–10 cm long and about 1–2.5 cm thick, often split longitudinally. The thick bark is pale brownish grey and wrinkled transversely above and longitudinally below. Fracture short and rather spongy; taste resembling that of Gentian (q.v.).

Part Used: Root.

Constituents: (i) Gentiopicroside (= gentiopicrin) (ii) Methoxyxanthones (iii) Tannins [2].

Medicinal Use: Tonic, stimulant. Used in a similar way to Gentian and Calumba Root (q.v.).

COMBRETUM

Combretum sundaicum Mig.
Fam. Combretaceae

Synonyms: Opium Antidote, Jungle Weed.
Habitat: China.
Description: Leaves 10–13 cm long and about 6 cm broad, with 8–10 lateral spreading veins, perforated in the axils, surface minutely scaly on the young leaves. Taste, slightly astringent and tea-like.
Part Used: Herb.
Constituents: Tannin, resin [2].
Medicinal Use: Has been used in China for the treatment of the opium habit but its action is uncertain.

COMFREY

Symphytum officinale L.
Fam. Boraginaceae

Synonyms: Blackwort, Nipbone, Knitbone, Consolida. Tuberous Comfrey is *S. tuberosum* L., and Russian Comfrey is *Symphytum* × *uplandicum*.
Habitat: Common in moist places in Britain, Europe and the USA.
Description: The plant grows up to 1 m in height, bearing large, bristly obovate or lanceolate leaves, which may reach up to 25 cm long and 10 cm broad. The stem is hollow and also bristly. The flowers are bell-like, occurring in forked spikes, they are white or mauve; or in the case of *S. tuberosum*, white only, and *S.* × *uplandicum*, purple only. The root is brownish black, deeply wrinkled. Fracture short, showing in transverse section a thick bark and broad medullary rays. Taste, sweetish, mucilaginous; odourless.
Part Used: Root, leaves.
Constituents: (i) Allantoin [4, 393] (ii) Pyrrolizidine alkaloids, including echimidine, symphytine, lycopsamine, symlandine, their acetyl and other derivatives and their N-oxides [394, 395, 396] and in *S.* × *uplandicum* at least, uplandicine and others [395]. The alkaloids are found in the fresh young leaves and in the root, but in two separate investigations were found to be absent in the dried herb [397, 398]. *S. tuberosum* has a much lower alkaloid content than the others [399]. (iii) Phenolic acids; rosmarinic, chlorogenic, caffeic and lithospermic acids [400, 401] (iv) Mucilage, about 29%, composed of a polysaccharide containing glucose and fructose [402] (v) Miscellaneous; choline, asparagine, volatile oil [2], tannins, steroidal saponins (in the root), triterpenes etc. [5].
Medicinal Use: Demulcent, astringent, antiinflammatory, vulnerary, antipsoriatic. Comfrey has been used for hundreds of years for pulmonary complaints, as a gastric sedative, and for rheumatism and painful joints. It is also used in the form of an ointment, oil, or poultice for psoriasis, eczema, ulcers and to promote wound healing. The antiinflammatory activity of extracts of Comfrey has been demonstrated *in vitro* and *in vivo* [400, 403]. This may be at least partially due to the presence of rosmarinic acid which has a similar effect [400]. An aqueous extract (comparable to a

herbal tea) stimulates the release of a prostaglandin-like material from rat gastric mucosa [403], possibly explaining its usefulness as a gastric sedative. The soothing and wound healing properties are probably due to the allantoin which is a well-known dermatological agent. The pyrrolizidine alkaloids are hepatotoxic in animals [389, 395, 405] and Comfrey has been implicated in causing in one instance a case of hepatic veno-occlusive disease after chronic use [406]. However in animal studies the alkaloids were poorly absorbed through the skin [396] and since they are not usually found in commercial samples of the herb [397, 398], toxicity does not appear to be a problem. It would be wise however to avoid using the fresh leaves in salads. Aqueous extracts of Comfrey leaves increase the survival times of mice bearing spontaneous tumours, and decrease tumour growth [407], and in an Ames test produced less mutants than the control [408], suggesting that Comfrey may have antimutagenic activity.

Preparations: Liquid Extract (root), dose: 2–4 ml.

Potter's Products: Comfrey Tablets; D4 Special Formula Stomach Tablets; Comfrey Oil; Comfrey Ointment; Pile Compound Herb; D1 Special Mild Formula Stomach Tablets.

Regulatory Status: GSL.

CONDURANGO

Marsdenia condurango Nich.
Fam. Asclepiadaceae

Synonyms: Eagle Vine, *Gonolobus condurango* (Nich.) Triana.

Habitat: Ecuador and Peru.

Description: Occurs in quilled pieces, 5–10 cm long, about 1–2 cm in diameter, and 2–6 mm thick. Outer surface brownish-grey, often warty, with patches of lichen; inner surface paler in colour, striated. Transverse fracture granular, yellowish-white, with scattered, fine, silky fibres. Taste, bitter and somewhat acrid, odour faintly aromatic.

Part Used: Bark.

Constituents: (i) Glycosides based on condurangogenins, which are esterified polyoxypregnanes; known as condurangoglycosides A, A_1, C, C_1, A_0, C_0 and B_0; and D_0 and its 20-O-methyl and 20-iso-O-methyl derivatives [409, 410, 411] (ii) Miscellaneous; essential oil (ca. 0.01%), phytosterols, sugars, starch and fat [2].

Medicinal Use: Alterative, stomachic, orexigenic. Used specifically for nervous dyspepsia, anorexia and as a gastric sedative. Some of the condurangoglycosides are antitumour *in vitro* in several systems; these are A_0, B_0, C_0, D_0 and its derivatives [409, 410].

Preparations: Powdered bark, dose: 1–4 g; Liquid Extract, dose: 2–4 ml.

Regulatory Status: GSL.

CONTRAYERVA

Dorstenia contrayerva L.
and other species of *Dorstenia*
Fam. Moraceae

Habitat: Mexico, Peru, W. Indies.

Description: Rhizome about 2–4 cm long, 1 cm thick, reddish brown, rough with leaf scars, nearly cylindrical, tapering suddenly at the end into a tail-like root with numerous curled, wiry rootlets. Taste, slightly aromatic then acrid.

Part Used: Rhizome.

Constituents: Unknown.

Medicinal Use: Diaphoretic, stimulant. The root is normally taken by infusion, and was said by Joseph Miller [3] to "resist the bites of venomous creatures". The name in Spanish means antidote, however no further information on this usage is available.

COOLWORT

Tiarella cordifolia L.
Fam. Saxifragaceae

Synonyms: Mitrewort.

Habitat: America.

Description: Leaves heart-shaped, 6–12 cm wide, with radiate veins and 5–12 pointed lobes which are irregularly toothed. Taste, faintly astringent; odourless.

Part Used: Herb.

Constituents: Unknown.

Medicinal Use: Diuretic, tonic. It has been used for most complaints of the urinary organs and for dyspepsia, taken mainly as an infusion.

COPAIBA

Copaifera langsdorffii Desf.
and other species of *Copaifera*
Fam. Leguminosae

Synonyms: Copaiva or Copaiba Balsam.

Habitat: Tropical S. America.

Description: The oleoresin is tapped from cavities in the tree-trunk, where it accumulates, by drilling holes in the wood. It varies considerably in viscosity and colour, from relatively fluid and pale yellowish in colour to a more resinous material with a red or fluorescent tint. Taste, unpleasant; odour characteristic.

Part Used: Oleoresin.

Constituents: (i) Volatile oil, 30–90%, which may be separated by vacuum distillation, containing α- and β-caryophyllene as the major component, with copaene, *l*-cadinene, γ-humulene, β-bisabolol [50, 412, 413] (ii) Resins and terpenic acids such as copalic, copaiferic, copaiferolic and others [5].

Medicinal Use: Carminative, antiseptic, stimulant, diuretic, used mainly for cystitis, bronchitis and leucorrhoea. The oil is reported to be antibacterial [26].

Preparations: Copaiba Oil BPC 1934, dose: 0.3–1.2 ml; Solution of Copaiba BPC 1934, dose: 4–8 ml; Solution of Copaiba, Buchu and Cubeb BPC 1934, dose: 4–8 ml; Solution of Copaiba and Sandalwood BPC 1934, dose: 4–8 ml.

CORIANDER
Coriandrum sativum L.
Fam. Umbelliferae

Habitat: Native to Europe, Africa, Asia, and naturalized in N. America.

Description: The fruits are globular, about 0.5 cm diameter, with fine longitudinal ridges, separable into two halves, each of which is concave internally and shows two brown, longitudinal oil glands or vittae. Taste, aromatic; odour, characteristic. Unripe fruits have an unpleasant fetid odour, resembling rubber.

Part Used: Fruits.

Constituents: (i) Volatile oil, about 0.5–1% but may vary widely, with the major component being *d*-linalool (= coriandrol) 55–74% [1, 5]. Other constituents are anethole, borneol, camphor, carvone, decyl acetate, elemol, geraniol, geranyl acetate, limonene and γ-terpinene [5, 50, 124] (ii) Flavonoids including quercetin, 3-O-methyl kaempferol, rhamnetin, apigenin and homoeriodictyol [414] (iii) Coumarins including psoralen, angelicin, scopoletin, umbelliferone etc. [5] (iv) Phthalides such as neocnidilide [415] (v) Phenolic acids including caffeic and chlorogenic [5] (vi) Miscellaneous; sterols, sugars, starch, fixed oil etc [5].

Medicinal Use: Aromatic, carminative, antispasmodic. Experiments have shown that Coriander is hypoglycaemic and antiinflammatory in animals [5, 403] and the oil is reported to be larvicidal and bactericidal [5]. Coriander seeds and fresh leaves are used widely in cookery, and the oil as an ingredient of carminatives and as a flavouring.

Preparations: Powdered fruit, dose: 0.3–1 g; Liquid Extract, dose: 0.5–2 ml; Coriander Oil BP, dose: 0.05–2 ml.

Regulatory Status: GSL.

Biblical References: Exodus 16:31; Numbers 11:7.

CORN ERGOT
Ustilago zeae (Beckm.) Unger
Fam. Ustilaginaceae

Synonyms: Cornsmut, Cornbrand, Ustilago, *U. maydis* Leveille.

Habitat: Wherever corn (maize) is grown.

Description: A blackish powder in irregular, globose masses, consisting of fungal spores with portions of the enclosing membrane. Taste and odour; unpleasant, heavy.

Part Used: Fungus.
Constituents: (i) Imidazole alkaloids (unspecified) (ii) Ustilagin, a choline sulphonic acid ester) (iii) Amino acids [2].
Medicinal Use: Emmenagogue, parturient. Has been used in the same way as Ergot (q.v.) after childbirth, for post-partum and other haemorrhage.
Regulatory Status: POM.

CORNFLOWER

Centaurea cyanus L.
Fam. Compositae

Synonyms: Bluebottle, Blueblow. According to Culpeper it was also called Hurtsickle as "it turns the edges of the sickles that reap the corn".
Habitat: Grows wild throughout Europe, especially in cornfields, naturalized elsewhere and cultivated in gardens.
Description: The flowerheads are globular with closely overlapping fringed scales and florets. The florets are usually bright blue, but other colours have been cultivated. They are tubular, and the outer ones trumpet shaped and seven-lobed.
Part Used: Flowers.
Constituents: (i) Flavonoids, including quercimetrin, and the anthocyanins pelargonin and cyanin [416, 386] (ii) Sesquiterpene lactones including cnicin (= centauriin) [2] (iii) Acetylenic compounds (iv) Coumarins, e.g. cichoriin (= esculetin-7-glucoside) [2].
Medicinal Use: Rarely used in medicine today but was formerly used as a tonic and stimulant, and for inflammation of the eye. Cnicin is weakly antibiotic. Nowadays Cornflowers are used as an ingredient of cosmetics such as hair shampoos and rinses and eye lotions.
Regulatory Status: GSL.

CORN SILK

Zea mays L.
Fam. Graminae

Synonyms: *Stigmata maydis,* Yumixu (Chinese).
Description: Fine, silky, yellowish threads, up to 20 cm long, consisting of the styles and stigmas from the female flowers of unripe maize. Taste, sweetish; odourless.
Part Used: Flower pistils.
Constituents: (i) Saponins (unspecified) [5, 417] (ii) Allantoin [417] (iii) Sterols, especially β-sitosterol and stigmasterol [417, 7] (iv) The alkaloid hordenine, in some samples [417] (v) Miscellaneous; vitamins C and K, sugars, cryptoxanthin, anthocyanins, plant acids etc. [5, 7, 417].
Medicinal Use: Demulcent, diuretic. Used mainly for urinary tract complaints such as cystitis, urethritis and prostatitis. The diuretic activity has been demonstrated in animals and clinically [5, 7]. It is also hypotensive in animals [418] and choleretic in humans as well as animals, and in China is used for oedema of various origins and for hepato-biliary disease [7].

Preparations: Liquid Extract BPC 1923, dose: 2–8 ml.
Potter's Products: Compound Elixir of Damiana and Saw Palmetto; Compound Elixir Prostitis.
Regulatory Status: GSL.

CORSICAN MOSS

Alsidium helminthocorton Kutz.
Fam. Rhodomelaceae

Synonyms: *Fucus helminthocorton* L.
Habitat: N. Atlantic Ocean.
Description: Occurs in tangled tufts of slender, brownish-white, cylindrical threads with a striated appearance. Taste, saline; odour, that of seaweed.
Constituents: (i) Floridoside, a glycoside (ii) Amino acids [2]. Active constituents unknown.
Medicinal Use: Anthelmintic, vermifuge. Taken with honey or treacle or as an infusion.

COTO

Nectandra coto L.
and other species of *Nectandra*
Fam. Lauraceae

Synonyms: Paracoto.
Habitat: Bolivia.
Description: Rarely found in commerce. The bark occurs as thick pieces 10–15 cm or more long, about 6 cm wide, and 1–1.5 cm thick. Outer surface brown, corky, sometimes with whitish patches, and a striated inner surface. Taste, hot and biting; odour aromatic.
Part Used: Bark.
Constituents: (i) Alkaloids; parastemine, cotoine [2] (ii) Tannins, essential oil, resin etc.
Medicinal Use: Antiseptic, astringent. Formerly used for catarrh, diarrhoea and dysentry, as a decoction.

COTTON ROOT

Gossypium herbaceum L.
and other species of *Gossypium*
Fam. Malvaceae

Habitat: Indigenous to India but cultivated in China, Southern Europe and the USA.
Description: Flexible or quilled strips, light reddish brown externally with faint, longitudinal ridges and small lenticels and occasionally attached rootlets. Cork often exfoliating and easily separated. The inner surface is paler in colour with a silky sheen. Fracture, very fibrous. Taste, faintly acrid and astringent; odour distinctive.
Part Used: Root bark.

Constituents: (i) Oil, containing the polyphenol gossypol 1–2%, 6-methoxygossypol, 6,6'-dimethoxygossypol [419, 420] and furfuraldehyde [33] (ii) Flavonoids including quercimetrin [421] (iii) Miscellaneous; phenolic acids, betaine, resin, catechol and sterols [33, 37].

Medicinal Use: Emmenagogue, oxytocic, male contraceptive. It is not certain whether the oxytocic activity is due to gossypol or an unknown constituent. Gossypol was first discovered in China when the oil used for cooking caused infertility in men; since then it has been extensively clinically tested there as a male contraceptive [422, 423, 424 and references therein]. It causes a marked decrease in sperm count, but also a degeneration of germ cells in the seminiferous tubules in men and animals. This means that gossypol is unlikely to be used clinically in other countries. It is reported to cause a transient weakness early in therapy, hypokalaemia, and changes in ECG among other side effects [425]. Its contraceptive effects are normally reversible. Gossypol also has antiviral and antibacterial activity both *in vitro* and *in vivo* [419, 420]. It has recently been shown to be a potent inhibitor of arachidonate 5- and 12-lipoxygenase [426] and to inhibit lung-strip contractions induced by histamine, PAF-acether and leukotrienes B_4 and D_4 [427]. This helps to explain the use of Cotton Root in dysmenorrhoea.

Preparations: Liquid Extract BPC 1934, dose: 2–4 ml; Tincture of Cotton Root BPC 1934, dose: 2–4 ml.

Regulatory Status: GSL.

COUCHGRASS
Agropyron repens (L.) Beauv.
Fam. Graminae

Synonyms: Twitchgrass, Quickgrass, Doggrass (in the USA), *Triticum repens* L.

Habitat: Grows in many parts of the world, including Britain. As Joseph Miller]3] says, ". . . and is too frequent in gardens, whence it is hard to extirpate it".

Description: Rhizome slender, tubular, about 2 mm diameter, pale yellow, stiff, smooth with nodes at intervals of 2–3 cm. Taste, slightly sweet; odourless.

Part Used: Rhizome.

Constituents: (i) Carbohydrates; triticin, a fructosan polysaccharide, about 8%, inositol, mannitol and mucilage [428] (ii) Volatile oil, up to about 0.05%, consisting mainly of agropyrene (1-phenyl-2,4-hexadiyne) [5] (iii) Miscellaneous; vanillin glucoside, vitamins A and some B, fixed oil, minerals including silica and iron [5, 428].

Medicinal Use: Diuretic, demulcent, aperient, anticholesteraemic. Used in urinary and bladder complaints, cystitis, nephritis etc., and for gout and rheumatism. Agropyrene is reported to have broad antibiotic properties [429], and extracts of Couchgrass are diuretic in rats [430] and sedative in mice [432].

Preparations: Liquid Extract BPC 1934, dose: 4–8 ml.
Potter's Products: Kasbah Remedy Compound herb; Alpine Herb Medicinal Tea Bags; Antitis Tablets.
Regulatory Status: GSL.

COWHAGE

Mucuna pruriens DC.
Fam. Leguminosae

Synonyms: Cowage, Cowitch, *Dolichos pruriens* L.
Habitat: India, Africa, S. America.
Description: The hairs are brown, about 2.5 mm long, and consist of a conical, sharply pointed cell less than 1 mm in diameter, barbed at the apex. They are extremely irritating to the skin and must be handled with caution.
Part Used: The hairs on the pod.
Constituents: (i) Amines such as 5-hydroxytryptamine (serotonin), *N,N*-dimethyltryptamine, bufotenine, a 5-oxindole-3-alkylamine derivative and the alkaloids mucunadine, mucunine, prurienine, mucuadine, mucuadinine [432, 433, 183] (ii) Mucuanain, a proteolytic enzyme [183].
Medicinal Use: Anthelmintic, rubefacient. The indole bases are reported to be spasmolytic and to depress respiration and blood pressure in animals [433]. The plant also reduces blood sugar and cholesterol [183].
Preparations: Powder, dose: 0.5–4 g.

COWSLIP

Primula veris L.
Fam. Primulaceae

Synonyms: Paigles, Peagles, *P. officinalis.*
Habitat: Common in Britain, Europe and temperate Asia.
Description: A short, hairy perennial, with oval, wrinkled leaves. The flowers are tubular, yellow, about 1 cm diameter, five-lobed and spotted with orange at the throat. Taste, sweetish; odour, apricot-like.
Part Used: Flowers, occasionally root.
Constituents: (i) Saponin glycosides, especially in the root, based on the triterpene aglycones primulagenin A, dehydroprimulagenin A, primverogenins A and B, including primulic acid (about 5–10%) primulaveroside, primveroside etc [386, 434] (ii) Flavonoids, particularly in the flowers, at least 19 of which have been isolated so far, consisting of quercetin, luteolin, kaempferol, isorhamnetin, and apigenin and their glycosides [435] (iii) Phenolic glycosides, such as methoxysalicylicacid methyl ester [2] (iv) Tannins; epicatechin and epigallotannin [435] (v) Essential oil, a trace [2].
Medicinal Use: Sedative, antispasmodic, mild diuretic and aperient. The flowers are particularly high in flavonoids and these may be considered to be the main active principles. The flavonoids are antiinflammatory and antispasmodic; they inhibit histamine release and act as free radical scavengers [436, 437].
Regulatory Status: GSL.

CRAMPBARK

Viburnum opulus L.
Fam. Caprifoliaceae

Synonyms: Guelder Rose, Snowball Tree.
Habitat: Europe, Britain and America.
Description: A large bush, growing to a height of about 2.5 m. The bark is about 0.5–2 mm thick, in curved pieces, greyish brown externally with scattered lenticels, and faintly cracked longitudinally. Inner surface paler brown, laminate. Fracture tough, with flat splinters. Taste, bitter, slightly astringent.
Constituents: (i) Hydroquinones; arbutin, methylarbutin and traces of free hydroquinone (ii) Coumarins, such as scopoletin and scopoline (iii) Tannins; mainly catechins [386].
Medicinal Use: Antispasmodic, astringent, sedative, nervine. As its name suggests, it is used for cramp, particularly of menstruation, and other uterine dysfunctions.
Preparations: Liquid Extract, dose: 2–8 ml.
Regulatory Status: GSL.

CRANESBILL, AMERICAN

Geranium maculatum L.
Fam. Geraniaceae

Synonyms: Alumroot, Storksbill, Wild Geranium.
Habitat: USA.
Description: Root about 3–5 cm long, 0.5–1 cm thick, dull brown, hard, knotty, with small protuberances. Fracture short, cut surface pale or reddish brown, with white dots. Taste, very astringent; odourless. English Cranesbill is *Geranium dissectum* L.; it is reputed to have similar properties.
Part Used: Root, herb.
Constituents: Tannins, up to 30%, including gallic acid [2]. No further information is available.
Medicinal Use: Styptic, astringent, vulnerary, tonic. The root is even more astringent than the herb. An infusion or decoction is taken for diarrhoea, internal or external bleeding. It may be taken in the form of a douche for leucorrhoea and topically for ulcers and haemorrhoids.
Preparations: Liquid Extract, dose: 2–8 ml.
Potter's Products: D4 Special Formula Stomach Tablets.
Regulatory Status: GSL.

CRAWLEY

Corallorhiza odontorhiza Nutt.
Fam. Orchidaceae

Synonyms: Coral Root, Dragon's Claw, Chicken Toe.
Habitat: USA.
Description: The rhizome appears in small, brown, coral-like, branched pieces, about 2–3 cm long and 2 mm in thickness, with minute warts and

transverse scars. Fracture short and horny. Taste, sweetish then bitter; odour, strong and peculiar when fresh.

Part Used: Rhizome.

Constituents: Unidentified.

Medicinal Use: Diaphoretic, febrifuge, sedative.

Preparations: Liquid Extract, dose: 0.5–1.5 ml.

CROSSWORT
Galium cruciatum L.
Fam. Rubiaceae

Synonyms: Yellow Bedstraw.

Habitat: A common wild plant in Britain and Europe, flowering in May.

Description: Stem slender, about 30–60 cm long, bearing whorls of four leaves, ellipsoidal, oblong, hairy. Flowers, yellow, in small clusters, about eight together in the axils of the upper leaves.

Part Used: Herb.

Constituents: (i) Coumarins, including umbelliferone, scopoletin, and cruciatin, a coumarin monoglucoside (ii) Flavonoids such as hyperoside and rutin (iii) Tannins [438].

Medicinal Use: Formerly used made into a salve for wounds.

CROTON SEEDS
Croton tiglium L.
Fam. Euphorbiaceae

Synonyms: Tiglium, *Tiglium officinale* Klotsch., Badou (Chinese).

Habitat: Widely distributed throughout Asia and China.

Description: The seeds have a brown, mottled appearance. The outer layer is easily removed, leaving a hard, black coat. The oil is yellowish or reddish brown and rather viscid, with an unpleasant odour. It is toxic and should be handled with extreme care.

Part Used: Oil expressed from seeds.

Constituents: (i) Diterpene esters of the tigliane type, at least 11 of which have been isolated. The most important of these is tetradecanoyl phorbol acetate (TPA); formerly known as phorbol myristate acetate (PMA) [439]. For full review and structures see [440].

Medicinal Use: Irritant, rubifacient, cathartic. Rarely used medicinally as the effects are drastic and modern research has shown it to be dangerous. Croton oil is tumour promoting (co-carcinogenic) [441]. TPA has a wide range of pharmacological effects in addition to tumour promotion; it causes erythema, vesication and hyperplasia of the skin, platelet aggregation, interference with prostaglandin metabolism and many other actions. It has recently been shown to activate the enzyme protein kinase C [442]. TPA and the other esters are currently the subject of worldwide biochemical research, using them as pharmacological probes to investigate carcinogenesis, inflammation and other cellular mechanisms. For review

see [443]. Croton seeds are still used in Chinese medicine in very small doses, to treat biliary colic, intestinal obstruction, malaria, mastitis and other conditions [7]. The side effects are; severe irritation, lacrimation, oedema, and blistering of skin and mucous membranes. Internally it is strongly purgative, causing hypotension, abdominal pain, rapid and weak pulse and even shock. 1 ml of oil is usually fatal.
Regulatory Status: POM.

CUBEB

Piper cubeba L.
Fam. Piperaceae

Synonyms: Tailed Pepper, *Cubeba officinalis* Miq.
Habitat: Native to Indonesia, but cultivated elsewhere.
Description: The fruit resembles black pepper in size and colour, but tapers sharply into the stalk. The seed has a minute embryo in a small cavity at the apex. Taste, warm, aromatic and rather like turpentine.
Part Used: Unripe fruit.
Constituents: (i) Volatile oil, 10–20%, consisting of mono- and sesquiterpenes including α- and β-cubebine, sabinene, α-thujene, α- and β-pipene, γ- and α-terpinene and others [444, 445] (ii) Lignans; mainly (−)-cubebine, about 2% [446], with (−)-cubebinin and kinokinin; and (−)-dihydrocubebinin, (−)-clusin, and derivatives [447] (iii) Miscellaneous; cubebic acid, resins gums etc [5].
Medicinal Use: Aromatic, diuretic, expectorant, carminative. Used for bronchitis, coughs and urinary tract infections. The ground fruits have been found to be effective in treating amoebic dysentery [5]. The oil is reputedly antiviral in rats and antibacterial *in vitro* [26].
Preparations: Powdered fruit, dose: 2–4 g; Liquid Extract, dose: 2–4 ml; Cubeb Oleoresin BPC 1949, dose: 0.3–2 ml; Cubeb Oil BPC 1949, dose: 0.3–1.2 ml; Cubeb Tincture BPC 1949, dose: 2–4 ml.
Potter's Products: Asthma and Chest Mixture.
Regulatory Status: GSL.

CUCKOOPINT

Arum maculatum L.
Fam. Araceae

Synonyms: Lords and Ladies, Wake Robin, Wild Arum, Starchwort, Ramp.
Habitat: Europe and the British Isles.
Description: The plant consists of a one-leafed, erect and pointed spathe, enclosing the flower. Inside the spathe is the club-shaped, purplish or buff-coloured spadix. The root is ovoid and about the size of a hazel nut, showing annular scars left by the leaves and rootlets. Taste, acrid; odourless.
Part Used: Root.

Constituents: (i) Saponin glycosides of unknown structure [79] (ii) Polysaccharides, four of which are acetylated mannans [448] (iii) Miscellaneous; polyphenols and basic volatile substances [448].

Medicinal Use: Diaphoretic, expectorant. Has been used locally for sore throats. Large doses cause gastric inflammation, and fatal effects have been recorded. An extract of the root was found to contain a factor or factors which react specifically with receptors on human spermatozoa, causing agglutination [449]; the usefulness or significance of which is unclear.

The plant has a long history of rather unusual uses; Dioscorides stated that the root has an effect against gout, "being laid on stamped with cow's dung"; and Gerard writes "Bears, after they have lain in their dens 40 days without any manner of sustenance but what they get from licking and sucking their own feet, do, as soon as they come forth eat the herb Cuckoo-pint; through the windy nature thereof, the hungry gut is opened and made fit enough to receive sustenance". The starch from the root was used to starch the ruffs worn in the days of Queen Elizabeth I, and Gerard also says that it was "the most pure white starch" but "it choppeth, blistereth and maketh the hands rough and rugged and withall smarting".

CUDWEED

Gnaphalium uliginosum L.
Fam. Compositae

Synonyms: Marsh Cudweed, Cottonweed, Cotton Dawes.
Habitat: A native British plant.
Description: The plant is densely woolly, with small, narrow leaves, about 3 cm long and 0.5 cm wide; the flowerheads are compositous, small yellow corymbs.
Part Used: Herb.
Constituents: Largely unknown. The herb contains volatile oil and tannins [2].
Medicinal Use: Astringent, stomachic. It is used particularly for tonsillitis and laryngitis as a gargle. Reputedly antidepressant and aphrodisiac [37]. In the USSR it is used clinically to treat hypertension, usually in combination with other herbs [450].
Preparations: Liquid Extract, dose: 2–4 ml.
Regulatory Status: GSL.

CUMMIN

Cuminum cyminum L.
Fam. Umbelliferae

Synonyms: Cumin.
Habitat: Cultivated widely along the Mediterranean and in India.
Description: Fruits about 6 mm long, 1 mm wide, longitudinally ribbed, often with pedicel attached, light brown in colour. Each mericarp has four dorsal and two commisural vittae. Odour and taste characteristic.

Part Used: Fruits.

Constituents: (i) Volatile oil, about 2–5%, composed mainly of cuminalde-hyde, 1,3- and 1,4-*p*-menthadien-7-al, 3-*p*-menthen-7-al, with α- and β-pinene, α- and β-phellandrene, limonene and many others [451] (ii) Flavonoids, including apigenin and luteolin glycosides [452] (iii) Miscellaneous; octadecenoic acid, protein, aminoacids etc. [5].

Medicinal Use: Antispasmodic, stimulant, carminative. The oil is reportedly larvicidal and antibacterial [5]. It is used more frequently in cookery than in medicine.

Regulatory Status: GSL.

Biblical References: Isaiah 28 : 25–27; Matthew 23 : 23.

CUPMOSS

Cladonia pyxidata Fries.
Fam. Cladoniaceae

Synonyms: Chin Cups.

Habitat: British Isles and Europe on barren ground.

Description: The plant is a lichen, not a moss as the name suggests. The scyphi are greyish-white, about 2.5 cm long, wineglass shaped, with hollow stems and a terminal cup. Taste, mucilaginous and slightly sweet; odourless.

Part Used: Scyphi.

Constituents: (i) Lichen acids such as fumaroprotocetraric, barbatic and psoromic acids (ii) An enzyme, emulsin [2].

Medicinal Use: Expectorant and antitussive. Formerly used for whooping cough (or Chin-Cough, hence the synonym) as a decoction, sweetened with honey.

CUP-PLANT

Silphium perfoliatum L.
Fam. Compositae

Synonyms: Indian Cup Plant, Ragged Cup.

Habitat: India.

Description: Rhizome cylindrical, crooked, elongated, pitted and rough, with small roots. The transverse section shows large resin canals.

Part Used: Rhizome.

Constituents: Unknown. The aerial parts contain triterpene glycosides based on oleanolic acid [453].

Medicinal Use: Tonic, diaphoretic, alterative.

D

DAMIANA
Turnera diffusa Will.
Fam. Turneraceae

Habitat: Southern USA, Mexico and parts of sub-tropical America and Africa.

Description: Leaves wedge-shaped, about 1–2.5 cm long, up to 6 mm broad, shortly stalked, with a few serrate teeth and recurved margins. Taste, bitter, aromatic, with a fig-like flavour.

Part Used: Leaves.

Constituents: (i) Volatile oil, about 0.5–1%, containing thymol, α-copaene, δ-cadinene and calamene, 1,8-cineole, α- and β-pinenes and calamenene [1, 5] (ii) Flavonoids such as 5-hydroxy-7,3′,4-trimethoxyflavone [454] (iii) The hydroquinone, arbutin [455] (vi) Miscellaneous; a cyanogenetic glycoside, a bitter substance of undetermined structure called damianin, resin, tannin [5].

Medicinal Use: Aphrodisiac, tonic, stomachic, antidepressant. The aphrodisiac activity has not yet been demonstrated experimentally, however this is very difficult to do. The leaves are reportedly antidepressant [456].

Preparations: Liquid Extract BPC 1934, dose: 2–4 ml; Damiana Extract BPC 1934, dose: 0.3–0.6 g; Compound Damiana Mixture BPC 1934, dose: 4–8 ml.

Potter's Products: Strength Tablets; Compound Elixir of Damiana and Saw Palmetto.

Regulatory Status: GSL.

DANDELION
Taraxacum officinale Weber.
Fam. Compositae

Synonyms: *Taraxacum dens-leonis* Desf., *Leontodon taraxacum* L.

Habitat: Widely distributed throughout most of the world as a troublesome weed.

Description: The Dandelion is so well-known it needs no description. The root is collected in the autumn.

Part Used: Leaves, root.

Constituents: (i) Sesquiterpene lactones; taraxacoside (an acylated γ-butyrolactone glycoside) [457] and at least four others of the eudesmanolide, germacranolide and tetrahydroridentin B types [458] (ii) Triterpenes; taraxol, taraxerol, ψ-taraxasterol, β-amyrin, stigmasterol and β-sitosterol [5] (iii) Phenolic acids; caffeic and *p*-hydroxyphenylacetic acids (iv) Polysaccharides; glucans and mannans [459] and inulin (v) Carotenoids such as lutein and violaxanthin [5] (vi) Miscellaneous; protein, sugars, pectin, choline etc. The vitamin A content is higher than in carrots [5].

The flowers contain carotenoids like those in the leaves and root, and others [5].

Medicinal Use: Diuretic, tonic, antirheumatic and mild aperient. Used chiefly in kidney and liver disorders, for rheumatism and as a general tonic. The antiinflammatory activity has recently been confirmed in animal studies [403]. The polysaccharides and aqueous extracts have antitumour activity in animals [459, 460]. The root, when roasted, is used as a coffee substitute or flavour additive, and the fresh young leaves may be used in salads. The flowers are used to make country-style wines.

Preparations: Liquid Extract BPC 1949, dose: 2–8 ml; Dandelion Juice BPC 1949, dose: 4–8 ml.

Potter's Products: Liver and Bile Medicinal Tea Bags; Stomach and Liver Medicinal Tea Bags; Diuretic Mixture No. 110; Boldo Aid to Slimming Tablets; Natural Herb Tablets.

Regulatory Status: GSL.

DEER'S TONGUE

Trilisia odoratissima (J F Gmel) Cass.
Fam. Compositae

Synonyms: Vanilla Leaf, Wild Vanilla, Hound's Tongue, *Liatris odoratissima* Michx., *Carphephorus odoratissimus* (J F Gmel) Heb.

Habitat: Eastern USA.

Description: Leaves obovate-lanceolate; those from the root are fleshy and taper at the base into a flattened stalk, stem leaves sessile. The dried leaves have a strong odour of new-mown hay.

Part Used: Leaves.

Constituents: (i) Coumarins; coumarin itself, about 1.6% [461], dihydrocoumarin [462] (ii) Triterpenes; lupeol, lupenone, β-amyrin etc. [461, 463] (iii) Sesquiterpenes; eudesmin and epieudesmin [461, 463].

Medicinal Use: Diuretic, stimulant, tonic. The medicinal effects are mainly due to the presence of coumarin, which also gives Deer's tongue its flavour.

DEVIL'S BIT

Succisa pratensis Moench.
Fam. Dipsacaceae

Synonyms: Devil's Bit Scabious, Ofbit.

Habitat: Damp grassy places throughout Europe.

Description: Leaves opposite, stalked, lanceolate-ovate, with scattered glands. Flowerheads blue-purple, florets four lobed, receptacle hairy.

Part Used: Herb.

Constituents: Saponin glycosides of unknown structure, including scabioside [2].

Medicinal Use: Diaphoretic, demulcent, febrifuge. It may be taken as an infusion for coughs and fevers. Culpeper states "The root was longer until the Devil bit it away, envying its usefulness to mankind".

DEVIL'S CLAW
Harpagophytum procumbens DC.
Fam. Pedaliaceae

Habitat: Indigenous to Southern and Eastern Africa.

Description: The plant bears a large, hooked claw-like fruit, hence the name. The tuber is up to about 6 cm in diameter, with a yellowish-brown longitudinally striated bark. In commerce it usually occurs cut, in circular or fan-shaped pieces. Fracture short, showing a light grey-brown concentric and radiate xylem in transverse section, with occasional cavities. Taste astringent; odourless.

Part Used: Tuber.

Constituents: (i) Iridoid glycosides, including harpagide, harpagoside and procumbide [464, 465, 466] (ii) Flavonoids, mainly kaempferol and luteolin glycosides [467] (iii) Phenolic acids; chlorogenic and cinnamic acid [467] (iv) A quinone, harpagoquinone [467] (v) Miscellaneous; triterpenes, oleanolic and ursolic acid derivatives and esters, sugars, especially stachyose [467].

Medicinal Use: Antiinflammatory, antirheumatic, analgesic, sedative. Methanolic extracts have shown *in vivo* antiinflammatory activity in the rat-paw oedema test [468], analgesic effects comparable to that of phenylbutazone in rabbits, and antiphlogistic effects in a variety of tests [469]; however other tests have not confirmed these results [470]. The extracts also cause a reduction in arterial blood pressure in rats, a decrease in heart rate in rabbits, and a protective effect against arrythmias caused by adrenaline and chloroform, and calcium chloride [470]. There is some doubt as to the main active constituent and at present whole plant extracts are being used. Devil's Claw is said to have oxytocic properties and should be avoided during pregnancy [471].

Preparations: Powdered tuber, dose: 0.1–0.25 g.

Regulatory Status: GSL.

DILL
Anethum graveolens L.
Fam. Umbelliferae

Synonyms: *Peucedanum graveolens* Benth.

Habitat: Indigenous to the Mediterranean region and the Southern USSR, cultivated widely elsewhere.

Description: Fruits normally separated into two mericarps; each ovoid, compressed, winged, about 2–3 mm wide with three longitudinal ridges on each side and four dorsal vittae. On the flat commisural surface there are two more vittae and the pale carpophore. Odour and taste, pleasant, aromatic and characteristic. Indian Dill is from *A. sowa* Roxb., and the fruits are narrower and more convex, with more pronounced ridges and narrower wings.

Part Used: Fruits; the herb is used in cookery.

Constituents: (i) Volatile oil, about 2.5–5% or more, consisting mainly of carvone (about 50%), with dihydrocarvone, limonene, α- and β-phellandrene, eugenol, anethole, myristicin, carveole, α-pinene and others

[1, 2, 5] (ii) Flavonoids; kaempferol and its glucuronide, vicenin and others [451, 472] (iii) Coumarins such as scopoletin, esculetin, bergapten, umbelliferone etc. [5] (iv) Xanthone derivatives such as dillanoside [473] (v) Miscellaneous; triterpenes, phenolic acids, protein, fixed oil etc. [1, 5]. The roots contain phthalides; butylphthalide, Z-ligustilide, neocnidilide and senkyunolide [474]. It is not known whether these occur in the aerial parts. Indian Dill contains volatile oil; it has similar components although it usually has higher concentrations of dillapiole and apiole [475] and a lower carvone content [4].

Medicinal Use: Carminative, stomachic. Used frequently in infants gripe waters for wind and colic. Dill oil has a demonstrated carminative and antifoaming action [268].

Preparations: Dill oil BP, dose: 0.05–2 ml; Concentrated Dill Water BPC 1973, dose: 0.3–1 ml.

Regulatory Status: GSL.

DODDER

Cuscuta epithymum Murr.
Fam. Convolvulaceae

Synonyms: Lesser Dodder, Dodder of Thyme, Hell-weed, Devil's Guts.
Habitat: A parasite growing in most parts of the world.
Description: Stem thread-like, curled and twisted, without leaves but with small, globular clusters of flowers. Taste, saline and slightly acrid; odourless.
Part Used: Herb.
Constituents: (i) Flavonoids; kaempferol, quercetin and its 3-glucoside (ii) Substituted *p*-hydroxycinnamic acids [476].
Medicinal Use: Hepatic, laxative. Has been used in urinary, spleen and liver disorders.

DOG-ROSE

Rosa canina L.
and other spp.
Fam. Rosaceae

Synonyms: Wild Briar, Rosehips, Cynosbatos.
Habitat: Europe, N. Africa and parts of Asia. Extensively cultivated.
Description: The fruits, or hips, are oval, fleshy, scarlet when fresh and blackish when dried, with the remains of the calyx teeth at the apex. Seeds angular, whitish, densely covered with hairs, taste, sweetish and acidulous.
Part Used: The ripe or nearly ripe fruit.
Constituents: (i) Vitamins, especially vitamin C, up to 1.25%, with Vitamin A, thiamine, riboflavine, niacin and Vitamin K (ii) Flavonoids such as rutin (iii) Tannins 2–3% (iv) Invert sugar, 10–14% (v) Miscellaneous; pectin, plant acids, polyphenols, carotenoids and traces of essential oil and vanillin [1, 2, 4, 5].

Medicinal Use: Astringent, antidiarrhoeal, source of vitamin C. A syrup made from the fruits is suitable for infants.
Preparations: Confection of Rose Fruit BPC 1934, Syrup of Rose-Hips.
Potter's Products: Rose-Hip Tablets.
Regulatory Status: GSL.
Biblical References: Words translated "briar" may refer to this.

DRAGON'S BLOOD

Daemonorops draco Blume
D. propinquus Becc.
Fam. Palmae

Synonyms: Dracorubin, Sanguis Dranconis.
Habitat: Malaysia, Indonesia.
Description: A red resin produced by the fruits, softened with water and pressed and dried. Occurs as lumps, tears or sticks.
Part Used: Resin.
Constituents: Red tannin derivatives called dracoresinotannols, with benzoic acid and its esters [2].
Medicinal Use: Astringent in diarrhoea, colouring agent.

DWARF ELDER

Sambucus ebulus L.
Fam. Caprifoliaceae

Synonyms: Ground Elder, Danewort, Wallwort.
Habitat: Europe, including the British Isles, where it is a troublesome weed.
Description: Leaves pinnate, leaflets longer than those of the common Elder (q.v.), often with stipules at the base. Flowers white with pink anthers. In the US the name Dwarf Elder is given to a different plant, *Aralia hispida* Vent., (Araliaceae).
Part Used: Leaves.
Constituents: Information not easily available. See [477].
Medicinal Use: Expectorant, diuretic. Aqueous extracts induced diuresis in rats and are hypotensive in cats. No toxic side effects were observed [477].
Regulatory Status: GSL.

DYER'S GREENWEED

Genista tinctoria L.
Fam. Leguminosae

Synonyms: Greenweed, Dyer's Weed, Dyer's Broom.
Habitat: Europe, cultivated elsewhere.
Description: Stems almost unbranched, about 15–20 cm long, angular, with erect lanceolate sessile, hairless leaves, about 2 cm long and 4 mm broad. Flowers, yellow, papilionaceaous, in terminal spikes. Taste, bitter; odourless.
Part Used: Twigs, leaves.
Constituents: (i) Isoflavone glycosides including genistein, its 7-O-glucoside and daidzein [478] (ii) Flavonoids, mainly luteolin glycosides [479] (iii) Alkaloids such as anagyrine, cytisine, N-methylcytisine and lupanine [2].
Medicinal Use: Diuretic, cathartic, emetic. It has been used for gout.

E

ECHINACEA   *Echinacea angustifolia* (D. C.) Heller
                                              E. pallida (Nutt.) Britt.
                                              E. purpurea Moensch.
                                                      Fam. Compositae

Synonyms: Coneflower, Purple Coneflower *(E. purpurea)*, Black Sampson, *Brauneria angustifolia, B. pallida.*

Habitat: Native to the northern USA, cultivated in Europe.

Description: The dried rhizome is greyish-brown, often twisted, longitudinally furrowed, up to about 1 cm in diameter. The transverse section shows a thin bark, and a yellowish porous wood flecked with black. Taste, slightly sweet then bitter, leaving a tingling sensation on the tongue; odour, faintly aromatic.

Part Used: Roots and rhizome.

Constituents: (i) Echinacoside, a triglycoside of a caffeic acid derivative, in *E. angustifolia* but not *E. purpurea* [480] (ii) Unsaturated isobutyl amides, including echinacin and others, in *E. angustifolia* and *E. pallida* [481, 482]. These are unstable. (iii) Polysaccharides; a heteroxylan and an arabinorhamnogalactan [483] (iv) Polyacetylenes, at least thirteen of which have been isolated [484]. It has been postulated that these are artifacts formed during storage, since they are found in dried but not fresh roots of *E. pallida* [485]. (v) Essential oil, containing humulene, caryophyllene and its epoxide, germacrene D, and methyl-*p*-hydroxycinnamate [480, 482] (vi) Miscellaneous; vanillin, linolenic acid derivatives, a labdane derivative [482], alkanes and flavonoids [480], and the alkaloids tussilagine and isotussilagine, in very small quantities (0.006%) [486].

Sesquiterpene esters which were originally identified in commercial samples of *E. purpurea* [487] have since been shown to be due to the presence of an adulterant, *Parthenium integrifolium* L. (American Feverfew) [488]. It appears that this adulteration may be widespread in commercial samples [488].

Medicinal Use: Antibacterial, antiviral, vulnerary, alterative. It is used especially for skin diseases; boils, carbuncles, septicaemia and to aid wound healing generally, and for upper respiratory tract infections such as tonsillitis and pharyngitis. It is usually taken internally but may also be applied externally as a poultice. The antibacterial and antiviral effects are well documented *in vitro* and clinically [480, 489, 490, 491]. One of the most important actions of Echinacea is its ability to stimulate the immune system. This property has been shown by total extracts and by the polysaccharide fraction in a number of *in vivo* and *in vitro* tests, including the stimulation of phagocytosis, and also clinically [483, 491, 492, 493]. The polysaccharide fraction activates macrophages, causing an increase in secretion of free radicals and interleukin I, possibly explaining its activity against infections and in some antitumour systems [480, 491]. Echinacin has been shown to inhibit the formation of hyaluronidase by bacteria; this helps to localize the infection and stop it spreading [480]. Extracts of *E. angustifolia* also inhibit *Trichomonas vaginalis* growth *in vitro* [495].

Preparations: Liquid Extract, dose: 2–4 ml.

Potter's Products: Antifect tablets, Skin Clear Tablets, Compound Elixir of Echinacea.

Regulatory Status: GSL.

ELDER

Sambucus nigra L.
Fam. Caprifoliaceae

Synonyms: Black Elder, European Elder.

Habitat: Europe, and the British Isles, commonly growing in hedges and on waste ground.

Description: The flowers, appearing in May, are small, creamy white with yellow anthers, four-petalled, in flat-topped umbel-like clusters. Taste mucilaginous, odour characteristic. The flowers are followed by small shiny purplish-black berries. Leaves pinnate, leaflets broad with serrate margins. Bark light grey, with wide fissures revealing the smooth white inner surface. Taste, sweetish, then nauseous.

Part Used: Flowers, berries, leaves, bark.

Constituents: Flowers (i) Triterpenes including ursolic acid, 30-β-hydroxy-ursolic acid, oleanolic acid, α- and β-amyrin and free and esterified sterols [496, 497] (ii) Fixed oil, containing free fatty acids; mainly linoleic, linolenic and palmitic acids, and alkanes [498] (iii) Flavonoids, including rutin, quercetin and kaempferol etc [5] (iv) Miscellaneous; phenolic acids, e.g. chlorogenic acid, pectin, sugars etc. [5]. Leaves: (i) Triterpenes similar to those found in the flowers [499] (ii) Cyanogenetic glycosides, e.g. sambunigrin [1] (iii) Flavonoids including rutin and quercetin [499] (iv) Miscellaneous, fatty acids, alkanes, tannins [5]. The bark contains phytohaemagglutinins [500].

Medicinal Use: Alterative, diuretic, antiinflammatory. The flowers are used most frequently, as an infusion or herbal tea. Their antiinflammatory action has been demonstrated recently in animals. It has been suggested that this is due to the ursolic acid content [403]. The flowers and berries are often used to make wine, for their flavour rather than medicinal effect, however the wine taken hot has long been used for colds and a mixture of Elder flowers and Peppermint is an old remedy for influenza.

Preparations: Dried flowers, dose: 2–4 g; Liquid Extract, dose: 2–4 ml.

Potter's Preparations: Elderflower and Peppermint with Composition Essence, Life Drops, Tabritis, Remedy for Arthritis.

Regulatory Status: GSL.

ELECAMPANE
Inula helenium L.
Fam. Compositae

Synonyms: Scabwort, Yellow Starwort, *Helenium grandiflorum* Gilib., *Aster officinalis* All., *A. helenium* (L.) Scop.

Habitat: Indigenous to Europe and temperate Asia, naturalized in the USA, and cultivated widely in Europe and also China.

Description: Roots light grey, hard, horny, in cylindrical pieces of varying length, usually 1–2 cm thick and often attached to large pieces of the crown of root. Fracture short, the transverse section showing a radiate structure with numerous dark oil glands. Taste, bitter, acrid; odour aromatic, sweet, and faintly camphoraceous.

Part Used: Root.

Constituents: (i) Volatile oil, about 1–4%, containing sesquiterpene lactones, mainly alantolactone (= helenalin or elecampane camphor), isoalantolactone and their dihydro derivatives, alantic acid and azulene [501, 502] (ii) Inulin; up to 44% [5] (iii) Miscellaneous; sterols, resin etc [5].

Medicinal Use: Diaphoretic, diuretic, expectorant, alterative, tonic. Used principally in combination with other herbs for coughs, bronchitis and other pulmonary disorders, and for nausea, diarrhoea and as an anthelmintic. Alantolactone is antiinflammatory in animals and has been shown to stimulate the immune system [147]; it is also anthelmintic and hypotensive in animals [5] and antibacterial and antifungal *in vitro* [503]. The infusion is sedative in mice [504].

Preparations: Powdered root, dose: 2–4 g; Liquid Extract, dose: 2–4 ml.

Potter's Products: Asthma and Chest Mixture, Asthma and Bronchitis Medicinal Tea Bags, Horehound and Aniseed Cough Mixture, Pile Compound Herb.

Regulatory Status: GSL.

ELM
Ulmus campestris L.
Fam. Ulmaceae

Synonyms: Common Elm, Field Elm, *Ulmus carpinifolia* Gled.

Habitat: A common tree in Britain and Europe.

Description: The inner bark only is used; it occurs in thin strips 2–3 mm thick, externally rusty brown colour but paler on the inner surface. Fracture laminate and fibrous. Taste, mucilaginous, astringent and faintly bitter; odourless.

Part Used: Bark.

Constituents: (i) Tannins, including phlobaphene (ii) Mucilage [2] The wood contains naphthaquinones such as mansinone C [218], but it is not known whether this occurs in the inner bark.

Medicinal Use: Astringent, demulcent, diuretic.

Regulatory Status: GSL.

Biblical References: Hosea 4:13, probably the terebinth *Pistachia terebinthus*.

EMBELIA
Embelia ribes Burm.
Fam. Myrsinaceae

Habitat: India.

Description: The fruits are small, globular, reddish-brown, with a small projection at the apex. Taste, astringent; odour, faintly aromatic.

Part Used: Fruit.

Constituents: Naphthaquinones, such as embelin (= embelic acid), rapanone and vilangin [218].

Medicinal Use: Taenicide, carminative, diuretic, reputed contraceptive. Embelin is being investigated as contraceptive agent, it has antifertility effects in animals and appears to act by preventing implantation [505, 506], without being blastotoxic [505]. It was found to be oestrogenic and weakly progestogenic at the minimum effective dose [505].

Preparations: Powdered fruit, dose: 2–4 g; Liquid Extract, dose: 2–4 ml.

Regulatory Status: P.

EPHEDRA
Ephedra sinica Stapf.
E. equisetina Bunge
E. gerardiana Wall.
and others
Fam. Ephedraceae

Synonyms: Ma Huang.

Habitat: China, *E. gerardiana* is Indian.

Description: Slender green stems jointed in branches of about 20 tufts about 15 cm long. Leaves reduced to sheaths surrounding the stems, which terminate in a sharp, recurved point.

Part Used: Stems.

Constituents: Alkaloids, up to about 3%, but widely varying. *E. sinica* usually has higher concentrations than the other species. The major alkaloid is *l*-ephedrine, with *d*-ψ-ephedrine, pseudoephedrine, nor-ephedrine, N-methylephedrine, benzylmethylamine etc. [1, 2, 4, 37].

Medicinal Use: Antiasthmatic, bronchodilator, sympathomimetic, CNS and cardiac stimulant. Ephedra has been used since ancient times in China for asthma and hay fever. It is now used by herbalists to treat in addition, enuresis, allergies, narcolepsy and other disorders. Ephedrine and pseudo-ephedrine are widely used in the form of nasal drops, tablets and elixirs as decongestants [4]. They should be avoided by patients with high blood pressure.

Preparations: Powdered Stems, dose: 1–4 g; Liquid Extract, dose: 1–3 ml.

Regulatory Status: P.

ERGOT
Claviceps purpurea Tul.
Fam. Clavicipitaceae

Synonyms: Ergot of Rye, Smut of Rye, Spurred Rye, *Secale cornutum* Nees.

Habitat: Grows on rye.

Description: The hard mycelium of the fungus is formed from the grains of rye; it is purplish, up to about 3 cm long, 0.5 cm diameter, cylindrical, compressed, with a longitudinal furrow down each side and tapering to rounded ends. Fracture short and horny; interior whitish with a purplish tinge. Odour, disagreeable.

Part Used: Fungus.

Constituents: (i) Indole alkaloids; including the ergometrine or ergonovine group which includes ergometrine and ergometrinine, the ergotamine group which includes ergotamine and ergotaminine, the ergotoxine group which includes ergocristine, ergocristinine, ergocryptine, ergocryptinine, ergocornine and ergocorninine [1, 4] (ii) Miscellaneous; histamine, tyramine and other amines, sterols and acetylcholine [1].

Medicinal Use: Oxytocic, vasoconstrictor, α-adrenergic blocker. The alkaloids ergotamine and ergometrine are normally used individually because of their potency and slightly different effects. Ergotamine is used to relieve migrainous headaches as it is a vasoconstrictor and has antiserotonin activity. Ergometrine is used after childbirth in the third stage of labour and for post-partum haemorrhage; it is a powerful uterine stimulant, particularly of the puerperal uterus. Both must be used only under careful medical supervision.

It is thought that the plagues of the Middle Ages referred to as St Anthony's Fire were due to contamination of flour with ergot, the toxic symptoms included hallucinations and gangrene and are known as ergotism. This was not as common in Britain where rye is not usually grown, however ergot of wheat was responsible for a similar outbreak. Ergot is the starting material for the illicit manufacture of the hallucinogen LSD and its supply is monitored.

Preparations: Prepared Ergot BPC 1968, dose: 150–500 mg, Liquid Extract BPC 1954, dose: 0.6–1.2 ml.

Regulatory Status: POM.

ERYNGO

Eryngium maritimum L.
Fam. Umbelliferae

Synonyms: Eringo, Sea Holly. Field Eryngo is *E. campestre* L. and may be substituted.

Habitat: Sandy soils near the sea in Britain and Europe.

Description: A hairless perennial with leathery blue-green spiny leaves showing whitish veins and margins. The flowers are blue, in tight umbels with spiny bracts. The root is up to about 8 cm long, transversely wrinkled, dark brown and crowned with the remains of the leaf-stalks. Fracture, spongy, coarsely fibrous, with a small, radiate, yellow centre. Taste, sweetish, mucilaginous; odour, faint.

Part Used: Root.

Constituents: (i) Saponins; these are haemolytic, based on the barrigenols esterified with angelic and tiglic acids and containing arabinose, glucose and xylose. Present in both species [507, 508] (ii) Coumarins, in *E.*

campestre at least, mainly dihydropyranocoumarins of the xanthyletin type, including aegelinol and its benzoate, agasyllin and grandivetin [509] (iii) Plant acids such as malic, malonic etc and polyphenolic acids such as rosmarinic and chlorogenic acids [508] (iv) Flavonoids (unspecified) [508].

Medicinal Use: Diuretic, antiinflammatory, expectorant. Mostly used for urinary tract conditions such as cystitis, urethritis, polyuria and renal colic, and for prostate trouble. The antiinflammatory activity is demonstrable in some animal models by a hydrophilic extract [510]. This is probably due in part to the rosmarinic acid which has a similar activity [400].

Preparations: Powdered root, dose: 2–4 g.

Regulatory Status: GSL.

ETERNAL FLOWER

Helichrysum stoechas D. C.
Fam. Compositae

Synonyms: Goldilocks, *Gnaphalium stoechas* L., *G. citrinum* Lam., *Stoechas citrina*.

Habitat: A garden plant in Britain and Europe.

Description: Flowerheads ovate, compositous, arranged in a crowded corymb; the outer florets are yellow and shiny. Taste, bitter, pungent; odour, faint.

Part Used: Tops.

Constituents: *Helichrysum* spp. contain volatile oil, the major components of which are nerol and neryl acetate; sesquiterpenes, triterpenes and flavonoids [5].

Medicinal Use: Formerly used as an expectorant.

EUCALYPTUS

Eucalyptus globulus Labill.
Fam. Myrtaceae

Synonyms: Blue Gum, Gum Tree. Other species used for oil production include *E. polybracteata* R. T. Baker, and *E. smithii* R. T. Baker. A lemon scented Eucalyptus is obtained from *E. citriodora*, which grows in Queensland.

Habitat: Victoria and Tasmania in Australia, cultivated in Southern Europe and elsewhere.

Description: The leaves are scimitar-shaped, 10–15 cm long and about 3 cm wide, shortly stalked and rounded at the base, with numerous transparent oil glands. Taste and odour, characteristic.

Part Used: Leaves and the oil distilled from them.

Constituents: (i) Volatile oil, up to about 3.5%, the major component of which is 1,8-cineole (= eucalyptol), 70–85%; with terpineol, α-pinene, *p*-cymene and small amounts of sesquiterpenes such as ledol, aromadendrene and viridoflorol; aldehydes, ketones and alcohols [511, 50, 5] (ii) Polyphenolic acids; caffeic, ferulic, gallic, protocatechuic and others [512] (iii) Flavonoids including eucalyptin, hyperoside and rutin [512].

Medicinal Use: Antiseptic, antispasmodic, expectorant, stimulant, febrifuge. Eucalyptus oil is taken internally in small doses, as an ingredient of cough mixtures, sweets and pastilles, and as an inhalation; and externally in the form of a liniment, ointment or "vapour rub" as a rubifacient, decongestant and antiseptic. It is used as a flavouring for dentifrices and in many other pharmaceuticals and cosmetics.

Preparations: Eucalyptus Oil BP, dose: 0.05–0.2 ml; Menthol and Eucalyptus Inhalation BPC.

Regulatory Status: GSL.

EUCALYPTUS KINO

Eucalyptus rostrata Schlecht
E. camadulensis and other spp.
Fam. Myrtaceae

Synonyms: Red Gum.

Habitat: Madras and Sri Lanka.

Description: Dark reddish brown irregularly shaped pieces of gum. Taste, astringent, adheres to the teeth and colours the saliva red.

Part Used: Dried juice of the tree.

Constituents: (i) Volatile oil, containing about 70% citronellal (ii) Tannins; about 40% kinotannic acid, catechol, pyrocatechol and "kino red" [2].

Medicinal Use: Astringent and tonic. Used for inflamed mucous membranes and for diarrhoea, and as a gargle or lozenge for sore throats.

Preparations: Powder, dose: 0.3–1.2 g; Tincture of Kino BPC 1949, dose: 2–4 ml, Lozenge of Eucalyptus Kino BPC 1949.

Regulatory Status: GSL.

EUPHORBIA

Euphorbia hirta L.
Fam. Euphorbiaceae

Synonyms: Pill-bearing Spurge, Asthma-weed, *E. pilulifera* Jaquin, *E. capitata* Lam.

Habitat: A widespread tropical weed.

Description: Stem slender, cylindrical, with bristly hairs and opposite leaves which are lanceolate, about 2 cm long and 1 cm wide, toothed at the margin. Flowers very small, in dense, round clusters in the axils of the leaves. Taste, bitter; odourless.

Part Used: Herb.

Constituents: (i) Flavonoids; quercetin, quercitrin, cyanidin 3,5-diglucoside and others [513] (ii) Terpenoids such as taraxerol, friedalin [513], sterols; campesterol etc [514] (iii) *n*-Alkanes, triacontane etc. [514] (iv) Phenolic acids e.g. gallic and ellagic acids [515] (v) Shikimic acid [515] (vi) Choline [515]. Diterpene esters similar to those found in other *Euphorbia* spp. have been reported to be present [516]; this work was discredited and the toxic esters have been shown conclusively to be absent [517, 518].

111

Medicinal Use: Anti-asthmatic, pectoral. Two of the active constituents are thought to be choline and shikimic acid, which affect isolated smooth muscle preparations [515].

Preparations: Euphorbia Liquid Extract BPC 1949, dose: 0.12–0.3 ml.

Potter's Products: Antibron Tablets, Asthma and Bronchitis Mixture No. 80A.

Regulatory Status: GSL.

EUPHORBIUM

Euphorbia resinifera Berg.
Fam. Euphorbiaceae

Habitat: Native to N. Africa.

Description: The plant has fleshy quadrangular stems, covered with spines and resembling a cactus. The latex is collected by incising the stem and allowing the milky juice to harden on exposure to the air. Tasting and inhaling are not advised, it is acrid and highly sternutatory.

Part Used: Dried latex.

Constituents: Diterpene esters; derivatives of 12-deoxyphorbol. For full review see [440, 518].

Medicinal Use: Euphorbium was formerly used as a drastic purgative, but it is irritant, vesicant and toxic and should not be taken in any form. The 12-deoxyphorbol esters are tumour promoting, proinflammatory and cause platelet aggregation [440, 518, 519, 520, 521]; they have recently been shown to activate protein kinase C, and at the present time a great deal of biochemical research is being carried out into their properties and mechanism of action. For review see [518].

EVENING PRIMROSE

Oenothera biennis L.
and other *Oenothera* spp.
Fam. Onagraceae

Synonyms: Tree Primrose, Sun Drop.

Habitat: USA, cultivated as a garden plant elsewhere and found as a garden escape on waste, especially sandy soil.

Description: The plants are medium or tall hairy perennials with alternate, lanceolate leaves and large, yellow, four-petalled flowers, followed by long elongated capsules.

Part Used: Leaves, oil from the seed.

Constituents: The oil contains about 70% *cis*-linolenic acid and about 9% *cis*-γ-linolenic acid (GLA).

Medicinal Use: The leaves were formerly used as a poultice and for a variety of "female" disorders. Recently the oil has been extensively investigated, and even more extensively advertised, for a vast number of uses. The wildly extravagant claims made for the oil have obscured the real therapeutic benefits, which are due mainly to the GLA content. Its main clinically proven uses are for: atopic eczema [522], especially in infants

[523], for mastalgia [524], and the most wide usage of all, premenstrual syndrome [525]. Claims that it is an antiobesity agent were disproven [526]. GLA appears to lower blood pressure and inhibit platelet aggregation [527] and has been shown to correct some of the defects, including restoring the motility of red cells, in the blood of patients with multiple sclerosis [528]. Other potential uses claimed for the oil are the treatment of schizophrenia, hyperactivity in children and arthritis; however these have not been adequately substantiated yet.

Evening Primrose oil is usually taken in conjunction with Vitamin E to prevent oxidation.

Preparations: Oil, dose: very variable, usually 250 mg upwards daily.
Regulatory Status: GSL.

EYEBRIGHT

Euphrasia officinalis L.
E. rostkoviana
and other spp.
Fam. Scrophulariaceae

Habitat: Meadows and grassy places in Britain and Europe.
Description: Stems about 10–15 cm long, often branched near the base, leaves opposite near the base and alternate above, about 1 cm long and 0.5 cm broad, lanceolate, with four or five teeth on each side. Flowers small, white, often tinged with purple or with a yellow spot, axillary, two-lipped, with four yellow stamens. Taste, saline, bitter; odourless.
Part Used: Herb.
Constituents: (i) Iridoid glycosides, including aucubin [529]. *E. rostkoviana* has been shown to contain at least 8 of these, including geniposide, catalpol, luproside and derivatives, as well as aucubin [530]. Also, in *E. officinalis* (ii) Tannins, both condensed and hydrolysable gallic acid types (iii) Phenolic acids including caffeic and ferulic (iv) Volatile oil, about 0.017% (v) Miscellaneous; an unidentified alkaloid or base, sterols, amino acids and choline [530].
Medicinal Use: Astringent, tonic. Used principally as a remedy in disorders of the eye such as conjunctivitis, as an eye lotion.
Preparations: Liquid Extract, dose: 2–4 ml.
Regulatory Status: GSL.

F

FENNEL

Foeniculum vulgare Mill.
Fam. Umbelliferae

Synonyms: Sweet Fennel is the variety generally used; it is sometimes referred to as var *dulce* and Bitter Fennel as var *vulgare*.

Habitat: Indigenous to the Mediterranean region but widely cultivated elsewhere.

Description: The fruit is about 1 cm long and 0.25 cm broad, oblong, cylindrical and slightly curved. Each half fruit has four longitudinal ridges, the two lateral thicker than the two dorsal. The colour varies from greenish to brown. Taste, sweet, aromatic; odour, characteristic.

Part Used: Fruit. The herb and fresh bulb are used in cooking.

Constituents: (i) Volatile oil, up to about 8%, consisting mainly of anethole; approximately 80% in sweet fennel and 60% in bitter fennel. Some varieties are anethole-free with up to 80% estragole [531], these are not suitable for normal use. The other major component of the oil is fenchone, higher in bitter than sweet fennel, about 10–30% [531, 532, 533]. Minor components include limonene, anisaldehyde, α- and β-pinene, α-phellandrene, myrcene, ocimene, α- and β-terpinene and apiole [5, 532, 533] and the polymers of anethole, dianethole and photoanethole [534] (ii) Flavonoids; mainly rutin, quercetin and kaempferol glycosides [452, 535] (iii) Coumarins; bergapten, imperatorin, xanthotoxin and marmesin [536] (iv) Miscellaneous; sterols, fixed oils and sugars [5].

The essential oil from the root contains a substantial amount of apiole and that from the aerial parts is similar in composition to the oil from the fruit [537].

Medicinal Use: Stomachic, carminative, antiinflammatory, orexigenic. Fennel is used particularly to treat flatulence and colic in infants. The volatile oil is spasmolytic, carminative [538, 269] and has been shown to increase liver regeneration in partially hepatectomized rats [539]. Fennel is antiinflammatory in rats and also reportedly slightly oestrogenic [534]. It is a popular flavouring in drinks, sweets and in cooking.

Preparations: Fennel Oil BPC 1949, dose: 0.03–0.2 ml; Concentrated Fennel Water BPC 1934, dose: 0.3–1 ml; Liquid Extract, dose: 0.5–2 ml.

Potter's Products: Lion Cleansing Herbs, Constipation Medicinal Tea Bags.

Regulatory Status: GSL.

FEVERBUSH

Garrya fremontii Torr.
Fam. Cornaceae

Synonyms: Skunkbush, California Feverbush.

Habitat: California, N. and Middle America.

Description: Leaves up to 8 cm long and nearly as broad, shortly stalked with an entire margin and pointed apex. Taste, bitter; odour, slight.
Part Used: Leaves.
Constituents: Unknown.
Medicinal Use: Tonic, bitter, febrifuge.

FEVERFEW   *Tanacetum parthenium* (L.) Schultz Bip.
Fam. Compositae
Synonyms: Featherfew, Featherfoil, Midsummer Daisy, *Chrysanthemum parthenium* (L.) Bernh., *Leucanthemum parthenium* (L.) Gren and Godron, *Pyrethrum parthenium* (L.) Sm.
Habitat: Grows wild in many parts of Europe and the British Isles.
Description: A perennial herb reaching up to 60 cm, with a downy erect stem. The leaves are yellowish-green, alternate, stalked, ovate and pinnately divided with an entire or crenate margin. The flowers, which appear in June to August, are up to about 2 cm in diameter and arranged in corymbs of up to 30 heads, with white ray florets and yellow disc florets and downy involucral bracts. Taste, bitter and nauseous; odour, strongly aromatic, characteristic.
Part Used: Herb.
Constituents: (i) Volatile oil, containing α-pinene and several pinene derivatives, bornyl acetate and angelate, costic acid, β-farnesine and spiroketal enol ethers [540] (ii) Sesquiterpene lactones; the major one being parthenolide [541] (a germacranolide), with santamarine (= balchanin) [542], and a number of others including esters of parthenolide, reynosin, artemorin and its epoxide, 3β-hydroxyparthenolide, 3β-hydroxycostunolide, 8α-hydroxyestafiatin, traces of canin and artecanin [540], partholide and chrysantholide [543]. Recently a new dimeric germacranolide, chrysanthemonin, has been isolated [543] (iii) Acetylene derivatives, mainly in the root [540].
Medicinal Use: Febrifuge, analgesic, antirheumatic, stomachic, anthelmintic. Used for rheumatism, headache and menstrual problems. For review see [544]. There has been a great resurgence of interest in Feverfew for rheumatism, and especially as a prophylactic treatment for migraine, where a recent clinical trial has shown it to be highly efficaceous [545]. The fresh leaves may be eaten, usually with other foods to disguise the nauseous taste, or standardized capsules or tablets taken daily to prevent migraine attacks. Pharmacological work carried out to discover the mode of action of Feverfew, thought to be due to the sesquiterpene lactones present, has shown that it inhibits prostaglandin production and arachidonic acid release, explaining at least part of its antiplatelet and antifebrile actions [546, 547]. Extracts also inhibit secretion of serotonin from platelet granules and proteins from polymorphonuclear leucocytes (PMN's) [548]. Since serotonin is implicated in the aetiology of migraine and PMN secretion is increased in rheumatoid arthritis, these findings

substantiate the use of Feverfew in these conditions [548]. The stomachic effect may be due to the spiroketal ethers which are spasmolytic (see German Chamomile). Parthenolide has been shown to reduce calcium secretion in animals, whch may be useful in the treatment of hypercalcuria and related conditions [549]. Like most potent substances Feverfew may have side effects in a few individuals; these are dermatitis and soreness or ulceration of the mouth [545], and more pleasantly, a mild tranquillising effect [544].

Preparations: Liquid Extract, dose: 4–8 ml.
Potter's Products: Feverfew Tablets.
Regulatory Status: GSL.

FIG

Ficus carica L.
Fam. Moraceae

Habitat: Cultivated in most Mediterranean countries, especially Greece, Turkey and Spain.

Description: The fig is fleshy inflorescence containing the minute ovaries of the female flowers. The male flowers occupy the small orifice at the apex.

Part Used: Fleshy inflorescence or "fruit".

Constituents: (i) Flavonoids; schaftoside and isoschaftoside, which are isomeric C-glycosides of apigenin [550] (ii) Miscellaneous; sugars, mainly glucose, vitamins A and C with minor amounts of B and D, plant acids and enzymes including ficin [1, 4].

Medicinal Use: Nutritive, emollient, demulcent, mild laxative. The fresh and dried fruits are used in constipation.

Preparations: Compound Fig Elixir BPC, dose: 2.5–10 ml.

Biblical References: Numbers 13:23 and 20:5; II Kings 20:7; Nehemiah 13:15; Song of Solomon 2:13; Isaiah 38:21; Jeremiah 24:1–8 and 29:17; Matthew 7:16; Mark 11:13; Luke 6:44; James 3:12; Revelation 6:13. Also 39 references to the tree.

Regulatory Status: GSL.

FIGWORT

Scrophularia nodosa L.
Fam. Scrophulariaceae

Synonyms: Rosenoble, Throatwort, Carpenter's Square, Scrofula Plant.

Habitat: A European and British wild plant.

Description: The stem is quadrangular, bearing opposite, stalked leaves which are 10–12 cm long and 3–5 cm broad, rounded but unequal at the base and tapering to a point at the apex. The margin is sharply serrate and the veins depressed above and prominent beneath. Taste, bitter; odour characteristic.

Part Used: Herb.

Constituents: (i) Iridoids, 0.1–15% of the dry weight, including aucubin, harpagide, acetyl harpagide and 6α-rhamnopyranosylcatalpol [551, 552] (ii) Flavonoids; diosmin and hesperidin [553] (iii) Phenolic acids; ferulic, isoferulic, *p*-coumaric, caffeic, vanillic and chlorogenic acids [554].

Medicinal Use: Diuretic, depurative, anodyne. Aucubine is a mild laxative [197] and has been shown to stimulate the excretion of uric acid from the kidneys [196] in animals. Figwort is usually taken as an infusion or applied as a poultice.
Preparations: Liquid Extract, dose: 4–8 ml.
Potter's Products: Liver and Bile Medicinal Tea Bags.
Regulatory Status: GSL.

FIVE-LEAF-GRASS

Potentilla reptans L.
Fam. Rosaceae

Synonyms: Cinquefoil, Fivefinger.
Habitat: A common British wild plant.
Description: Slender creeping stems with five leaflets, bluntly serrate, about 3 cm long, with scattered hairs on the veins and margins. Flowers small, bright yellow, five-petalled with numerous stamens. Taste, astringent; odourless.
Part Used: Herb, root.
Constituents: Tannins [2].
Medicinal Use: Astringent, febrifuge. The herb is normally taken as an infusion for diarrhoea and externally as an astringent lotion.

FLEABANE

Erigeron canadense L.
Fam. Compositae

Synonyms: Canada Fleabane, Coltstail, Prideweed.
Habitat: Europe and the USA..
Description: Stem unbranched, lower leaves oblanceolate and short stalked. with five teeth, upper leaves becoming linear with an entire margin, 2.5–5 cm long. Flowerheads numerous, bell-shaped, about 0.5 cm long and broad, whitish. Taste, astringent, aromatic and bitter; odour slight.
Part Used: Herb, seeds.
Constituents: (i) Volatile oil, about 0.3–0.6%, containing *d*-limonene, terpineol, linalool and dipentene [2] (ii) Flavonoids, including apigenin (iii) Terpenes such as α-spinasterol and β-sitosterol (iv) Plant acids; vanillic, caffeic, succinic [555] (v) Tannins; gallic acid [2].
Medicinal Use: Astringent, diuretic, tonic. Formerly used for diarrhoea and kidney disorders, often as an infusion. An aqueous extract has a transient hypotensive effect in rats [556].
Preparations: Liquid Extract, dose: 4–8 ml; Oil, dose: 0.01–0.25 ml.

FLUELLEN

Kickxia elatine (L.) Dum.
K. spuria (L.) Dum.
Fam. Scrophulariaceae

Synonyms: Fluellin. Sharp-leaved Fluellen is *K. elatine* (= *Linaria elatine* L.) Mill., Round-leaved Fluellen is *K. spuria* (= *Linaria spuria* L.) Mill.
Habitat: A British and European wild plant.
Description: A partly recumbent, much branched annual. Leaves greyish-green, round or oval and, in *K. elatine*, somewhat pointed. Flowers yellow, two-lipped, the lower lip is three-lobed and the upper two-lobed.
Part Used: Herb.
Constituents: *K. spuria* has been shown to contain the flavonoids salvigenin and sinensetin [557].
Medicinal Use: Astringent. Taken as an infusion or applied externally for nasal and other bleeding.
Regulatory Status: GSL.

FOENUGREEK

Trigonella foenum-graecum L.
Fam. Leguminosae

Synonyms: Fenugreek.
Habitat: N. Africa, India, cultivated worldwide.
Description: The seeds are brownish yellow, 4–7 mm long, oblong or rhomboid, with a deep longitudinal furrow almost dividing the seed. Taste and odour characteristic.
Part Used: Seeds.
Constituents: (i) Volatile oil, in small quantities, containing 3-hydroxy-4,5-dimethyl-2-furanone, dihydrobenzofuran, dihydroactinidiolide, ϵ-muurolene, β-elemene, β-selinene [558] (ii) Alkaloids, including trigonelline, gentianine and carpaine [4, 5] (iii) Saponins, based mainly on the sapogenins diosgenin and its isomer yamogenin, gitogenin and tigogenin [559, 560] (iv) Flavonoids, including vitexin and its glycosides and esters, isovitexin, orientin, vicenins 1 and 2, quercetin and luteolin [561, 562] (v) Mucilage; mostly a galactomannan [5] (vi) Miscellaneous; protein, ca. 25%, fixed oil, up to 8%, vitamins A, B_1 and C and minerals [5].
Medicinal Use: Demulcent, nutritive, laxative, digestive, antipyretic and expectorant. Saponin-rich extracts of Foenugreek are antidiabetic in animal models [563, 564, 565] and reduce blood levels of cholesterol [565]. The fibrous fraction also causes a reduction in blood lipids [565]. Aqueous and alcoholic extracts have been reported to be oxytocic in animals [566]. The aqueous extract promotes healing of gastric ulcers produced experimentally in rats, and exhibits a mild smooth muscle relaxant effect in rabbits without affecting either the heart or blood pressure [567], which substantiates its claim as a demulcent and aid to digestion. Trigonelline has been shown to significantly inhibit liver carcinoma in mice, and is used in China to treat cancer of the cervix, as pessary [7]. Foenugreek is a useful source of sapogenins and new varieties are undergoing field trial [1]. It is an ingredient of curry powders and is used as a flavouring.
Regulatory Status: GSL.

FOOL'S PARSLEY
Aethusa cynapium L.
Fam. Umbelliferae

Synonyms: Dog Parsley, Dog Poison.

Habitat: A British and European wild plant.

Description: Resembles parsley somewhat, may be distinguished by the three long slender bracts hanging from the base of the flowers.

Part Used: Herb.

Constituents: (i) Alkaloids such as cynapine, with traces of coniine [2, 79] (ii) Volatile oil (iii) Polyines; aethusin, aethusanol A and B [2].

Medicinal Use: Sedative, stomachic in small doses. Its use is not advisable as it is poisonous; it has been mistaken for parsley with unfortunate results.

FOXGLOVE
Digitalis purpurea L.
Fam. Scrophulariaceae

Synonyms: Purple Foxglove. The Woolly Foxglove, *D. lanata* L., and other species are also used.

Habitat: British Isles and Europe.

Description: Leaves ovate, about 10–30 cm long and up to 10 cm wide, with a subacute apex and a crenate margin; petiolate with a decurrent base. The veins are prominent on the undersurface and depressed on the upper surface, anastomosing near the margin. Taste, very bitter; odour faint.

Part Used: Leaves.

Constituents: (i) Cardenolides; glycosides based on digitoxigenin, gitoxigenin and gitaloxigenin. There are many, but the most important ones are digitoxin and gitoxin. *D. lanata* contains related glycosides, including digoxin and lanatosides. It is the main source of digoxin for the pharmaceutical industry [1, 2, 4]. (ii) Anthraquinones such as alizarin derivatives and others, in both species [1] (iii) Miscellaneous; flavonoids and saponins [1].

Medicinal Use: Cardiac tonic. Digitalis glycosides increase the force of contraction of the heart without increasing the oxygen consumption, and slow the heart rate when auricular fibrillation is present. They are used to treat congestive heart failure. Digitalis leaf, even in the standardized form, is rarely used. Due to their potency and different onset of action it is preferable to use the isolated glycosides and only under close medical supervision. Digoxin is the glycoside of choice since it is the least cumulative and most rapidly excreted; it is very widely prescribed and very valuable therapeutically. Due to their cumulative effect the glycosides can easily exhibit toxic symptoms; these include nausea, vomiting and anorexia. For reviews see [568, 569].

Preparations: Prepared Digitalis BP; Prepared Digitalis Tablets BP.

Regulatory Status: POM.

FRINGETREE

Chionanthus virginicus L.
Fam. Oleaceae

Synonyms: Old Man's Beard, Snowdrop Tree.
Habitat: Southern USA.
Description: The root bark occurs in irregular, quilled pieces up to about 8 cm long and about 3 mm thick, externally dull brown with concave scars. The inner surface is quite smooth and buff coloured. Fracture short, dense, showing projecting bundles of stone cells.
Part Used: Rootbark.
Constituents: Largely unknown. Chionanthin, a haemolytic saponin glycoside has been reported [2].
Medicinal Use: Alterative, hepatic, cholagogue, diuretic, tonic. Fringetree is highly thought of particularly for liver disorders, jaundice and for gallstones.
Preparations: Liquid Extract, dose: 0.3–1.5 ml.
Potter's Products: Elixir of Chelidonium.
Regulatory Status: GSL.

FROSTWORT

Helianthemum canadense Michx.
Fam. Cistaceae

Synonyms: Rock Rose, Frostweed, *Cistus canadense* L.
Habitat: Europe and the USA.
Description: Twigs, slender, purplish-green, with opposite leaf scars. Leaves linear, up to 1.5 cm long, greyish-green, downy. Flowers apetalous in small clusters. Taste, astringent and bitter; odourless.
Part Used: Herb.
Constituents: (i) Tannins, about 10% (ii) Helianthinin, a glycoside [2].
Medicinal Use: Astringent, alterative, tonic. It may be taken internally as an infusion or applied externally as a wash for ulcers etc.
Preparations: Liquid Extract, dose: 2–4 ml.
Regulatory Status: GSL.

FUMITORY

Fumaria officinalis L.
Fam. Fumariaceae

Synonyms: Common Fumitory, Earthsmoke.
Habitat: Common in Europe and the British Isles, especially in cultivated fields, flowering throughout the summer.
Description: Leaves pinnate, glabrous. Flowers slender, tubular, two-lipped, pink with darker tips, in short spikes. Fruit, globular, containing one seed. Taste, bitter and saline; odour, faint.
Part Used: Herb.
Constituents: Isoquinoline alkaloids, including bulbocapnine, canadine, coptisine, corydaline, dicentrine, cryptopine, fumaricine, fumariline, fumaritine, N-methylhydrastine, protopine, sanguinarine, sinactine and others [112, 174].

Medicinal Use: Tonic, mild diuretic and laxative, antiinflammatory. Used mainly in stomach disorders, liver complaints and skin infections. Culpeper wrote "The juice of the Fumitory and Docks mingled with vinegar and the places gently washed therewith, cures all sorts of scabs, pimples, blotches, wheals and pushes which arise on the face or hands and any other part of the body". At least some of these actions are due to the presence of sanguinarine, which is antiseptic. See Bloodroot.

Preparations: Liquid Extract, dose: 2–4 ml.

Potter's Products: Blood Purifying Compound Herb.

Regulatory Status: GSL.

G

GALANGAL

Alpinia officinarum Hance
Fam. Zingiberaceae

Synonyms: Galanga, East India Root, Lesser Galangal. Greater Galangal is *A. galanga* Willd.

Habitat: S. E. Asia, cultivated in India.

Description: The rhizome is dark reddish brown, cylindrical, about 1–2 cm diameter and 3–6 cm long, marked at short intervals with raised rings which are the scars of the leaf bases. Fracture hard and tough, showing a paler inside with a darker central column. Taste, pungent and spicy; odour, aromatic, rather like ginger. Greater Galangal is larger and paler and is less pungent.

Part Used: Rhizome.

Constituents: Volatile oil, about 1%, containing α-pinene, cineole, linalool and the sesquiterpenes galangol and galangin [50, 37]. *A. galanga* contains 1′-acetoxychavicol and 1′-acetoxyeugenol [570].

Medicinal Use: Carminative, stimulant, used mainly for dyspepsia. A paste containing galangal and bloodroot has been used for peridontal diseases such as gingivitis, and also for skin cancer [176]. *A. galanga* has anti-ulcer activity in animals [571] and the 1′-acetoxy derivatives mentioned show antitumour effects *in vitro* [570].

Preparations: Powdered rhizome (root), dose: 1–2 g; Liquid Extract, dose: 2–4 ml.

Regulatory Status: GSL.

GALBANUM

Ferula gummosa Boiss.
and other species.
Fam. Umbelliferae

Synonyms: *F. galbaniflua* Boiss. et Buhse.

Habitat: Middle East and the Levant.

Description: The gum-resin occurs in translucent, yellowish or bluish-green masses of tears. Soft Galbanum (Levant) is more viscous and may contain small pieces of root; Hard Galbanum (Persian) is friable and may contain pieces of stem. Odour; rather like musk or turpentine.

Part Used: Gum-resin.

Constituents: (i) Volatile oil, from 5-30%, the highest being in the soft variety, containing mono- and sequiterpenes, alcohols and acetates including α- and β-pinene, carene, limonene, terpinolene, linalool, terpineol, borneol, myrcene, cadinene, guaiol, galbanol, 10-epijunenol and others [445, 572, 573]; azulenes such as guiazulene [574]; thiol esters such as S-isopropyl-3-methylbutanethioate and S-sec-butyl-3-methyl-butanethioate [574]; undecatrienes including *n*-1,3,5-undecatriene [575] (ii) Resinic acids, 30–40% (iii) Gums (iv) Umbelliferone [576, 5].

Medicinal Use: Carminative, stimulant, expectorant, vulnerary, it may be taken internally or applied as an ointment or ingredient of plasters.
Preparations: Compound Galbanum Pill, dose: 1 or 2 pills.
Regulatory Status: GSL.
Biblical References: Exodus 30:34 an ingredient of incense.

GALE, SWEET

Myrica gale L.
Fam. Myricaceae

Synonyms: Bog Myrtle, Dutch Myrtle.
Habitat: Native to Britain, Scandinavia, France, Portugal, N. America and parts of Russia.
Description: Leaves leathery, lanceolate-obovate, about 2–3 cm long and 1 cm wide, with small resinous glands. Taste, astringent; odour, aromatic, recalling that of bay leaves.
Part Used: Shrub.
Constituents: (i) Essential oil, about 0.4%, containing cineole, germacrone and dipentene [2] (ii) Dihydrochalcones; 2'-hydroxy-4,6'-dimethoxy-3'methyldihydrochalcone and others [577] (iii) Flavonoids such as myricitrin (iv) Esters of fatty acids [2].
Medicinal Use: Aromatic, astringent. The methylated dihydrochalcones are bacteriostatic and fungistatic *in vitro* [577].
Regulatory Status: GSL.

GALLS

Quercus infectoria Olivier.
Fam. Fagaceae

Synonyms: Nutgalls, Blue Galls, Oak Galls, *Gallae ceruleae.*
Habitat: Mediterranean countries, the Middle and Far East.
Description: Galls are formed as a result of the bark being punctured by an insect for laying eggs, after which an excrescence grows. The plant itself is of the oak family but rarely grows to more than a shrub. Taste, very astringent and slightly acid, then sweetish; odourless.
Part Used: Gall.
Constituents: 60–70% Gallotannic acid, a complex mixture of glycosides of phenolic acids, mainly gallic acid polymers. Varies widely in composition but is generally regarded as pentadigalloylglucose [5].
Medicinal Use: Astringent. Formerly used for diarrhoea and dysentery but may have cytotoxic effects as well as its antiviral, antimicrobial and other properties. These are probably due to the ability of tannins to precipitate proteins.
Preparations: Powder, dose: 0.5–1.2 g; Gall Ointment BPC 1954; Gall and Opium Ointment BPC 1963.
Biblical References: The biblical word refers to a bitter herb, Matthew 27:34; Acts 8:23.

GAMBOGE

Garcinia hanburyi Hook, F.
Fam. Guttiferae

Synonyms: Camboge, Gutta Cambodia, Gutta Gamba. Indian Gamboge is derived from *Garcinia morella* Desf.

Habitat: S. E. Asia.

Description: Usually in the form of cylindrical sticks, deep orange brown and opaque. The transverse fracture should be smooth and conchoidal. Taste, very acrid; the powder is strongly sternutatory.

Part Used: Gum-resin.

Constituents: (i) Resins, 70–75%, consisting mainly of α- and β-garcinolic acids, with gambogic and neogambogic acids [2, 578] (ii) Gum, about 20–25% [2]. *G. manni* contains biflavanones such as maniflavone [327].

Medicinal Use: Purgative; usually in combination with other laxatives. Maniflavone is an aldose reductase inhibitor and has been used in medicines to treat vascular permeability and fragility [327].

Regulatory Status: GSL. Maximum dose 10 mg.

GARLIC

Allium sativum L.
Fam. Liliaceae

Habitat: Cultivated worldwide.

Description: The bulb is well-known, creamy-white, composed of a number of small bulbs or "cloves" covered with membranous bracts.

Part Used: Bulb.

Constituents: (i) Volatile oil, about 0.2%, consisting of sulphur-containing compounds, including allicin (= S-allyl-2-propenthiosulphinate), allyl-methyltrisulphide, diallyldisulphide, diallyltrisulphide, diallyltetrasulphide, allylpropyldisulphide [579, 580, 581], ajoene (= 4,5,9-trithiododeca-1,6,11-triene 9-oxide) [581], 2-vinyl-4*H*-1,3-dithiin [582], and alliin, which breaks down enzymatically to allicin [578]; with citral, geraniol, linalool and α- and β-phellandrene [5] (ii) Miscellaneous; enzymes including allinase, vitamins of the B group, minerals flavonoids etc. [5, 33].

Medicinal Use: Antibiotic, expectorant, diaphoretic, hypotensive, anti-thrombotic, antidiabetic. Used most frequently at present for colds, flu, bronchitis and asthma, but the great revival of interest in garlic will probably lead to a much wider usage soon. The antibiotic effects are normally attributed to the action of allicin, which has been shown to be active *in vitro* against *Candida albicans, Trichomonas* spp., *Staphylococcus aureus, Escherischia coli* [583], *Salmonella typhi,* and *paratyphi, Shigella dysenterica,* and *Vibrio cholerae* [7]. Allicin and allylpropyldisulphide are hypoglycaemic in humans and animals [584, 585]; however garlic also contains hyperglycaemic compounds [585] which may account for the discrepancies in earlier publications. It has been suggested that the active hypoglycaemic compounds have an insulin-sparing effect due to the thiol groups competing for insulin with the inactivating compounds [586]. It is also hypolipidaemic [587, 588]. One of the main fields of interest currently is the antithrombotic activity of garlic. Extracts have been shown to inhibit platelet aggregation [589]. This is now known to be due at least in part to ajoene, which is a potent antithrombotic agent [581], as well as the less potent 2-vinyl-4*H*-1,3-dithiin [582].

Garlic has been used in Chinese medicine for many years, for indigestion, oedema, diarrhoea, whooping cough, abscesses and other skin conditions. It has been tested clinically there for bacillary and amoebic dysentery, giving success rates of 67% and 88% respectively, and for appendicitis where the improvement was said to be high in a number of different studies. Preparations of the bulb were found to lead to a significant reduction in blood lipid and cholesterol levels. In deep fungal infections, whooping cough, treatment of lead poisoning and carcinoma results were encouraging but rather equivocal [7].

Preparations: Garlic Juice BPC 1949, dose: 2–4 ml; Garlic Syrup BPC 1949, dose: 2–8 ml.

Potter's Products: Antifect Tablets, Garlic Tablets.

Regulatory Status: GSL.

Biblical References: Numbers 11:5.

GELSEMIUM
Gelsemium sempervirens (L.) Ait.
Fam. Loganiaceae

Synonyms: Yellow Jasmine, Wild Jasmine, Yellow Jessamine, Wild Jessamine, Wild Woodbine, *Bignonia sempervirens* L., *Gelsemium nitidum*.

Habitat: Southern USA, cultivated elsewhere as an ornamental.

Description: The root is tortuous, brown and smooth, with a thin bark and woody centre showing broad medullary rays. The rhizome is less tortuous and is distinguished by the distinct pith and purplish longitudinal lines on the bark. Fracture, short and woody, showing a few silky fibres in the bark. Taste, slightly bitter; odour, faintly aromatic. The plant should not be confused with the yellow flowering Jasmine cultivated in Britain and elsewhere.

Part Used: Root, rhizome.

Constituents: (i) Alkaloids, consisting mainly of gelsemine, with gelsedine, gelsemicine, gelsemidine, gelsevirine and others [589, 5] (ii) Iridoids; gelsemide and its 7-glucoside, gelsemiol and its 1- and 3-glucosides, 9-hydroxy-semperoside, semperoside and brasoside [590] (iii) Coumarins such as fabiatin [590] and scopoletin (= gelsemic acid) [5] (iv) Tannins, fatty acids etc. [5].

Medicinal Use: Sedative, diaphoretic, antispasmodic and febrifuge. It is used in small doses for neuralgia, nervous excitement, insomnia, inflammation of the bowels and diarrhoea. The alkaloids are CNS depressants and Gelsemium must be used with caution. Toxic effects include respiratory depression, giddiness, double vision and even convulsions. It has been known to be fatal [4].

Preparations: Gelsemium Tincture BPC 1973, dose: 0.3–1 ml.

Regulatory Status: POM or P in restricted dose.

GENTIAN
Gentiana lutea L.
Fam. Gentianaceae

Synonyms: Yellow Gentian. Stemless Gentian is G. acaulis L. and English or Field Gentian is G. campestris L.

Habitat: Mountainous parts of Europe.

Description: Occurs in commerce as cylindrical pieces, 2–4 cm in diameter, yellowish-brown or brown externally. The upper part, or rhizome, often bears encircling leaf scars and the lower part is longitudinally wrinkled. Fracture short and hard, showing a transverse surface which is orange-brown with a dark ring of cambium. Taste, initially sweet and then bitter; odour characteristic.

Part Used: Root and Rhizome.

Constituents: (i) Iridoids, including amarogentin, gentiopicroside (= gentiopicrin) and swertiamarin [591, 592, 593] (ii) Xanthones such as gentisein, gentisin, isogentisin, 1,3,7-trimethoxyxanthone and others [594, 595] (iii) Alkaloids; mainly gentianine and gentialutine [596, 597] (iv) Phenolic acids including gentisic, caffeic, protocatechuic, syringic and sinapic acids [598] (iii) Miscellaneous; sugars such as gentianose and gentiobiose, traces of volatile oil etc. [5]. G. acaulis contains the xanthone derivatives gentiacauloside and gentisin, and probably similar constituents to G. lutea [5]. The constituents of G. campestris are not known but are probably similar to the other two species.

Medicinal Use: Bitter, tonic. The most popular of all gastric stimulants and very widely used to improve digestion, stimulate the appetite and treat all types of gastrointestinal disorders including dyspepsia, gastritis, heartburn, nausea and diarrhoea. Gentiopicroside has been shown to stimulate gastric secretion in animals [7] and Gentian extract is reported to be choleretic [5].

In Chinese medicine other species of Gentiana are used, these are referred to as "Longdan" and have similar constituents. They are used for the same indications as well as for jaundice, hepatitis, conjunctivitis, urinary tract infections, pruritis and eczema [7].

Preparations: Powdered root, dose: 0.5–2 g; Alkaline Gentian Mixture BPC, dose: 10–20 ml; Acid Gentian Mixture BPC, dose: 10–20 ml; Concentrated Compound Gentian Infusion BP, dose: 1.5–4 ml; Compound Gentian Tincture BPC 1973, dose: 2–5 ml.

Potter's Products: Neurelax Tablets, Valerian and Scullcap Compound Tablets No. 337, Tonic and Nervine Essence, Stomach and Liver Medicinal Tea Bags.

Regulatory Status: GSL.

GERMANDER
Teucrium chamaedrys L.
Fam. Labiatae

Synonyms: Wall Germander.

Habitat: A common European wild plant, rare in Britain.

Description: Leaves dark green, shiny, rather leathery, up to 3 cm long and 1 cm broad, oval, pointed, with rounded teeth. Flowers purplish-red, two-lipped, with the upper lip deeply bifid, and projecting stamens. Taste, bitter; odourless.

Part Used: Herb.

Constituents: (i) Iridoid glycosides, including harpagide and acetyl harpagide [599] (ii) Clerodane and neoclerodane diterpenes; the teucrins A-G, teucvin, teucvidin, teuflin, teuflidin and isoteuflidin [600, 601] (iii) Phenylpropanoids such as teucroside [602] (iv) Volatile oil, containing about 60% caryophyllene [603] (v) Tannins and polyphenols [2]

Medicinal Use: Gastric stimulant, tonic, diuretic, diaphoretic and anti-rheumatic. It is also used topically as an antiseptic and vulnerary.

Preparations: Liquid Extract, dose: 2–4 ml.

Regulatory Status: GSL.

GINGER

Zingiber officinale Rose.
Fam. Zingiberaceae

Habitat: Native to S. E. Asia but cultivated in India, China, the West Indies, Nigeria and elsewhere in the tropics.

Description: The appearance is well-known. The rhizome is freed from rootlets and may be peeled before drying. Some types are sun-bleached to improve appearance; bleaching with lime is no longer considered desirable. African ginger is usually unpeeled. Fracture, short and fibrous; odour and taste, characteristic, aromatic and pungent.

Part Used: Rhizome.

Constituents: (i) Volatile oil, 1–2% or occasionally more, containing mainly zingiberene and bisabolene, with zingiberol, zingiberenol, curcumene, camphene, citral, cineole, borneol, linalool, methylheptenone and many other minor components [5, 37] (ii) Pungent principles; a mixture of phenolic compounds with carbon side chains consisting of 7 or more carbon atoms, referred to as gingerols, gingerdiols, gingerdiones, dihydrogingerdiones and shogaols [604, 605]. The shogaols are produced by dehydration and degradation of the gingerols and are formed during drying and extraction. The shogaols are twice as pungent as the gingerols [604], which accounts for the fact that dried ginger is more pungent than fresh.

Medicinal Use: Carminative, antiemetic, spasmolytic, antiflatulent, anti-tussive. (6)-Gingerol and (6)-shogaol have been shown to suppress gastric contractions [606], and in a recent study capsules containing the dried rhizome (940 mg) were found to be superior to an antihistamine (dimenhydrinate 100 mg) in preventing the gastrointestinal symptoms of motion sickness [607]. Both fresh and dried rhizome suppress gastric secretion and reduce vomiting [608]. Gingerols and shogaols also have sedative, antipyretic, analgesic and transient hypotensive actions [609] and inhibit the synthesis of $PGF_{2\alpha}$ in the bowel, this is thought to reduce bowel activity [610]. They are also hepatoprotective, the activity depending on the chain length with the gingerols being more active than the homologous shogaols [68]. Ginger is anticonvulsant and hypocholesterolaemic [611, 612]. Reports of antibacterial activity are contradictory [605].

In Oriental medicine ginger is so highly regarded that it forms an ingredient of about half of all multi-item prescriptions. A distinction is made between the indications for the fresh rhizome (vomiting, coughs, abdominal distension and pyrexia) and the dried or processed rhizome (abdominal pain, lumbago and diarrhoea). This is probably justifiable since the constituents are present in different proportions. Clinical work in China has confirmed the usefulness of an injected preparation of ginger in treating rheumatic pain and lumbago. It was also demonstrated in animal tests [7].

Ginger is an important culinary spice, both fresh and dried.

Preparations: Powdered root, dose: 0.3–1 g; Ginger Oleoresin BPC 1968, dose: 15–60 mg; Ginger Syrup BPC 1973, dose: 2.5–5 ml; Strong Ginger Tincture BP, dose: 0.25–0.5 ml; Weak Ginger Tincture BP, dose: 1.5–3 ml.

Potter's Products: Elder Flowers and Peppermint with Composition Essence, Stomach and Liver Medicinal Tea Bags No. 42, Hydrastis Compound Digestive Tablet No. 24. Ginger Root Capsules.

Regulatory Status: GSL.

GINGER, WILD

Asarum canadense L.
Fam. Aristolochiaceae

Synonyms: Indian Ginger, Canadian Snakeroot.
Habitat: N. America, Canada.
Description: Rhizome slender, hardly branched, about 10 cm long and 3 mm thick, wrinkled, greyish or purplish-brown. Rootlets whitish, occurring on the nodes. Fracture, short. Taste, bitter and pungent; odour aromatic.
Part Used: Rhizome.
Constituents: (i) Volatile oil, 3.5–4.5%, containing methyleugenol [2] (ii) Aristolochic acid [613].
Medicinal Use: Expectorant, carminative, stimulant. It has been used for amenorrhoea. For details of the actions of aristolochic acid, see Birthwort. This plant is not a substitute for Ginger.

GINKGO

Ginkgo biloba L.
Fam. Ginkgoaceae

Synonyms: Maidenhair-Tree.
Habitat: A dioeceous fossil tree, indigenous to China and Japan and cultivated elsewhere.
Description: Leaves petiolate, glabrous, bilobed; each lobe triangular, up to about 6 cm long and 4 cm wide, with fan-like, fine, prominent, radiate veins and an entire margin. Only recently found in commerce.

Part Used: Leaves.

Constituents: (i) Lignans; the ginkgolides A, B and C, with bilobalide and possibly others [614, 615, 616, 2] (ii) Flavonoids, mainly flavone glycosides and including ginkgetin and quercitin and kaempferol derivatives [617, 618, 619, 2] (iii) Miscellaneous; terpenes such as bilobanone, traces of essential oil, tannins, nonacosane and nonacosanol (= ginnol), uroshiols [2].

Medicinal Use: Antiasthmatic, bronchodilator and platelet activating factor (PAF) antagonist. It is also used to improve the circulation. The ginkgolides, particularly ginkgolide B, known commercially as BN 52021, are PAF antagonists; this has useful and far-reaching effects. PAF is involved in allergic inflammation, anaphylactic shock and asthma [614, 620, 621 and references therein]. A recent study has found it to be effective in treating asthma in children [622]. BN 52021 also inhibits the other pharmacological effects produced by PAF, such as platelet aggregation and the wheal-and-flare response [621]. Ginkgo extracts have complex vasoactive effects on isolated blood vessels [623]. The flavonoid extract is used to improve the circulation in the brain and to treat haemorrhoids [618]. The extract was shown to protect normal healthy males against hypoxia in one study [619], and Ginkgo extract improved the mental performance in geriatric patients where this was impaired, but had no effect on normal subjects [624], thus substantiating its use in cerebral insufficiency.

Ginkgo has been reported to cause dermatitis [625] and toxic effects, though rare and mainly due to overdosage, include irritability, restlessness, diarrhoea and vomiting [48].

GINSENG

Panax ginseng C. A. Meyer
Fam. Araliaceae

Synonyms: Chinese Ginseng, Korean Ginseng, *P. schinseng* Nees. American ginseng is *P. quinquefolius* L. Japanese ginseng is *P. japonicus* C. A. Meyer (= *P. pseudo-ginseng* Wall.) var *japonicus* C. A. Meyer. Himalayan ginseng is *P. pseudo-ginseng* Wall. San-chi ginseng is *P. notoginseng* Burk. Siberian ginseng is *Eleutherococcus senticosus* Maxim (= *Acanthopanax senticosus*). Many other species and varieties are used [626].

Habitat: *P. ginseng* is native to China and cultivated extensively in China, Korea, Japan and Russia.

Description: *P. ginseng:* The root is spindle-shaped, pale brownish yellow, about 1–2 cm in diameter, ringed above and divided into two or three equal branches which are longitudinally wrinkled. Fracture short, mealy, showing a thin bark containing numerous reddish resin glands; wood wedges narrow, yellowish, with broad medullary rays. Taste, sweetish; odour faintly aromatic.

Part Used: Root.

Constituents: (i) Saponin glycosides. These are referred to as the ginsenosides by Japanese workers and panaxosides by Russian workers. At least 13 ginsenosides have been isolated; these are designated ginsenosides R_a, R_b... R_{g-1}, R_{g-2} etc. The panaxosides are described by the suffixes A–F, these do not correspond with those of the ginsenosides. In *Eleutherococcus* the saponins are chemically different, they are the eleutherosides A–F [626, 627 and references therein]. (ii) Glycans: the panaxans A–E, isolated only so far from *P. ginseng* [628] (iii) Volatile oil, about 0.05%, containing β-elemene, a diene panaxynol, and two acetylenic compounds, panaxydol and panaxytriol, falcarinol and falcarintriol [629, 630, 631].

Medicinal Use: Tonic, stimulant. Ginseng is taken to improve stamina and concentration, for debility, ageing, sexual inadequacy, diabetes, insomnia, stress and many other real or imaginary ailments. Extensive research is being carried out into the pharmacological effects of ginseng, which will be summarized briefly. The ginsenosides have immunomodulatory activity [632, 633]; they stimulate the biosynthesis of proteins in rat liver and kidney and increase plasma levels of ACTH and corticosterone [634]; and inhibit thrombin induced conversion of fibrinogen to fibrin, preventing platelet aggregation in experimental disseminated coagulation in rats [635]. They control homoeostasis by acting on the endocrine system [636]. Ginsenoside R_{b-1} acts as a CNS sedative and R_{g-1} has antifatigue and stimulant properties [637]. In animals, an extract increases the capacity of skeletal muscle to oxidize free fatty acids in preference to glucose to produce cellular energy [638], which would help to explain the antifatigue activity seen in conventional exhaustion tests. For review see [626]. The glycans, panaxans A–E, are hypoglycaemic in mice and are probably responsible for at least some of the effects of ginseng on carbohydrate metabolism. Although ginseng is taken so widely, fatalities are unknown. However despite it being so safe, side effects are well documented and include oestrogenic effects, hypertension, irritability and related symptoms. For further details see [639].

Preparations: Powdered root, dose: 0.5–1 g.

Regulatory Status: GSL.

Biblical References: Ezekiel 27:17.

GLADWIN
Iris foedidissima L.
Fam. Iridaceae

Synonyms: Stinking Iris, Gladwine, Stinking Gladdon, Roastbeef Plant.

Habitat: Woods and shady places in Britain and parts of Europe.

Description: Long narrow leaves; flowers bluish-purple, shaped like the common Iris but smaller; bright orange seeds. Odour when bruised, sickly, unpleasant.

Part Used: Rhizome.

Constituents: Unknown. A resin, glycoside named irisin or iridin, and myristic acid are reported to be present [79].

Medicinal Use: Antispasmodic, cathartic, anodyne.

Preparations: Powdered rhizome, dose: 0.3–2 g.

GOA
Andira araroba Ag.
Fam. Leguminosae

Synonyms: Araroba, Bahia Powder, Brazil Powder, Chrysarobin.

Habitat: S. America, mainly Brazil.

Description: The yellowish powder is scraped out of longitudinal fissures in the tree after felling, and purified by sifting and solvent extraction. It is very irritating to the eyes and mucous membranes.

Constituents: A complex mixture of anthraquinone derivatives known as "chrysarobin" [218].

Medicinal Use: Taenifuge, antiparasitic. It has been used externally as an ointment for ringworm and other parasitic infections. It is irritant and should not be used internally.

Preparations: Chrysarobin BPC 1949, Chrysarobin Ointment BPC 1949.

GOAT'S RUE
Galega officinalis L.
Fam. Leguminosae

Synonyms: French Lilac.

Habitat: Grows wild in Europe, naturalized in Britain.

Description: An erect, branched plant reaching 1.5 m. The leaves have 6–8 pairs of elongated leaflets and the tip terminates in a small point. Flowers pale bluish-purple, or more rarely pink or white, borne on short stalks in an erect spike. Pods almost cylindrical.

Part Used: Herb.

Constituents: (i) Galegine (= isoamyleneguanidine), its 4-hydroxy derivative and peganine [79, 2] (ii) Flavonoids (iii) Saponins [2].

Medicinal Use: Galactagogue, diuretic, vermifuge.

Preparations: Powdered herb, dose: 0.3–1.2 g; Liquid Extract, dose: 1–2 ml.

GOLDEN ROD
Solidago virgaurea L.
Fam. Compositae

Habitat: A common garden and wild plant in Britain and Europe.

Description: A tall upright perennial herb, with oblong-lanceolate leaves, pointed and finely serrate. The flowers which appear in July to September, are golden yellow, compositous, shortly rayed and on branched spikes. Taste, acrid and bitter; odour, when dry, agreeable and slightly aromatic.

Part Used: Leaves.

Constituents: (i) Saponins based on polygalic acid [640] (ii) Clerodane diterpenes, at least 12 of which have been isolated; these include solidagolactones I–VII and elongatolides C and E [641] (iii) Phenolic glucosides, including leicarposide [642] (iv) Miscellaneous; acetylenes, cinnamates, flavonoids such as rutin and quercitrin, hydroxybenzoates, polysaccharides, phenolic acids and tannins [2, 641 and references therein].

Medicinal Use: Diaphoretic, antiinflammatory, antiseptic, carminative, diuretic. Leicarposide has antiinflammatory effects in animals [642]. The saponins are antifungal against *Candida* species [640]. An extract of the leaves and flowers showed a transient hypotensive effect in rats [643].

Preparations: Liquid Extract, dose: 2–4 ml.

Potter's Products: Liver and Bile Medicinal Tea Bags.

Regulatory Status: GSL.

GOLDEN SEAL

Hydrastis canadensis L.
Fam. Ranunculaceae

Synonyms: Orange Root, Yellow Root.

Habitat: Native to N. America; mostly cultivated.

Description: The rhizome is yellowish-brown, about 5 cm long and 1 cm thick, knotty and twisted, wrinkled longitudinally and encircled by leaf scars. Rootlets frequently present in abundance. Fracture short, showing a dark yellow cut surface, thick bark, large pith and broad medullary rays. Taste, very bitter; odour, strong, characteristic and disagreeable.

Part Used: Rhizome, gathered in the Autumn.

Constituents: (i) Isoquinoline alkaloids, mainly hydrastine, berberine and canadine (= tetrahydroberberine), with lesser amounts of related alkaloids [644] (ii) Miscellaneous; fatty acids, resin, polyphenolic acids and a small amount of volatile oil [5].

Medicinal Use: Tonic, mild laxative, alterative, haemostatic, antiinflammatory. Used internally for dyspepsia, gastritis, peptic ulceration, colitis, menorrhagia and other menstrual disorders; and topically for conjunctivitis, eczema and inflammation of the ear. The alkaloids are reported to have anticonvulsant activity on the mouse small intestine and uterus [645]. Berberine and hydrastine have similar actions, including stimulating bile in humans, and hypotensive and sedative effects in animals [646]. Berberine is antibacterial, amoebicidal and is effective against diarrhoea (see Barberry).

Preparations: Powdered root, dose: 0.5–1.2 g; Liquid Extract BPC 1949, dose: 0.3–1 ml; Tincture, dose: 2–4 ml.

Potter's Products: Hydrastis Compound Digestive Tablet No. 24, Special Formula Stomach D4 Tablet, Special Formula Stomach D1 Tablet, Indigestion Mixture.

Regulatory Status: GSL.

GOLD THREAD

Coptis trifolia L. (Salis.)
C. groenlandica (Oed.) Fern.
Fam. Ranunculaceae

Synonyms: Mouth Root, Vegetable Gold.

Habitat: *C. trifolia* is Indian in origin and *C. groenlandica* is from the USA and Canada.

Description: Rhizomes thread-like, golden yellow, matted, with very small roots. Taste, very bitter; odour, slight.

Part Used: Rhizome.

Constituents: (i) Isoquinoline alkaloids; both species contain berberine, coptisine and others [2].

Medicinal Use: Bitter tonic. Used to promote digestion and for similar indications as Barberry and Golden Seal (q.v.).

Preparations: Powdered rhizome, dose: 0.5–1.2 g; Liquid Extract, dose: 2–4 ml.

GOUTWORT
Aegopodium podagraria L.
Fam. Umbelliferae

Synonyms: Ground Elder, Goutweed, Gout Herb, Ashweed, Ground Ash, Herb Gerarde.

Habitat: A troublesome weed in Britain and Europe. Gerard, in the 16th century, said that "it groweth of it selfe in gardens without setting or sowing and is so fruitful in his increase, that where it hath once taken root, it will hardly be gotten out againe, spoiling and getting every year more ground, to the annoying of better herbs".

Description: A creeping perennial with white typically umbelliferous flowers and 1–2 trefoil leaves.

Part Used: Herb.

Constituents: Not investigated. A small amount of volatile oil [2].

Medicinal Use: Diuretic, sedative. Formerly used externally as a poultice and internally for gout; Culpeper said "the very carrying of it about in the pocket will defend the bearer from any attack of the aforesaid complaint".

Preparations: Liquid Extract, dose: 2–4 ml.

GRAINS OF PARADISE *Aframomum melegueta* (Rosc.) K. Schum.
Fam. Zingiberaceae

Synonyms: Guinea Grains, Melegueta Pepper.

Habitat: Tropical West Africa.

Description: The seeds are red-brown, small, hard, shiny and oyster-shaped. Taste and odour, aromatic and pungent.

Part Used: Seeds.

Constituents: (i) Volatile oil, 0.3–0.75 % [2] (ii) Pungent principles including paradol [1] (iii) Miscellaneous; tannin, starch, fixed oil [2].

Medicinal Use: Stimulant.

GRAVEL ROOT
Eupatorium purpurea L.
Fam. Compositae

Synonyms: Gravelweed, Joe-Pye Weed, Queen of the Meadow Root.

Habitat: USA.

Description: Rhizome up to 3 cm diameter, very hard and tough, with a thin, greyish-brown bark and thick, whitish wood, often hollow in the centre and with wide medullary rays. The short lateral branches usually have crowded, tough, slender, woody roots attached. Taste, bitter, astringent and slightly acrid.

Part Used: Rhizome and root.

Constituents: This species is not well investigated compared to other spp. of *Eupatorium*. (i) Volatile oil, about 0.07%, of unknown composition (ii) Flavonoids, including euparin (iii) Resin [37].

Medicinal Use: Diuretic, stimulant, tonic, antirheumatic. Used principally in the treatment of gravel stones in the bladder and other kidney and urinary disorders, including cystitis and urethritis.

Preparations: Liquid Extract, dose: 2–4 ml.

Potter's Products: Back and Kidney Tablets No. 252.

Reglatory Status: GSL.

GRINDELIA

Grindelia camporum Green
G. squarrosa Nutt.
Fam. Compositae

Synonyms: Gum Plant, Gum Weed, Tar Weed, *G. robusta* (= *G. camporum*).

Habitat: The USA and S. America.

Description: Leaves lanceolate, glabrous, those of *G. camporum* being broader at the base, leathery, brittle, serrated at the margins, about 6–10 cm long and 1–3 cm broad. Flowerheads globular, about 2 cm in diameter, with yellow florets and reflexed, linear, pointed involucral scales. Taste, bitter; odour faint, aromatic, balsamic.

Part Used: Herb.

Constituents: (i) Diterpenes of the grindelane type, including grindelic acid and its 17-hydroxy derivative, 13-isogrindelic acid, 17-grindeloxy-grindelic acid and many others, in both spp. [647] (ii) Flavonoids; including acacetin, kumatakenin, quercetin and its 3,3′-dimethyl ether derivative, in both spp. [647] (iii) Resins [1, 37].

Medicinal Use: Antispasmodic, expectorant, antiasthmatic. Used mainly for asthma and bronchitis, cystitis and as a lotion for dermatitis. An aqueous extract has recently been shown to have antiinflammatory activity in the rat paw oedema test [403].

Preparations: Liquid Extract, BPC 1949, dose: 0.05–1.2 ml.

Regulatory Status: GSL.

GROUND IVY

Glechoma hederacea L.
Fam. Labiatae

Synonyms: *Nepeta hederacea* (L.) Trev., *N. glechoma* Benth.

Habitat: A common wild plant in Europe and the British Isles.

Description: Stems quadrangular, unbranched, often purplish, hairy, bearing opposite leaves, which are kidney-shaped, hairy, bluntly serrate and long-stalked. Flowers blue, two-lipped, in groups of two or three in the axils of the leaves. Taste, bitter; odour, aromatic.

Part Used: Herb.

Constituents: (i) Sesquiterpenes, including glechomafuran, a furano-germacrane [2] (ii) Flavonoids; isoquercitin, hyperoside, and apigenin and luteolin glycosides [648] (review) (iii) Miscellaneous; essential oil, about 0.03–0.06%, a bitter substance glechomine, saponin, resin, choline and tannins [2].

Medicinal Use: Astringent, tonic, diuretic, expectorant. Used mainly for bronchitis and catarrh, but also for haemorrhoids. Externally it may be used to soothe inflammation. The antiinflammatory activity has been demonstrated in rats [403].

Preparations: Liquid Extract, dose: 2–4 ml.

Regulatory Status: GSL.

GROUND PINE, AMERICAN

Lycopodium complanatum L.
Fam. Lycopodiaceae

Habitat: USA, Europe, Russia.

Description: Stem long, creeping, yellowish-green, scaly, about 2 mm in diameter, giving off at intervals erect, fan-shaped, forked branches with minute, scale-like leaves, and bearing stalked tufts of four to five cylindrical spikes of spore cases in the axils of minute bracts. Taste and odour, aromatic, slightly terebinthinate.

Constituents: Alkaloids; including lycopodine, complanatine and nicotine [362, 363].

Medicinal Use: Little used here although it is used in Chinese medicine as a tonic and for skin disorders. Lycopodine produces uterine contractions and increases peristalsis in the small intestine of animals [363]. Lycopodium alkaloids are toxic.

GROUND PINE, EUROPEAN

Ajuga chamaepitys Schreb.
Fam. Labiatae

Habitat: Grows in bare, sparse, stony places in Britain and parts of Europe.

Description: A low greyish annual, with narrow, erect, deeply trifid leaves with single yellow two-lipped flowers in the axils. Taste and odour, terebinthinate.

Part Used: Leaves.

Constituents: (i) Iridoid glycosides, including acetyl harpagide [62] (ii) Phytoecdysterols; ajugalactone, cyasterone, makisterone and β-ecdysone [649].

Medicinal Use: Stimulant, diuretic, emmenagogue. Used for gout and rheumatism and female disorders, combined with other herbs, often as an infusion.

Preparations: Liquid Extract, dose: 2–8 ml.

GROUNDSEL

Senecio vulgaris L.
Fam. Compositae

Synonyms: Grounsel.

Habitat: A common weed worldwide.

Description: A low annual, with pinnately lobed leaves and ray-less, brush-like yellow flowerheads, about 6 mm long and 3 mm broad, in loose clusters, with black-tipped sepal-like bracts. Taste, saline; odour, imperceptible.

Part Used: Herb.

Constituents: (i) Pyrrolizidine alkaloids; senecyphylline, senecionine, retrorsine and others [650, 651], mainly as the N-oxides [652] (ii) Volatile oil, the main component of which is β-caryophyllene, with myrcene, α-copaene, β-farnesine and germacrene D [653] (iii) Flavonoids; glucuronides of quercetin and isorhamnetin [654].

Medicinal Use: Formerly used as a diuretic and diaphoretic and to relieve bilious pains. Due to the high concentration of hepatotoxic alkaloids, internal use is not recommended.

GUAIACUM

Guaiacum officinale L.
G. sanctum L.
Fam. Zygophyllaceae

Synonyms: Guaiac, *Lignum vitae, Lignum sanctum.*

Habitat: W. Indies, Florida and S. America.

Description: The wood is normally sold as shavings. The heart-wood is greenish brown, heavier than water and with an aromatic and irritating taste. The resin, which accounts for about 20%, is produced by firing the logs, and collected when melted.

Part Used: Wood, resin.

Constituents: (i) Lignans; furoguaiacidin, guaiacin, furoguaiacin, furoguaiaoxidin and others [655, 656, 657] (ii) Resin acids; (−)-guaiaretic, (−)-hydroguaiaretic, guaiacic and α- and β-guaiaconic acids [658, 37] (iii) Miscellaneous; vanillin, terpenoids including guaiagutin, guaiasaponin etc. [37].

Medicinal Use: Antirheumatic, antiinflammatory, diuretic, diaphoretic, mild laxative. Used mainly for rheumatic pain and gout.

Preparations: Liquid Extract, dose: 2–4 ml; Ammoniated Guaiacum Tincture BPC 1949, dose: 2–4 ml; Guaiacum Tincture BPC 1949, dose: 2–4 ml; Compound Confection of Guaiacum BPC 1949, dose: 4–8 g; Concentrated Compound Decoction of Sarsaparilla BPC 1949, dose: 8–30 ml.

Potter's Products: Gout and Rheumatism Tablet No. 31, Guaiacum Compound Tablet No. 215, Rheumatic Pain Tablet No. 372.

Regulatory Status: GSL.

GUARANA

Paullinia cupana Kunth ex H.B.K.
Fam. Sapindaceae

Synonyms: Brazilian Cocoa *Paullinia sorbilis* Mart.

Habitat: Brazil and Venezuela.

Description: The paste is formed from the pulverized and roasted seeds, formed into rolls or bars and dried. These have an astringent, bitter then sweet taste; and an odour recalling that of chocolate.

Part Used: Seeds.

Constituents: (i) Caffeine, up to 7%, with theobromine, theophylline, xanthine and other xanthine derivatives (ii) Tannins, about 12%, including *d*-catechin (iii) Miscellaneous; saponins, starch, fats, choline, pigments [5].

Medicinal Use: Stimulant, astringent. The pharmacological effects are mainly due to the caffeine content.

Preparations: Powdered Guarana, dose: 0.5–4 g.

H

HAIR CAP MOSS

Polytrichum juniperum Willd.
Fam. Polytrichaceae

Synonyms: Ground Moss.
Habitat: A common British and European moss. It is said that this moss is found growing on human skulls.
Description: Stems slender, unbranched, 5–8 cm long, with small, short, awl-shaped, red-tipped "leaves", overlapping and crowded in the upper part of the stem. Fruit stalks terminate in a quadrangular capsule containing the spores.
Part Used: Whole plant.
Constituents: Tannins [2].
Medicinal Use: Diuretic, styptic. Extracts have been shown to have weak antitumour effects in mice [156].

HARTSTONGUE

Scolopendrium vulgare Sm.
Fam. Polypodiaceae

Synonyms: Asplenium scolopendrium L., *Phyllitis scolopendrium* Green.
Habitat: It grows in gardens and woodlands in parts of Europe, the USA, S. W. and E. Asia.
Description: Fronds stalked, up to about 60 cm long and 5 cm wide, with transverse simple veins and on the reverse side, lines of spore cases in transverse series. Taste, unpleasant; odourless.
Part Used: Herb.
Constituents: Tannins, mucilage, flavonoids including leucodelphidin [2].
Medicinal Use: Diuretic, laxative, pectoral. It may be taken as a decoction.
Regulatory Status: GSL.

HAWTHORN

Crataegus oxycanthoides Thuill.
C. monogyna Jacq.
Fam. Rosaceae

Synonyms: Haw, May, Whitethorn.
Habitat: A common British and European hedge plant.
Description: A hairless, thorny, deciduous shrub with 3–5 lobed leaves, bearing white, dense clusters of flowers followed by deep red false fruits containing one seed (in *C. monogyna*,) or two seeds (in *C. oxycanthoides*). The flowers appear in early summer and the berries or "haws" in September.
Part Used: Berries, leaves, flowers.
Constituents: (i) Amines; phenethylamine, *o*-methoxyphenethylamine and tyramine, in the flowers [659] (ii) Flavonoids; vitexin, vitexin-4-rhamnoside, quercetin and quercetin-3-galactoside, in the flowers, leaves and buds

[660] (iii) Phenolic acids including chlorogenic, 2-phenylchromone derivatives in the flowers, leaves and buds [661] (iv) Miscellaneous: tannins, ascorbic acid [2, 37].

Medicinal Use: Cardiac tonic, hypotensive, antisclerotic. Animal studies have shown beneficial effects on coronary blood flow, blood pressure and heart rate [662]; at least some of these properties are thought to be due to the amines present [659]. A recent clinical study of 80 patients in Japan showed statistically significant improvement in cardiac function, oedema and dyspnoea in patients treated with a preparation made from the fruits and leaves [663]. *Crataegus* species have been described as sedatives [664], however the method of testing for this has been disputed [665] so evidence is not yet available.

Preparations: Liquid Extract, dose: 0.5–1 ml.

Potter's Products: Cardivallin Tablets, Heart Drops.

Regulatory Status: P.

HEARTSEASE

Viola tricolor L.
Fam. Violaceae

Synonyms: Wild Pansy.

Habitat: A common British wild and garden plant.

Description: Leaves oval to broad lanceolate; stipules leafy, pinnately lobed. Flowers 1–2.5 cm, blue-violet, yellow or all three, with a spurred calyx. Taste, insipid; odourless.

Part Used: Herb.

Constituents: (i) Flavonoids, including violanthin (which is a di-glucoside of apigenin), rutin, violanthin, violaquercitrin [666, 50, 5] (ii) Methyl-salicylate, traces [50] (iii) Miscellaneous; mucilage, gums, resin, saponin [37, 50].

Medicinal Use: Expectorant, diuretic, antiinflammatory. Used for bronchitis, rheumatism, skin eruptions and eczema, often as an infusion.

Regulatory Status: GSL.

HEDGE-HYSSOP

Gratiola officinalis L.
Fam. Scrophulariaceae

Synonyms: Gratiola.

Habitat: A British and European wild plant found in damp places.

Description: A medium hairless perennial, with opposite, lanceolate, sessile leaves about 3 cm long and 0.5 cm broad, with a toothed margin near the tip. Flowers white or pale pink, tubular, with five stamens. Taste, acrid and bitter; odourless.

Part Used: Herb, root.

Constituents: (i) Glycosides; gratiotoxin and gratioside (ii) Cucurbitacins; elatineride (iii) Triterpenes including gratiolone [2].

Medicinal Use: Diuretic, emetic, cathartic. The glycosides are said to have digitalis-like action (see Foxglove) and the cucurbitacins are cathartic and cytotoxic (see Bryony, White). The use of this plant is therefore not recommended.

HEDGE MUSTARD

Sisymbrium officinale L.
Fam. Cruciferae

Habitat: Common throughout Europe.

Description: The flowers are about 3 mm diameter, with pale yellow petals in the shape of a cross, followed by the pods which are 6–20 mm long and pressed to the stem. The stems long and spreading and the rosette leaves deeply pinnately lobed. Odour and taste, mustard-like.

Part Used: Herb.

Constituents: Glucosinolates; sinigrin, glucoputranjivin, glucocochlearin, glucocheirolin, glucobrassicin and neoglucobrassicin [667, 668].

Medicinal Use: Formerly used for hoarseness, weak lungs and to help the voice.

Preparations: Liquid Extract, dose: 2–4 ml.

HELLEBORE, AMERICAN

Veratum viride Ait.
Fam. Liliaceae

Synonyms: Green Hellebore, American Veratrum, Indian Poke. White Hellebore is *V. album.*

Habitat: N. America and Canada. *V. album* is from Central Europe.

Description: The rhizome is blackish, obconical, 5–8 cm long and 1–3 cm diameter, with tufts of stem leaf remains at the top and numerous shrivelled yellowish-brown rootlets. Internally it is whitish with a ring of air spaces in the cortex and the endodermis and vascular bundles visible in the centre. It closely resembles that of White Hellebore. Taste, bitter and acrid; odourless but sternutatory.

Part Used: Rhizome.

Constituents: (i) Steroidal alkaloids, classified into the jerveratrum type, which are present as glycosides or free alkamines and include pseudo-jervine and veratrosine; and the ceveratrum type which are usually found as esters and include protoverine and veracevine esters; and some unclassified alkaloids [669]. *V. album* contains similar alkaloids [669] (ii) Chelidonic acid [2].

Medicinal Use: Hypotensive, cardiac depressant. Formerly used for high blood pressure, especially toxaemia of pregnancy. The ceveratrum-type alkaloids are hypotensive; they cause peripheral vasodilatation, probably by inhibition of the vasomotor centre and stimulation of the vagus. When taken by mouth overdosage causes immediate vomiting, and poisoning in this way is very rare despite the toxicity of the plant.

Preparations: Tincture BPC 1934, dose: 0.3–2 ml.

Regulatory Status: POM.

HELLEBORE, BLACK

Helleborus niger L.
Fam. Ranunculaceae

Synonyms: Christmas Rose, Melampodium.

Habitat: Native to sub-alpine woods in Southern and Eastern Europe, cultivated in Britain as an ornamental. The plant flowers in mid-winter, hence the synonym.

Description: The rhizome is blackish, occurring as a tangled mass of short branches, bearing straight, slender, rather brittle black rootlets with a central cord. Taste, bitter and acrid; odour faint, fatty.

Part Used: Rhizome.

Constituents: Cardiac glycosides; helleborin, helleborein hellebrin and others based on helleborigenin [79, 1].

Medicinal Use: Cardiac tonic, purgative, abortifacient. The glycosides have digitalis-like action (see Foxglove). They are dangerous and should be used only under medical supervision. The plant was formerly used to treat lice, however it has caused abortion in a pregnant woman using it for this purpose [79].

Regulatory Status: P.

HELLEBORE, FALSE

Adonis vernalis L.
Fam. Ranunculaceae

Synonyms: Yellow Pheasant's Eye.

Habitat: N. Europe and Asia.

Description: Stem about 15–25 cm long, bearing feathery 2–3 pinnate leaves and a single large yellow flower, 40–80 mm across with ten or more petals and numerous stamens. Taste, slight; odourless.

Part Used: Herb.

Constituents: (i) Cardiac glycosides, including adonitoxin, 16-hydroxy-strophanthidin and others based on the aglycones adonitoxigenin and adonitogenin [670, 671] (ii) 2,6-dimethoxybenzoquinone [672].

Medicinal Use: Cardiac tonic, diuretic. The glycosides have digitalis-like action (see Foxglove). They stimulate the vagus and increase the contractility and work output of the heart [670]. This plant should be used only under medical supervision.

Regulatory Status: P.

HEMLOCK

Conium maculatum L.
Fam. Umbelliferae

Habitat: Great Britain and Europe.

Description: Typically umbelliferous in appearance. Leaves hairless, repeatedly pinnate; stem hollow with purplish spots. Fruits ovate, plano-convex, indented on the flat surface with five ridges on the back. Taste and odour, unpleasant, foetid.

Part Used: Leaves, unripe fruits.

Constituents: (i) Alkaloids; mainly coniine, with γ-coniceine, methyl-coniine, conhydrin, pseudoconhydrin and N-methylpseudoconhydrin

[673, 674] (ii) Volatile oil (very low in some varieties), the major component of which is myrcene [674].

Medicinal Use: Sedative, anodyne. The alkaloids are very toxic and should be used only under medical supervision, if at all.

Preparations: Powdered Leaf, dose: 0.12–0.5 g; Extract BPC 1949, dose: 0.12–0.4 g.

Regulatory Status: POM or P in restricted strength.

Biblical References: Hosea 10:4; Amos 6:12 where wormwood is meant (q.v.).

HEMP AGRIMONY

Eupatorium cannabinum L.
Fam. Compositae

Synonyms: Water Hemp.

Habitat: A common European and British wild plant found in damp places.

Description: Stem angular, often reddish, striated, rough; leaves palmate, 3–5 lobed, the segments lanceolate, irregularly serrate. Flowerheads slender, tubular, pinkish, with all the florets rayless. Taste, sweetish, then bitter; odour, faintly aromatic.

Part Used: Herb.

Constituents: (i) Volatile oil, about 0.5%, containing α-terpinene, *p*-cymene, thymol, an azulene, neryl acetate, germacrene D and many others [675] (ii) Sesquiterpene lactones, the major one being eupatoriopicrin [676] (iii) Flavonoids (unspecified) [675] (iv) Pyrrolizidine alkaloids; supinine, and amabiline [677] (v) Polysaccharides; 4-*o*-methylglucuronoxylans [678] (vi) Miscellaneous; euparin, eupatopicrin, lactucerol [2].

Medicinal Use: Diuretic, alterative. The polysaccharides have immunostimulatory activity; they enhance phagocytosis in a number of immunological test systems [678]. Eupatoriopicrin has recently been shown to be cytostatic as well as cytotoxic; it delayed transplanted tumour growth in mice in a dose dependent manner [676]. Internal administration is not advised unless the hepatotoxic alkaloids are shown to be absent from the sample.

Preparations: Liquid Extract, dose: 2–5 ml.

HENBANE

Hyoscyamus niger L.
Fam. Solanaceae

Habitat: Grows in waste places in Britain and Europe.

Description: A slightly sticky, hairy, annual or biennial, with alternate leaves. In the annual plant these are smaller and usually sessile. In the biennial they are larger in the first year, up to 30 cm long, ovate or lanceolate, petiolate; and in the second year, 10–20 cm long with a deeply dentate margin and much more hairy. The flowers are five-lobed, tubular, creamy yellow with purplish veins. Taste and odour, unpleasant, characteristic.

Part Used: Leaves and flowering tops.

Constituents: Tropane alkaloids, 0.045–0.14%, the principal ones being hyoscyamine and hyoscine (= scopolamine) [1, 4]. Egyptian Henbane, *H. muticus*, contains higher concentrations of the alkaloids, this and other species of *Hyoscyamus* are used as a source of hyoscine.

Medicinal Use: Antispasmodic, anodyne, sedative, mydriatic. The alkaloids are parasympatholytic, with similar actions to Belladonna (q.v.). although with less cerebral excitement. Henbane is used mainly for its antispasmodic effect on the digestive and urinary tracts, and to counteract griping due to purgatives. It is an ingredient of some antiasthmatic smoking mixtures and herbal cigarettes. The alkaloid hyoscine is used very widely, as a pre-operative medication, to prevent travel sickness and for many other purposes.

Preparations: Hyoscyamus Dry Extract BPC, dose: 15–60 mg; Hyoscyamus Liquid Extract BPC, dose: 0.2–0.5 ml; Hyoscyamus Tincture BP, dose: 2–5 ml.

Regulatory Status: POM or P with restrictions.

HENNA
Lawsonia inermis L.
Fam. Lythraceae

Synonyms: Henne, *L. alba* Lam.

Habitat: Egypt, the Middle East, India.

Description: Leaves shortly stalked, smooth, lanceolate, up to 5 cm long, with revolute, entire margins and a mucronate apex. Taste, astringent; odour, tea-like.

Part Used: Leaves.

Constituents: (i) Naphthaquinones, such as lawsone [679, 680] (ii) Coumarins; laxanthone I, II, and III [680, 681] (iii) Flavonoids; luteolin and its 7-O-glucoside, acacetin-7-O-glucoside [680] (iv) Miscellaneous; β-sitosterol-3-O-glucoside, tannins etc. [680, 33].

Medicinal Use: Astringent, antihaemorrhagic. It has been used to treat skin infections such as *Tinea* and lawsone is known to be antibacterial [679]. It is also oxytocic [33]. Henna is used more often as a dye for the hair and in some Eastern countries to stain the hands and feet orange-red.

Biblical References: In Song of Solomon 1:4 & 4:13 as "camphire".

HOLLY
Ilex aquifolium L.
Fam. Aquifoliaceae

Synonyms: Holm, Hulm.

Habitat: Grows freely in Britain and Europe.

Description: The bush is well-known; the leaves are shiny, leathery and with a spiny margin; the berries appear in early winter and are globular and bright red.

Part Used: Leaves, berries.

143

Constituents: (i) Ilicin, a bitter substance [2, 79] (ii) Ilexanthin, a yellow pigment (iii) Theobromine (in the leaf) (iv) Caffeic acid [2].

Medicinal Use: Diuretic, febrifuge, cathartic. Rarely used medicinally. An extract caused a fatal drop in blood pressure in rats [643].

HOLLYHOCK
Althaea rosea L.
Fam. Malvaceae

Habitat: A well-known garden plant.

Description: The dried flowers are deep purplish black, about 6 cm in diameter. The corolla is united with the stamens which form a tube; the anthers, which are reniform, are free.

Part Used: Flowers.

Constituents: Anthocyanidins.

Medicinal Use: Emollient, demulcent, diuretic. Used in a similar way to Marshmallow (q.v.).

HOLY THISTLE
Cnicus benedictus Gaertn.
Fam. Compositae

Synonyms: Blessed Thistle, *Carbenia benedicta* Berul. *Carduus benedictus* Steud.

Habitat: Coastal regions of the Mediterranean.

Description: Leaves greyish-green, thin and brittle, with prominent, pale veins and irregularly toothed margins, each tooth ending in a spine. Flowerheads about 2 cm long and 4 cm broad, with bristly involucral scales. Taste, very bitter; odourless.

Part Used: Herb.

Constituents: (i) Lactonic lignans; arctigenin, trachelogenin, nortracheloside, 2-acetylnortracheloside, salonitenolide [682], and in the fruit, arctiin [683] (ii) Sesquiterpene lactones, e.g. cnicin [683] (iii) Lithospermic acid [684] (iv) Volatile oil, of unknown constitution [50] (v) Miscellaneous; tannins, mucilage, potassium and manganese salts [184].

Medicinal Use: Stomachic, bitter, antihaemorrhagic, expectorant, antiseptic, vulnerary. It is used internally for anorexia, dyspepsia and catarrh; and externally for wounds and ulcers. Cnicin has some antibiotic activity [683].

Preparations: Liquid Extract, dose: 2–4 ml.

Potter's Products: Natural Herb Tablets.

Regulatory Status: GSL.

HONEYSUCKLE
Lonicera caprifolium L.
Fam. Caprifoliaceae

Synonyms: Dutch Honeysuckle.

Habitat: Widespread in many parts of the world.

Description: The dried flowers are yellowish brown, mostly tubular flowerbuds mixed with the stalked heads of young fruits. Leaves, thin, up to 5 cm long and about 2–3 cm broad, oval and shortly stalked. Taste, sweet and mucilaginous; odour, imperceptible when dried.
Part Used: Flowers, leaves.
Constituents: Unknown.
Medicinal Use: Expectorant, laxative. Rarely used.
Regulatory Status: GSL.

HOPS
Humulus lupulus L.
Fam. Cannabinaceae

Habitat: Native to Europe, parts of Asia and N. America, and extensively cultivated.
Description: The female flower or strobile is yellowish-green, cone-like, about 2.5–3 cm long and 2–2.5 cm broad, formed from two membranous scales, one of which bears the small seed-like fruit at the base. It is scattered with shining yellow glands; these can be separated by sifting and are then known as lupulin. Taste, bitter; odour, aromatic and characteristic.
Part Used: Strobiles.
Constituents: (i) Volatile oil, about 0.4–0.85%, composed mainly of humulene (= α-caryophyllene), with β-caryophyllene, myrcene, farnesene, 2-methylbut-3-ene-2-ol, 3-methylbut-2-ene-1-al, 2,3,5-trithiahexane and similar compounds; with traces of acids such as 2-methylpropanoic and 3-methylbutanoic, which increases significantly in concentration in stored extracts [685, 686, 687] (ii) Flavonols; mainly glycosides of kaempferol and quercetin [688] (iii) Resin, about 3–12%, composed of α-bitter acids such as humulone, cohumulone, adhumulone and others; and β-bitter acids such as lupulene, colupulone, adlupulone etc [5] (iv) Oestrogenic substances of undetermined structure; two of these have molecular weights of approx. 66-80,000 and 80,000 respectively [688] (v) Miscellaneous; tannins, lipids, the chalcone xanthohumol and others [5].
Medicinal Use: Sedative, tranquillizer, hypnotic, tonic, diuretic, anodyne and aromatic bitter. The sedative and tranquillizing activity is well established in a variety of animal tests [689, 690]; it is due at least in part to the 2-methylbut-3-ene-2-ol. This substance, which is present in fresh extract, has been found to be absent from many commercial preparations; however these preparations are still efficaceous and it is thought that the compound may be formed in the body from the α-bitter acids [690, 691]. Hop pillows are a popular remedy for sleeplessness. Other pharmacological actions of hops include spasmolytic and antimicrobial activity; the bitter acids are antimicrobial [692] and an extract of hops is strongly spasmolytic on isolated smooth muscle preparations [693]. Most of the hops grown are used to produce beer – whether the useful pharmacological effects of hops survive the brewing process is of course arguable.

Preparations: Powder, dose: 0.5–1 g; Liquid Extract, dose: 0.5–4 ml; Tincture, dose: 2–4 ml; Lupulin, dose: 120–300 mg.
Potter's Products: Anased, Neurelax, Blood Pressure Tablets, Nervine Medicinal Tea Bags.
Regulatory Status: GSL.

HOREHOUND
Marrubium vulgare L.
Fam. Labiatae

Synonyms: White Horehound, Hoarhound.
Habitat: Found growing wild throughout Europe, cultivated in Britain.
Description: A downy perennial. Leaves cordate-ovate, bluntly serrate, wrinkled and stalked; flowers small, white, in dense whorls, the calyx having ten hooked teeth. Taste, bitter, aromatic; odour, characteristic.
Part Used: Herb.
Constituents: (i) Marrubiin, a diterpene lactone, with premarrubiin [694, 695, 696] (ii) Diterpene alcohols such as marrubiol, marrubenol, sclareol, peregrinin and dihydroperegrinin [697, 698, 699] (iii) Volatile oil, containing α-pinene, sabinene, limonene, camphene, *p*-cymol, fenchene and α-terpinolene [700] (iv) Alkaloids; traces of betonicine and its isomer turicine [701] (v) Miscellaneous; choline, alkanes, phytosterols, tannins etc. [701, 702, 703].
Medicinal Use: Expectorant, bitter tonic, antiseptic. Horehound is used particularly for bronchitis and asthma. Marrubiin is considered to be responsible for the expectorant activity. It has also been shown to normalize extrasystolic arrhythmias, and when the lactone ring is open the corresponding acid is strongly choleretic [5]. The oil has antimicrobial properties and is reported to be vasodilatory and hypotensive [700]. Extracts of horehound are antiinflammatory in the rat paw oedema test and have antiserotonin activity [403, 704]. Horehound is an ingredient of some tonics and has been made into a candy and brewed into an ale. It may be taken as an infusion.
Preparations: Powder, dose: 1–2 g; Liquid Extract, dose: 2–4 ml; Syrup BPC 1949, dose: 2–4 ml; Concentrated infusion BPC 1934, dose: 2–4 ml.
Potter's Products: Asthma and Bronchitis Medicinal Tea Bags, Asthma and Chest Mixture, Horehound and Aniseed Cough Mixture.
Regulatory Status: GSL.

HOREHOUND, BLACK
Ballota nigra L.
Fam. Labiatae

Synonyms: *Marrubium nigrum* Crantz.
Habitat: Similar to Horehound.
Description: Lower leaves cordate, upper leaves ovate; downy, with a crenate margin. Flowers purplish, labiate; calyx with five spreading, broadly ovate teeth. Taste and odour, unpleasant.
Part Used: Herb.

Constituents: Diterpenoids, including marrubiin, ballonigrin, ballotinone (= 7-oxomarrubiin), ballotenol and 7α-acetoxymarrubiin [705, 706]. Iridoids have been shown to be absent [62].

Medicinal Use: Stimulant, antiemetic, antispasmodic. Also used for similar indications to Horehound (q.v.) although not so widely because of the unpleasant taste.

HORSE CHESTNUT

Aesculus hippocastanum
Fam. Hippocasanaceae

Synonyms: Hippocastanum vulgare Gaertn.

Habitat: Native to Northern Asia but widely cultivated, common in Britain.

Description: Bark thick, greyish brown externally, with elongated warts; pinkish brown and finely striated internally; fracture finely fibrous and laminate. Taste, bitter and astringent; odourless. The fruits are well-known, the spiny capsule has three compartments containing the shiny brown roundish seeds or "conkers".

Part Used: Bark, seeds.

Constituents: Saponins, a complex mixture known as "aescin", composed of acylated glycosides of protoaesigenin and barringtogenol-C and including hippocaesculin and many others. The acyl groups are usually tiglic, angelic or acetic acids. [707, 48].

Medicinal Use: Antiinflammatory, febrifuge, astringent. Extracts of horse chestnut, or more usually, preparations of aescin, are used for rheumatism, venous congestion, haemorrhoids, and in cosmetics. Aescin has been shown to eliminate oedema and reduce exhudation, it antagonizes the effects of bradykinin although it is not a direct bradykinin antagonist [708]. It has antiinflammatory activity and causes an increase in plasma levels of ACTH, corticosterone and glucose in rats [709]. Aescin is also active against the influenze virus *in vitro* [710]. Hippocaesculin and barringtogenol-C-21-angelate have antitumour activity *in vitro* [707]. For a review of the cosmetic applications see [711].

Preparations: Liquid Extract (fruit), dose: 0.5–1.2 ml; Liquid Extract (bark), dose: 2–4 ml.

Regulatory Status: GSL.

HORSEMINT

Monarda punctata L.
Fam. Labiatae

Synonyms: American Horsemint.

Habitat: USA.

Description: Leaves opposite, lanceolate, smooth. The flowers occur in axillary tufts, the corolla is yellow with purple spots and two stamens and the sessile bracts yellow and purple. Taste, pungent and bitter; odour, rather like thyme.

Part Used: Leaves, tops.

Constituents: Volatile oil, the major component of which is thymol [2].

Medicinal Use: Stimulant, carminative, emmenagogue.

HORSEMINT, ENGLISH

Mentha longifolia (L.) Huds.
Fam. Labiatae

Synonyms: Mentha sylvestris L.
Habitat: Throughout Britain and Europe.
Description: Leaves opposite, nearly sessile, ovate-lanceolate, serrate and downy on the undersurface. Flowers lilac, labiate, in axillary clusters or a terminal spike. Taste and odour recalling that of garden mint.
Part Used: Herb.
Constituents: Volatile oil, the major component of which is epoxypulegone [2].
Medicinal Use: Carminative, stimulant.

HORSENETTLE

Solanum carolinense L.
Fam. Solanaceae

Synonyms: Bullnettle, Sandbrier.
Habitat: Eastern USA, growing on sandy soil
Description: Root cylindrical, smooth with a few slender rootlets, with a thin pale brown bark which is easily abraded, showing white underneath. Fracture, tough, woody. Taste, bitter then sweetish; odourless.
Part Used: Root, berries.
Constituents: Alkaloids; anabasine, cuscohygrine, solanine, solasodine, solamine and solaurethine [712].
Medicinal Use: Antispasmodic, sedative. An aqueous extract is antibacterial [712].

HORSERADISH

Armoracia rusticana (Gaertn) Mey. and Scherb.
Fam. Cruciferae

Synonyms: A. lapathifolia Gilib.
Habitat: Eastern Europe, but cultivated in Britain and the USA.
Description: Root yellowish-white, cylindrical, about 2 cm thick, with a fleshy consistency. Usually sold fresh. Taste and odour when crushed or scraped, pungent, mustard-like.
Part Used: Root.
Constituents: (i) Glucosinolates, mainly sinigrin, which releases allyl isothiocyanate on contact with the enzyme myrosin during crushing, and 2-phenylethylglucosinolate [1, 124] (ii) Miscellaneous; vitamin C, asparagine, resin, sugar, B vitamins [2].
Medicinal Use: Stimulant, diaphoretic, diuretic. Used more often in cooking, as horseradish sauce.

HORSETAIL

Equisetum arvense L.
Fam. Equisetaceae

Habitat: Common on wet ground and waste places all over Britain.
Description: A perennial herb reaching up to 80 cm but usually less. Stems hollow, grooved, green, bearing whorls of branches at the nodes, leaves reduced to sheaths above the nodes. Taste and odour slight.

Part Used: Herb.
Constituents: (i) Alkaloids, including nicotine, palustrine and palustrinine [713] (ii) Flavonoids such as isoquercitrin and equicetrin [2] (iii) Sterols including cholesterol, isofucosterol, campesterol and others [714] (iv) Silicic acid, 5–8% [2] (v) Miscellaneous; a saponin equisitonin, dimethyl-sulphone, thiaminase and aconitic acid [2, 715].
Medicinal Use: Haemostatic, astringent. Horsetail is used for genito-urinary complaints such as cystitis, prostatitis, urethritis and enuresis. It may be used internally as an antihaemorrhagic and externally as a styptic and vulnerary. The haemostatic substance has been shown to act orally, it has no effect on blood pressure and is not a vasoconstrictor [716].
Preparations: Liquid Extract, dose: 2–4 ml.
Potter's Products: Kasbah Remedy Medicinal Tea Bags, Antitis Tablets.
Regulatory Status: GSL.

HOUNDSTONGUE

Cynoglossum officinale L.
Fam. Boraginaceae

Synonyms: Dogstongue.
Habitat: Grows in dry grassy places and dunes.
Description: A greyish biennial, softly downy, with alternate, long, lanceolate leaves and dark red, funnel shaped flowers. Odour, like mice.
Part Used: Herb.
Constituents: (i) Pyrrolizidine alkaloids; cynoglossine, consolidine, heliosupine, echinatine [79] (ii) Allantoin (iii) Miscellaneous; tannin 8–9%, choline, mucilage, resin [2].
Medicinal Use: Anodyne, demulcent, astringent. Due to the toxic alkaloids its use is not recommended.

HOUSELEEK

Sempervivum tectorum L.
Fam. Crassulaceae

Habitat: A common garden plant in Britain and Europe.
Description: Leaves forming a rosette 5–8 cm in diameter, fleshy, sessile, oblong-ovate, incurved, pointed and hairy at the margin. Taste, saline, astringent and acid; odourless.
Part Used: Fresh leaves.
Constituents: Tannin, mucilage, malic acid [2].
Medicinal Use: Refrigerant, astringent. The fresh leaves have been bruised and applied as a poultice for burns and stings etc.

HYDRANGEA

Hydrangea arborescens L.
Fam. Saxifragaceae

Synonyms: Wild Hydrangea, Seven Barks.
Habitat: USA.

Description: Root pale fawn coloured, smooth with tapering branches; bark very thin. Fracture hard and woody, showing a radiate structure and in larger pieces a distinct pith. Taste, sweetish then pungent; odourless.

Part Used: Root.

Constituents: Largely unknown (i) Flavonoids; kaempferol and quercetin [717] (ii) Other reported constituents include hydrangin (of undetermined structure), saponin, volatile oil etc [5]. Tannins are absent [717].

Other species of *Hydrangea* contain hydrangeol, hydrangeic acid, stilbene derivatives, umbelliferone etc. See [5].

Medicinal Use: Diuretic, nephritic. Used particularly for urinary complaints including kidney and bladder stones, and as a prophylactic. The extract has been shown to be non-toxic in animals [718].

Preparations: Liquid Extract, dose: 2–4 ml.

Potter's Products: Antiglan Tablets, Back and Kidney Tablets.

Regulatory Status: GSL.

HYDROCOTYLE

Centella asiatica (L.) Urban.
Fam. Umbelliferae

Synonyms: Indian Pennywort, *Hydrocotyle asiatica* L.

Habitat: Indian and Pakistan, above an altitude of about 600 m.

Description: A small umbelliferous plant with kidney-shaped leaves up to 2 cm wide and 1 cm long, with a crenate margin and rounded apex. Taste and odour, slight.

Part Used: Leaves, herb.

Constituents: (i) Terpenoids; the saponins asiaticoside, oxyasiaticoside, brahminoside, brahmoside, centelloside, madecassoside and thankuniside; and free asiatic, brahmic, centellinic, isobrahmic, madecassic and betulic acids [719, 721, 722, 4] (ii) Volatile oil, containing β-caryophyllene, β-farnesine, germacrene D, β-elemene, bicycloelemene and other minor components [723] (iii) Miscellaneous; flavonoids, an alkaloid hydrocotyline (unconfirmed), tannin, sugars etc. [2].

Medicinal Use: Vulnerary, dermatic, antileprotic, antiinflammatory. *Centella asiatica* is enjoying a resurgence of interest at present, for the treatment of certain skin conditions, particularly ulcers, wounds and for keloid and hypertrophic scars. It has been shown to improve subjective and objective clinical findings in a trial of patients with venous disorders of the lower limbs [724] and to prevent and treat scarring after burns and postoperatively [725]. It was thought then to act on abnormal fibroblasts, and has since been shown to inhibit the growth of human fibroblasts *in vitro* [726]. An extract stimulated phagocytosis in mice [727]. A recent clinical trial has demonstrated the healing properties of a tincture of Hydrocotyle on wounds [728]. It may be taken orally, often as an infusion, and applied topically.

Preparations: Powdered leaves, dose 600 mg.

HYSSOP
Hyssopus officinalis L.
Fam. Labiatae

Habitat: A common garden plant.

Description: Leaves linear-lanceolate, nearly sessile, about 2 cm long and 2–3 mm broad, hairy on the margin. Flowers small, blue, labiate, in axillary tufts arranged on one side, with a calyx of five uneven teeth. Taste, bitter; odour, aromatic and camphoraceous.

Part Used: Herb.

Constituents: (i) Terpenoids, including marrubiin, oleanolic and ursolic acids [5] (ii) Volatile oil, composed mainly of camphor, pinocamphone, thujone and isopinocamphone, with α- and β-pinene, α-terpinene, linalool, bornyl acetate and many others [729, 5] (iii) Flavonoids, including diosmin and hesperidin [5] (iv) Miscellaneous; hyssopin (a glucoside), tannins 5–8%, resin etc. [5].

Medicinal Use: Stimulant, carminative, pectoral, sedative. Hyssop is used for bronchitis, coughs and colds. It contains marrubiin, which is an expectorant (see Horehound) and ursolic acid, which has antiinflammatory activity. The extracted oil is non-toxic and non-photosensitizing to the skin [730]. Hyssop may be taken as an infusion.

Preparations: Liquid Extract, dose: 2–4 ml.

Potter's Products: Asthma and Bronchitis Mixture.

Regulatory Status: GSL.

Biblical References: Exodus 12:22; Leviticus 14:4, 6, 49, 51, 52; Numbers 19:6, 18; Psalm 51:7 probably Syrian majoram *Origanum syriacum*. Also John 19:29 and Hebrews 9:19.

I

ICELAND MOSS

Cetraria islandica (L.) Ach.
Fam. Parmeliaceae

Synonyms: Iceland Lichen.

Habitat: Grows in most Northern countries.

Description: Thallus smooth, greyish or olive-brown, about 6 cm long, curled or channelled, terminating in spreading, flattened lobes which are fringed with small papillae. The under surface is paler with minute, depressed, white spots. Taste, bitter; odour, when wet, recalls that of seaweed.

Part Used: Lichen.

Constituents: (i) Lichen acids (depsidones); mainly fumarprotocetraric, protocetraric, cetraric, protolichesteric, lichesteric and usnic acids [731, 1, 386] (ii) Polysaccharides, about 50%; mainly lichenin and isolichenin [386, 50] (iii) Miscellaneous; furan derivatives, fatty acid lactones and terpenes [50].

Medicinal Use: Demulcent, expectorant, antiemetic, nutritive. These properties are due mainly to the polysaccharides, however the lichen acids have antibiotic properties [731, 1]. It is normally used as a decoction.

IGNATIUS BEANS

Strychnos ignatii Berg.
Fam. Loganiaceae

Synonyms: *S. cuspida* A. W. Hill, *S. lanceolaris* Miq., *S. ovalifolia* Wall ex G. Don.

Habitat: The Phillipinnes and other parts of S. E. Asia.

Description: Seeds ovoid, irregularly angular, about 2.5 cm long and 2 cm across, with a distinct hilum at one end. Externally dull grey, with occasional fragments of brown epidermis still adhering. Fracture hard, horny. Taste, intensely bitter; odourless.

Part Used: Seeds.

Constituents: Indole alkaloids; brucine and its N-oxide, α- and β-colubrine, diaboline, icajine, novacine, strychnine and its N-oxide, and 12-hydroxyderivatives, vomicine and others [732].

Medicinal Use: Stimulant, tonic. Its properties are similar to those of Nux Vomica (q.v.), including its highly poisonous nature.

Regulatory Status: Schedule 1 Poison. P.

INDIAN HEMP

Cannabis sativa L.
Fam. Cannabinaceae

Synonyms: Cannabis, Marihuana, Hashish, Ganja, Bhang, Dagga, *C. indica* Lamk.

Habitat: Indigenous to India and the Middle East, cultivated widely elsewhere, mostly illicitly.

Description: The flowering tops or "herb" consists of the female flowers, seeds and upper leaves. The leaves are long stalked, bearing usually five to seven lanceolate, pointed, sharply serrate leaflets. The seeds are globular, about 2 mm in diameter, often covered with the small leafy bracts; the whole head may be matted with resin. The resin itself, which may be separated from the rest, is found in greenish, yellowish or reddish-brown or black masses; it is usually hard and brittle. Taste and odour, characteristic.

Part Used: Flowering tops, resin.

Constituents: (i) Cannabinoids, about 60 of which have been isolated, the most important being Δ^9-tetrahydrocannabinol (THC); with other isomers of TCH, cannabinol, cannabidiol, cannabigerol, cannabichromene, cannabipinol, cannabidivarin and others, and their corresponding carboxylic acids, such as THC-acid, which easily decarboxylate at high temperatures (e.g. when smoked). The constituents vary widely depending on climate, cultivar, soil etc. [733, 734, 735, 736] (ii) Flavonoids; flavocannabiside, flavosativaside, glycosides of vitexin and isovitexin and others [734, 737, 738, 1] (iii) Essential oil, composed of olivetol, cannabene (a sesquiterpene) etc. [734, 1] (iv) Alkaloids; cannabisativine muscarine and trigonelline [734] (v) Stilbene derivatives, e.g. 3,4'-dihydroxybibenzyl and others [739] (vi) Miscellaneous; choline, calcium carbonate. For full review see [734].

Medicinal Use: Analgesic, antiinflammatory, hypnotic, sedative, cataleptic, hallucinogenic. The herb and resin have been used for centuries both medicinally and recreationally, however the use is illegal in most countries except for certain medical and scientific purposes. Recently the constituents of cannabis have been reinvestigated as therapeutic agents and pharmacological probes; they and their derivatives are being suggested for treating glaucoma, as antiinflammatory and analgesic agents and cannabinoid derivative is in clinical use as an antiemetic in cancer chemotherapy. The cataleptic, hypotensive and analgesic effects have been confirmed in animals [740, 741, 742] and further work is continuing into their mode of action. Biochemical work has shown the basis for the analgesic and antiinflammatory activity to be the interaction of some of the constituents with the enzymes involved in the inflammatory process, particularly cyclooxygenase, lipoxygenase and phospholipase A_2 [733, 744, 745, 746]. Although THC is the major psychoactive agent, it is not as potent in some of its other effects, such as antiinflammatory activity, as for example the cannabinoids cannabigerol and cannabidiol, and the non-cannabinoids olivetol and some of the flavonoids [747]. Flavocannabiside and flavosativaside are lens aldose reductase inhibitors which may help to explain some of the effects on the eye [737]. For further actions of *Cannabis*, including hormonal effects, see [733]; and for the latest research on the complex interactions of the constituents see [740–747].

Regulatory Status: CD. (Misuse of Drugs Act 1973). POM.

INDIAN PHYSIC

Gillenia trifoliata Moensch.
G. stipulacea Pursh.
Fam. Rosaceae

Synonyms: Indian Hippo, *Spiraea trifoliata* L., *S. stipulata* Muhl.
Habitat: USA.
Description: The roots are cylindrical, usually fissured transversely, 2–4 mm in diameter and up to 15 cm long. The external surface is blackish, and the transverse section shows a thick reddish bark which easily separates from the white woody centre. Taste, pleasantly bitter; odourless.
Part Used: Root bark.
Constituents: No information available.
Medicinal Use: Expectorant, cathartic, emetic. The American Indians used it in a similar way to Ipecacuanha (q.v.)

IPECACUANHA

Cephaelis ipecacuanha (Brotero) A. Rich.
C. acuminata Karsten
Fam. Rubiaceae

Synonyms: Ipecac. Rio, Matto Grosso or Brazilian Ipecac, *Psychotria ipecacuanha* Stokes apply to *C. ipecacuanha* and Cartagena, Nicaragua or Panama Ipecac and *U. granatensisto* to *C. acuminata.*
Habitat: *C. ipecacuanha* is native to tropical S. America, including Brazil, and cultivated in southern Asia; *C. acuminata* is from Central America.
Description: *C. ipecacuanha* root is slender, tortuous, reddish brown, up to about 4 mm in diameter, with a characteristic annular appearance. *C. acuminata* has fewer annulations and is larger, up to 7 mm diameter, and externally greyish brown. Taste, bitter; odour slight but the powder is sternutatory.
Part Used: Root, rhizome.
Constituents: (i) Isoquinoline alkaloids; usually about 2–3%, consisting mainly of emetine and cephaeline, with psychotrine, O-methylpsychotrine, emetamine and protoemetine [1, 5] (ii) Tannins; ipecacuanhin and ipecacuanhic acid [1] (iii) Glycosides such as ipecoside (a monoterpene isoquinoline derivative) and saponins [1, 5] (iv) Allergens, a mixture of glycoproteins of mol. wt. 35,000–40,000 [748] (v) Miscellaneous; starch, choline, resins [5].
Medicinal Use: Expectorant, emetic, stimulant, diaphoretic, amoebicide. Ipecac extract is an ingredient of a great many cough preparations because of its expectorant activity. In larger doses it is an emetic and is used to induce vomiting in cases of drug overdose, particularly in children. The alkaloids are clinically useful in the treatment of amoebiasis and although active in a number of antitumour systems *in vitro*, have not proved effective in treating leukaemia [749].
Preparations: Ipecacuanha Liquid Extract BP, dose: 0.25–1 ml; Ipecacuanha and Morphine Mixture BP, dose: 10 ml; Ipecacuanha Tincture BP, dose: 0.25–1 ml; Ipecacuanha and Opium Powder or Tablets (Dover's Powder and Tablets) BPC 1973, dose: 300–600 mg; Prepared Ipecacuanha BP, dose: 25–100 mg.
Potter's Products: Potter's Balm of Gilead, Vegetable Cough Remover.
Regulatory Status: GSL.

IRISH MOSS

Chondrus crispus (L.) Stackh.
Fam. Gigartinaceae

Synonyms: Carrageenan, Carragheen. Other related spp. of the order Gigartinales (red algae), including *Euchema* and *Gigartina* may be used.

Habitat: The Atlantic coast of Europe and N. America.

Description: The seaweed has a cylindrical base and a flat, forked frond with a fan-shaped outline, reaching up to 25 cm long, 0.3–1.25 cm wide and 1–2 mm thick. Taste, mucilaginous and saline.

Part Used: Seaweed.

Constituents: Polysaccharides. The extract, also known as carrageenin, consists of sulphated, straight chain galactans. There are two different types, a gelling fraction known as *k*-carrageenin and a non-gelling fraction known as λ-carrageenin. They are both composed of *o*-galactose and 3,6-anhydrogalactose residues with a high proportion of sulphate esters, but are differentiated by the relative proportions and the number, type and position of the sulphate esters [750]. There is a variety of grades of different molecular weight, including a food grade which has a molecular weight of about 100,000 to 500,000.

Medicinal Use: Demulcent, antitussive, nutritive. Used for coughs, bronchitis and for irritations of the kidney and bladder. The carrageenins of low molecular weight (around 20,000), including degraded forms, have been reported to have toxic effects in animals when injected and ingested [750, 751] but no toxicity has been observed in humans. Food grades of high molecular weight are not normally absorbed through the gut and are considered to be non-toxic [750]. Irish Moss is used extensively in the production of manufactured foods.

Regulatory Status: GSL.

IVY

Hedera helix L.
Fam. Araliaceae

Habitat: A common European and British climbing plant.

Description: Leaves dark green, paler beneath, leathery, shiny, long-stalked, about 5–10 cm wide, radiate veined with three to four triangular lobes. The upper leaves may be ovate. The berries are purplish-black, globular, 4–8 mm in diameter, with the calyx ring visible at the apex. Taste, bitter and nauseous; odour, aromatic and slightly resinous when rubbed.

Part Used: Leaves, berries.

Constituents: (i) Saponins; based on oleanolic acid and hederagenin, including hederosaponins (hederacosides) B and C, β-hederin and α-hederin which is produced on hydrolysis of leaf extracts [386, 752, 753, 754] (ii) Alkaloids: emetine has been isolated [756] (iii) Polyacetylenes such as falcarinone [631].

Medicinal Use: Cathartic, febrifuge, diaphoretic, anthelmintic. The saponins kill liver flukes *in vitro* and *in vivo* and antifungal and molluscicidal *in vitro* [753, 754, 755]. Emetine is amoebicidal (see Ipecacuanha). Ivy extracts are used in some cosmetic preparations.

IVY, AMERICAN
Parthenocissus quinquefolia Wild.
Fam. Vitaceae

Synonyms: Virginian Creeper, Woodvine, *Cissus hederacea* Ross, *C. quinquefolia* Desf., *Vitis quinquefolia* Lam.

Habitat: USA, but cultivated as an ornamental in Europe and elsewhere.

Description: The bark occurs in quilled pieces, externally brown, with enlarged, transverse lenticels. The fracture shows a whitish bark with coarse, flattened fibres in the inner portion. Taste, insipid; odour, faintly aromatic.

Part Used: Bark, twigs.

Constituents: Anthocyanins [2]. Active constituents unknown.

Medicinal Use: Tonic, expectorant, astringent; as a decoction.

Preparations: Liquid Extract, dose: 2–4 ml.

J

JABORANDI

Pilocarpus microphyllus Stapf.
and other spp. of *Pilocarpus*
Fam. Rutaceae

Synonyms: Maranham Jaborandi. Pernambuco Jaborandi is from *P. jaborandi* Holmes, and Paraguay Jaborandi from *P. pinnatifolius* Lemaire.
Habitat: Brazil.
Description: Leaflets dull green, up to 5 cm long and 3 cm wide, with entire, slightly recurved margins and an unequal base. The veins are prominent on the upper surface and oil cells are visible. The other species are larger, with only minor differences. Taste, bitter; odour, slightly aromatic.
Part Used: Leaves.
Constituents: (i) Imidazole alkaloids; pilocarpine, isopilocarpine, pilosine, isopilosine, epiisopilosine [757] (ii) Volatile oil, containing limonene, sabinene, α-pinene and caryophyllene [758]. The other two species have a lower alkaloid content than *P. microphyllus*.
Medicinal Use: Stimulant, expectorant, diaphoretic, miotic. Jaborandi has also been used in hair tonics to stimulate hair growth. Pilocarpine is a sympathomimetic agent, causing salivation, tachycardia and other effects; however its main use is in ophthalmic preparations as a miotic, in open angle glaucoma and to contract the pupil after the use of atropine.
Preparations: Jaborandi Liquid Extract BPC 1949; Jaborandi Tincture BPC 1949, dose: 0.6–2 ml; Pilocarpine Eye Drops BPC.
Regulatory Status: POM or P or GSL in restricted strengths.

JACOB'S LADDER

Polemonium coeruleum L.
Fam. Polemoniaceae

Synonyms: Greek Valerian, English Greek Valerian.
Habitat: Northern Europe, rare in Britain.
Description: Leaves pinnate, alternate; flowers in a cluster, purplish-blue, open, with five petal-lobes. Taste, slightly bitter; odourless.
Part Used: Herb.
Constituents: Unknown. Saponins with a high haemolytic index, volatile oil, resins and organic acids have been reported.
Medicinal Use: Diaphoretic, astringent. Similar in effect to Abscess Root (q.v.).

JALAP

Ipomoea purga Hayne
Fam. Convolvulaceae

Synonyms: Mexican Jalap, Vera Cruz Jalap, *I. jalapa* Scheide and Deppe, *Convolvulus jalapa* L., *C. purga* Wend., *Exogonium purga* Benth.
Habitat: Mexico.

Description: Roots usually ovoid, up to about 15 cm long, very hard and heavy. Externally dark brown, wrinkled, with paler, transverse lenticels. Fracture, hard, horny, showing a greyish interior.

Part Used: Tuberous root.

Constituents: Resin, about 10–18%, known as "convolvulin" and containing glycolipids of complex, only partially determined structure, such as jalapine (= convolvuline). The resins are composed of short chain fatty acids, e.g. valeric, tiglic and exegonic acid, and sugars such as quinovosides [759, 760].

Medicinal Use: Cathartic, purgative. Usually used with carminatives and other laxatives to prevent griping.

Preparations: Jalap Resin BPC 1963, dose: 60–300 mg; Jalap Tincture BPC 1949, dose: 2–4 ml.

JAMAICA DOGWOOD

Piscidia erythrina L.
Fam. Leguminosae

Synonyms: Fish Poison Tree.

Habitat: W. Indies, S. America.

Description: The bark occurs in quilled pieces, up to about 15 cm long and 3–6 mm thick, dark grey-brown externally with thin, longitudinal and transverse ridges, roughish and wrinkled, and somewhat fissured. Fracture tough, fibrous, showing blue-green or brownish-green patches. Taste, bitter and acrid; odour, characteristic.

Part Used: Bark.

Constituents: (i) Isoflavones; lisetin, jamaicin, ichthyone, and the rotenoids rotenone, milletone, isomilletone and others [761, 762, 763] (ii) Organic acids, including piscidic acid, its mono- and diethyl esters, fukiic acid and its 3'-O-methyl ester [764, 765] (iii) Miscellaneous; β-sitosterol, tannins etc [5].

Medicinal Use: Analgesic, sedative, antispasmodic. Used particularly for neuralgia, migraine, insomnia, female complaints, whooping cough and asthma. An extract has been demonstrated to have antispasmodic, antitussive, antipyretic, antiinflammatory and sedative actions in animals, with very low toxicity [766].

Preparations: Liquid Extract BPC 1934, dose: 2–8 ml.

Potter's Products: Headache and Nervous Exhaustion Mixture No. 101A, Anased Tablets.

Regulatory Status: GSL.

JAMBUL

Syzygium cumini (L.) Skeels.
Fam. Myrtaceae

Synonyms: Java Plum, *S. jambolanum* DC, *S. jambos* Alston.

Habitat: Indonesia, Australia.

Description: The seeds are subcylindrical, about 6 mm long and rather less in diameter; one end truncated and with a central depression. Externally hard and tough, blackish-brown; internally pinkish-brown. Taste, faintly astringent and aromatic; odour, slight.

Part Used: Seeds.

Constituents: (i) Phenols, including methylxanthoxylin and 2,6-dihydroxy-4-methoxyacetophenone [767] and tannins, including ellagic and gallic acids [2, 33] (ii) Jambosine, an alkaloid [33] (iii) Antimellin, a glycoside [2, 33] (iv) Triterpenes, such as Eugenia triterpenes A and B [768] (v) Essential oil [33].

Medicinal Use: Antidiabetic, astringent, diuretic. An extract of fruit ·and seeds produces a pronounced hypoglycaemic effect in animals, in some cases comparable to that of tolbutamide, and abolishes glycosuria in rats [769, 770, 771].

Preparations: Powdered seeds, dose: 0.3–2 g; Liquid Extract, dose: 4–8 ml.

Regulatory Status: GSL.

JEQUIRITY

Abrus precatorius L.
Fam. Leguminosae

Synonyms: Indian Liquorice, Wild Liquorice, Prayer Beads, Crab's Eyes.

Habitat: India, S. America, W. Africa.

Description: Seeds oval, rounded at the ends, about 3 mm diameter, hard and polished, vermilion red with the upper third black; very hard and tough.

Part Used: Seeds.

Constituents: (i) Abrin, a toxalbumin, and other proteins [772, 773] (ii) Indole derivatives; *N*-methyltryptamine, *N*-methyltryptophan and hypaphorine [774] (iii) Anthocyanins; xyloglucosyldelphinidin and (*p*-coumaryl-galloyl)-glucosyldelphinidin [775] (iv) Miscellaneous; oil, sterols, terpenes etc [33].

The leaves and roots contain the sweetening agent glycyrrhizin (see Liquorice) [773].

Medicinal Use: Irritant, abortifacient. Jequirity has been used to treat chronic granular conjunctivitis but its use has been abandoned; it has also been used as a contraceptive but this cannot be recommended as it is so poisonous. The seeds are teratogenic and abortifacient [774]. Abrin is the toxic agent; it causes agglutination of erythrocytes, haemolysis and enlargement of the lymph glands [33] and has caused fatalities.

JEWEL WEED

Impatiens aurens Muhl.
I. biflora Walt.
Fam. Balsaminaceae

Synonyms: Balsam Weed, Pale Touch-Me-Not, *I. pallida* Nutt., (*I. aurea*); Spotted Touch-Me-Not, Speckled Jewels, *I. fulva* (*I. biflora*).

Habitat: Indonesia, N. America.

Description: Leaves grey-green, thin, ovate, more or less dentate; stem jointed. Flowers axillary, solitary, slipper-shaped with a long, recurved spur. Those of *I. aurea* are pale yellow and those of *I. biflora* are orange-yellow and spotted. The valves of the fruit curl up when dehisced.
Part Used: Herb.
Constituents: Unknown.
Medicinal Use: Aperient, diuretic; as a decoction. The fresh plant has been made into an ointment for the treatment of haemorrhoids, and the juice is reputed to remove warts and corns and to cure ringworm.

JUJUBE
Zyzyphus jujube Mill.
Fam. Rhamnaceae

Synonyms: The closely related *Z. vulgaris* Lamk. is also used.
Habitat: Africa, Middle East, Far East.
Description: Fruits of variable size, depending on origin, usually up to 3 cm long and 1.5 cm in diameter, red, smooth and shiny when fresh, brownish-red and wrinkled when dried; fleshy and containing one or two seeds. Taste, sweet and mucilaginous.
Part Used: Berries.
Constituents: (i) Saponins of the dammarane type, known as the zyzyphus saponins I, II and III, jujubosides A and B, zizybeosides I and II, and zizyvyosides I and II, together with at least 11 pentacyclic triterpenoids [776, 777, 778, 779,]. In *Z. vulgaris* similar saponins have been found [780] (ii) Flavonoids; naringenin glycosides, vomifoloil and roseoside [778]. In *Z. vulgaris* spinosin (2′-O-β-glucosylswertisin) and derivatives of spinosin and swertisin are present [781] (iii) Sugars, mucilage etc.
Medicinal Use: Emollient, sedative, antitussive, anti-allergic and nutrient. In the Far East it is taken to improve muscular strength, increase body weight, protect the liver and prevent stress ulcer formation. Recent work there has shown that extracts of the fruit increase levels of cyclic AMP in leucocytes, and that the fruit itself contains very high levels of both cyclic AMP and cyclic GMP [782, 783, 784], which may help to explain the antiallergic activity [284]. An aqueous extract has been shown to inhibit experimental anaphylaxis in the skin of rats. It has no antibacterial activity but sedative activity and *in vitro* antitumour activity has been shown [284]. *Z. vulgaris* seed extract produces a transient fall in blood pressure and a prolongation of thiobarbital-induced sleeping time in animals [785].

JUNIPER
Juniperus communis L.
Fam. Cupressaceae

Habitat: Widely distributed throughout the world, particularly Europe.
Description: The fruit, usually called a "berry" which it resembles, is about 0.5–1 cm in diameter, globular, purplish-black with a grey bloom, and three lines or furrows joined at the apex, indicating the junction of the three seeds. Taste and odour, characteristic.

Part Used: Fruit.

Constituents: (i) Volatile oil, about 1–2%, containing mainly myrcene, sabinene and α-pinene, with 1,4-cineole, *p*-cymene, camphene, limonene, β-pinene, terpin-4-ol, γ-terpinene, α-thujene and others [5] (ii) Condensed tannins; (+)-afzelechin, (−)-epiafzelechin, (+)-catechin, (−)-epicatechin, (+)-gallocatechin and (+)-epigallocatechin [786] (iii) 1,4-dimethyl-3-cyclohexen-1-yl methyl ketone [787] (iv) Diterpene acids; myrceocommunic, communic, sandaracopimaric, isopimaric, torulosic acids [788] and other diterpenes such as geijerone [789] (v) Miscellaneous; sugars, resin, vitamin C [5].

Medicinal Use: Diuretic, antiseptic, carminative, antiinflammatory. Juniper is used for acute and chronic cystitis and rheumatism. The antiinflammatory effects have been demonstrated *in vivo* [403]. It is normally avoided during pregnancy, mainly because of the notorious reputation of gin, of which Juniper is the main flavour ingredient.

Preparations: Juniper Oil BPC 1949, dose: 0.03–0.2 ml; Juniper Spirit BPC 1949, dose: 0.3–1.2 ml.

Potter's Products: Sciargo Medicinal Tea Bags, Sciargo Tablets, Rheumatism Mixture, Cystitis Mixture No. 111A, Lumbago Mixture No. 117A.

Regulatory Status: GSL.

Biblical References: 1 Kings 19:4–5; Job 30:4; Psalm 120:4.

K

KAMALA

Mallotus philippinensis Mull. Arg.
Fam. Euphorbiaceae

Synonyms: Kameela, *Rottlera tinctoria* Roxb.
Habitat: Eastern Africa, India, Saudi Arabia.
Description: The hairs and glands covering the fruit are obtained by sifting; they form a red mobile powder which floats on water. Tasteless and nearly odourless.
Part Used: Capsule hairs and glands.
Constituents: (i) Phloroglucinol derivatives; rottlerin, isorottlerin, isoallo-rottlerin (the "red compound") and methylene-bis-methylphloroaceto-phenone (the "yellow compound") [790, 791] (ii) Kamalins I and II of undetermined structure [790].
Medicinal Use: Taenifuge, purgative. Used in India and elsewhere for the treatment of tapeworm infestation.
Preparations: Powder, dose: 2–10 g; Liquid Extract, dose: 8–14 ml.
Regulatory Status: P.

KAVA KAVA

Piper methysticum Forst.
Fam. Piperaceae

Synonyms: Kava, Kawa.
Habitat: South Sea Islands.
Description: Root large, externally blackish-grey, internally whitish. Fracture mealy and somewhat splintery, central portion porous, with irregularly twisted thin woody bundles, separated by broad medullary rays, forming meshes beneath the bark. Taste, pungent, numbing; odour reminiscent of lilac.
Part Used: Root.
Constituents: (i) Pyrone derivatives; kawain, dihydrokawain, dihydro-methysticin and yangonin [792] (ii) Pipermethysticine, a piperidine alkaloid [793].
Medicinal Use: Stimulant, tonic, diuretic. Has been used in bronchitis, rheumatism and gout, but is used more frequently for its diuretic and antifatigue properties. Large doses cause intoxication.
Preparations: Powder, dose: 2–4 g; Liquid Extract, dose: 2–4 ml.
Potter's Products: Antiglan Tablets.
Regulatory Status: GSL.

KINO

Pterocarpus marsupium Roxb.
Fam. Leguminosae

Habitat: India and Sri Lanka.
Description: The gum appears in commerce as small, blackish, shining fragments or as a coarse powder. Taste, very astringent. It adheres to the teeth when chewed.

Part Used: Juice.
Constituents: Polyphenolic compounds which are diverse but structurally
  related: (i) Tannins, such as (−)-epicatechin [794] (ii) Stilbenes; such as
  pterostilbene (iii) Flavonoids; liquiritigenin, isoliquiritigenin, 7-hydroxy-
  flavanone, 7,4-dihydroxyflavanone, 5-deoxykaempferol and pterosupin
  [795] (iv) Marsupsin, a benzofuranone (v) Others; propterol, *p*-hydroxy-
  benzaldehyde etc. [795, 796].
Medicinal Use: Astringent. Used mainly for diarrhoea and dysentery and as
  a local application for sore throats and leucorrheoa. In India it is also used
  for diabetes and pterostilbene is responsible for this activity [794].
Preparations: Powdered Gum, dose: 0.3–1 g; Kino Tincture BPC 1949,
  dose: 2–4 ml.
Regulatory Status: GSL.

KNAPWEED
Centaurea nigra L.
Fam. Compositae

Synonyms: Black Knapweed, Star Thistle, Black Ray Thistle, Ironweed.
Habitat: A native European wild plant.
Description: Globular flowerheads, about 5 cm long, the outer scales of
  which have blackish appendages at the apex with comb-like teeth. Florets
  purplish, tubular. Taste, bitter, slightly saline.
Part Used: Herb.
Constituents: Unidentified.
Medicinal Use: Diuretic, diaphoretic, tonic.

KNOTGRASS
Polygonum aviculare L.
Fam. Polygonaceae

Habitat: Britain, Middle and Eastern Europe, Russia.
Description: Stem slender, cylindrical, striated. Leaves narrowly lanceolate,
  about 1 cm long; stipules lanceolate. Taste, astringent; odourless.
Part Used: Herb.
Constituents: (i) Tannins, including catechin and gallic acid (ii) Flavonoids,
  mainly glycosides based on quercetin (iii) Polyphenolic acids; caffeic and
  chlorogenic acids (iv) Silicic acid, sugars, mucilage etc. [2].
Medicinal Use: Astringent, as an infusion, for diarrhoea.

KOLA
Cola acuminata (Beauv.) Schott et Endl.
C. nitida (Vent.) Schott et Endl.
and other spp. of *Cola*
Fam. Sterculiaceae

Synonyms: Cola, Guru Nut *Sterculia acuminata* Beauv.
Habitat: Native to W. Africa, extensively cultivated in the tropics,
  particularly Nigeria, Brazil, Sri Lanka and Indonesia.

Description: The seed is found in commerce as the dried, fleshy cotyledons with the testa removed. They are red-brown, often irregular in shape, usually oblong, convex on one side and flattened on the other, up to 5 cm long and about 2.5 cm in diameter.

Part Used: Seed.

Constituents: (i) Caffeine, up to 2.5%, with traces of theobromine [5, 33] (ii) Tannins and phenolics; *d*-catechin, *l*-epicatechin, kolatin, kolatein, kolanin, and in the fresh nut, catechol and (−)-epicatechol [5, 33, 183] (iii) Miscellaneous; phlobaphene, an anthocyanin pigment known as "kola red", betaine, protein, starch etc. [5, 33].

Medicinal Use: Stimulant, diuretic, cardiac tonic, astringent, antidepressive. Kola extracts are an ingredient of many tonics for depression, tiredness and to stimulate the appetite. The main active ingredient is caffeine. It is also effective in diarrhoea. One of the major uses is as a flavouring in the manufacture of soft drinks.

Preparations: Powder, dose: 1–3 g; Kola Liquid Extract BPC 1949, dose: 0.6–1.2 ml; Kola Tincture BPC 1934, dose: 1–4 ml.

Potter's Products: Strength Tablets, Debility Mixture.

Regulatory Status: GSL.

KOUSSO
Hagenia abyssinica J. J. Gmel.
Fam. Rosaceae

Synonyms: Kooso, Kusso, *Brayera anthelmintica* Kunth.

Habitat: North-east Africa.

Description: Flowers about 1 cm across, petals minute, linear; ten veined leaf-like sepals in two rows. The female inflorescence is normally used and occurs in commerce in the form of a cylindrical roll.

Part Used: Dried flowers.

Constituents: Butyrophenone derivatives; α- and β-kosin [25].

Medicinal Use: Anthelmintic. Used as an infusion and powder, in conjunction with purgatives such as castor oil (q.v.).

Regulatory Status: GSL.

KUMARHOU
Pomaderris elliptica L.
Fam. Rhamnaceae

Synonyms: Papapa, Gumdiggers Soap, Poverty Weed.

Habitat: New Zealand.

Description: It is a branching shrub, up to 3 m in height, leaves 5–8 cm long, shiny above and downy on the undersurface. The inflorescence is a many-flowered cyme; petals and sepals yellowish-white.

Part Used: Herb.

Constituents: Unknown.

Medicinal Use: Used by Maoris for asthma, bronchitis, kidney troubles and as a blood purifier.

L

LABRADOR TEA
Ledum latifolium Jacq.
Fam. Ericaceae

Synonyms: St. James's Tea. *L. palustre* is also referred to as Labrador Tea, or more frequently as Marsh Tea or Wild Rosemary.
Habitat: N. America and Canada. *L. palustre* grows in Northern Europe, Asia and America.
Description: Leaves linear-lanceolate, with a revolute margin, alternate, almost sessile, up to 5 cm long and 0.5 cm broad. The upper surface is dark green and smooth, the undersurface coated with red-brown hairs. Taste, bitter and camphoraceous; odour, aromatic.
Part Used: Leaves.
Constituents: Unidentified.
Medicinal Use: Pectoral, expectorant, diuretic.

LACHNANTHES
Lachnanthes tinctoria Ell.
Fam. Haemodoraceae

Synonyms: Spiritweed, Red Root, Paint Root, Wool Flower.
Habitat: W. Indies.
Description: Rhizome about 3 cm long, surrounded by long, slender, deep-red roots. Leaves scythe-shaped, somewhat succulent, 0.5–1.5 cm long, in a basal rosette, reddish-brown when dried. Flowers arranged in a woolly cyme. Taste, acrid; odourless.
Part Used: Root, herb.
Constituents: Unknown.
Medicinal Use: Tonic, narcotic. Has been used for coughs, pneumonia etc., but large doses produce vertigo, headache and other unpleasant symptoms.

LADY'S BEDSTRAW
Galium verum L.
Fam. Rubiaceae

Synonyms: Yellow Bedstraw, Cheese Rennet.
Habitat: A common herb growing in dry grassy places in Britain, throughout Europe and parts of N. America.
Description: Stems slender, angular, bearing whorls of 8–12 linear leaves with downy undersurfaces and revolute margins. Flowers very small, bright yellow, in terminal panicles. Taste, astringent, slightly bitter and acid; odourless.
Part Used: Herb.
Constituents: (i) Iridoids, including asperuloside and galioside [355,797]
(ii) Flavonoid glycosides; quercetin-3-glucoside, quercetin-7-glucoside,

quercitin-3-rutinoside, luteolin-7-glucoside and others [798] (iii) Anthra-quinone derivatives, such as alizarin, in the root [356] (iv) *n*-alkanes, mainly C_{31} and C_{29} [355].

Medicinal Use: Diuretic, alterative. Contains similar compounds to Clivers (q.v.) and used for similar purposes. The flowers have been used to make cheese instead of rennet, hence the synonym.

LADY'S MANTLE

Alchemilla vulgaris L.
Fam. Rosaceae

Synonyms: Lion's Foot.
Habitat: A common British and European wild plant.
Description: A variable group of similar microspecies, usually hairy but sometimes glabrous. Leaves up to about 5 cm in diameter, having 7–11, rounded, serrate, palmate lobes. Flowers green, apetalous, in small clusters, borne on a forked stem which has small three-lobed leaves and broad stipules at the base of each fork. Taste, slightly astringent; odourless.
Part Used: Herb.
Constituents: (i) Tannins, about 6–8%, consisting mainly of glycosides of ellagic acid [2] (ii) Salicylic acid, a trace [2]. No recent information is available.
Medicinal Use: Astringent, styptic. Used for excessive menstruation and diarrhoea, and topically for leucorrhoea and pruritis vulvae.
Preparations: Liquid Extract, dose: 2–4 ml.
Regulatory Status: GSL.

LADY'S SLIPPER

Cypripedium calceolus var *pubescens* R Br.
Fam. Orchidaceae

Synonyms: Nerve Root, American Velerian, *C. pubescens* Willd., *C. hirsutum* Mill., *C. parviflorum* Salisb.
Habitat: Indigenous to Canada and the USA, cultivated in Europe.
Description: Rhizome up to 8 cm long, 0.5 cm in diameter, reddish-brown, with numerous cup-shaped bud scars and a few buds on the upper surface, and many slender, matted roots on the lower surface. Fracture, short; taste, bitter and pungent; odour, characteristic, slightly valerianic.
Part Used: Rhizome.
Constituents: Largely unknown. There is an unidentified glycoside, essential oil, tannin and resin [2].
Medicinal Use: Antispasmodic, nervine, sedative, mild hypnotic. Used for anxiety states, headache, neuralgia and emotional tension.
Preparations: Powder, dose: 2–4 g; Liquid Extract, dose: 2–4 ml.
Regulatory Status: GSL.

LARCH
Larix dedidua Miq.
Fam. Pinaceae

Synonyms: European Larch, *L. europea* D.C., *Pinus larix L.*
Habitat: Europe, including the British Isles.
Description: The inner bark of the tree, deprived of the grey, outer, inert bark, is preferred for medicinal use. The external surface is reddish-brown, the inner surface with a pinkish or yellowish tint. Fracture short, slightly fibrous. Taste, astringent, bitter; odour, terebinthinate.
Part Used: Bark.
Constituents: (i) Lignans; lariciresinol, liovil, and *secoiso*lariciresinol [799] (ii) Resins, 60–80%, consisting of the resin acids larinolic and laricinolic acids and others [2] (iii) Essential oil, containing α- and β-pinene, limonene, phellandrene, borneol etc. [2].
Medicinal Use: Astringent, balsamic, diuretic. Larch has been used as a tincture to treat bronchitis and urinary inflammation.
Regulatory Status: GSL.

LARKSPUR
Delphinium consolida L.
Fam. Ranunculaceae

Synonyms: Lark's Claw, Knight's Spur.
Habitat: A common garden plant.
Description: Seeds black, tetrahedral, flattened, up to about 2 mm in diameter, with acute edges and pitted surface. Taste, bitter and acrid; odourless.
Part Used: Seeds.
Constituents: Diterpene alkaloids, of the aconitine type (see Aconite) including anthranoyllycoctomine, lycoctonine, delcosine and delsoline [800].
Medicinal Use: Parasiticide, insecticide, antispasmodic. A tincture has been used to destroy nits and lice in the hair. It should be used with great care.

LAUREL
Laurus nobilis L.
Fam. Lauraceae

Synonyms: Bay, Sweet Bay, Bay Laurel
Habitat: Native to the Mediterranean region, cultivated widely.
Description: The leaves are leathery, dark green with a paler undersurface, up to about 7 cm long and 2.5 cm across, elliptic-lanceolate, with an entire or slightly wavy margin. Taste and odour, characteristic, aromatic.
Part Used: Leaves, essential oil.
Constituents: Volatile oil, up to about 3%, containing cineole as the major component, 30–50%, with linalool, α-pinene and α-terpineol acetate; and in minor concentrations sabinene, limonene, methyleugenol, *p*-cymene, thuj-2-en-4-ol and the sesquiterpenes costunolide and laurenolide [801, 802, 803, 804].

Medicinal Use: Stomachic, cholagogue, diaphoretic and stimulant. The oil has been used as an external application for rheumatism and in hair dressings for dandruff. Bay leaves are an important culinary spice. Should not be confused with Myrcia, often called Bay or West Indian Bay, from *Pimenta racemosa* (Mill) J W Moore, which is an ingredient of Bay Rum.

LAVENDER
Lavendula angustifolia Mill.
Fam. Labiatae

Synonyms: Garden Lavender, *L. officinalis,* Chaix., *L. vera* D. C. Spike Lavender is *L. latifolia Medic., (= L. spica* D.C.). Lavandin is a hybrid of these.

Habitat: Native to the Mediterranean region.

Description: The flowers are usually met with in commerce separated from the spikes. The calyx is tubular, veined, purplish-grey, and five-toothed, one tooth being larger than the others. The corolla is tubular, blue or mauve, two-lipped, the upper lip having two lobes and the lower having three. Taste and odour; pleasant, characteristic.

Part Used: Flowers.

Constituents: Volatile oil, about 0.5–1%, containing linalyl acetate (up to 40%), with linalool, lavandulyl acetate, borneol, camphor, limonene, cadinene, caryophyllene, 4-butanolide, 5-pentyl-5-pentanolide and similar compounds [5, 805, 806, 807, 808, 809] (ii) Coumarins; Umbelliferone, herniarin, coumarin, dihydrocoumarin [5, 810] (iii) Miscellaneous; triterpenes e.g. ursolic acid, flavonoids e.g. luteolin [5]. Spike Lavender oil has 1,8-cineole and camphor as the major constituents, with only small amounts of linalyl acetate.

Medicinal Use: Carminative, spasmolytic, tonic, antidepressant. The oil is reported to have CNS depressant activity in mice, to be antimicrobial and of low toxicity [5]. Lavender is used extensively in perfumery, and Spike Lavender is used as an insect repellent.

Preparations: Compound Lavender Tincture BPC 1949, dose; 2–4 ml; Lavender Spirit BPC 1934, dose: 0.3–1.2.

Regulatory Status: GSL.

LAVENDER COTTON
Santolina chamaecyparissus L.
Fam. Compositae

Habitat: Mediterranean countries.

Description: Leaves linear, about 2.5–5 cm long and 6 mm broad, with short obtuse teeth. The flowerheads are sub-globular, borne on long, leafless stalks, yellow with lanceolate, pointed outer bracts and membranous inner bracts. Stems white, with cottony hairs. Taste, bitter; odour, strong and aromatic, recalling that of chamomile.

Part Used: Herb.

Constituents: Flavonoids, particularly 6-methoxy flavones; pectolinarigenin, hispidulin, nepetin and others [811].
Medicinal Use: Antiinflammatory, stomachic, emmenagogue, anthelmintic. In recent experiments the antiinflammatory effects were demonstrated in rats without ulcerogenicity or toxicity [812]. Used as an infusion.

LEMON

Citrus limon (L.) Burm.
Fam. Rutaceae

Synonyms: Limon.
Habitat: Native to Asia, cultivated widely, in Italy, Cyprus, USA etc.
Description: The fruit is too well-known to require description.
Part Used: Fruit, juice, peel and essential oil.
Constituents: (i) Essential oil, about 2.5% of the peel, consisting of mainly monoterpenes such as limonene, the major component (ca. 70%), with α-terpinene, α- and β-pinene, myrcene, sabinene; aldehydes, mainly citral; sesquiterpenes such as bisabolene and caryophyllene [1, 5] (ii) coumarins including limettin, bergamottin and imperatorin [5] (iii) Flavonoids, known as citroflavonoids or bioflavonoids; mainly hesperidoside, naringoside and eryodictyoside [33] (iv) Vitamin C, mucilage, calcium oxalate [1].
Medicinal Use: The citroflavonoids are used in vascular disorders where venous insufficiency results in haemorrhoids and varicose veins etc., since they control vascular permeability to liquids and proteins by decreasing porosity. They are also reportedly antiinflammatory (probably due to the bisabolol content), antihistaminic and diuretic [813, 814]. Lemons are a well-known source of vitamin C and are more usually used as a food and flavouring.
Preparations: Lemon Oil BP, Lemon Tincture BP 1958.
Regulatory Status: GSL.

LETTUCE, WILD

Lactuca virosa L.
Fam. Compositae

Synonyms: Lettuce Opium, Lactucarium.
Habitat: Indigenous to Central and Southern Europe and Northern Asia, cultivated elsewhere.
Description: Similar to garden lettuce, however the leaves are much narrower, with bristles on the undersurface of the midrib. The dried juice is less commonly used nowadays, it is dark reddish brown externally and waxy internally. Odour, characteristic, heavy; taste, very bitter.
Part Used: Leaves, dried juice.
Constituents: (i) Lactucin, a sesquiterpene lactone [815] (ii) Flavonoids; mainly based on quercetin [816] (iii) Coumarins; cichoriin and aesculin [816] (iii) N-methyl-β-phenethylamine [817] (disputed) [818] (iv) Hyoscyamine, a tropane alkaloid, (disputed) [818].

Medicinal Use: Mild sedative, hypnotic, anodyne, expectorant. Wild lettuce is used for bronchitis, irritable coughs, for insomnia and as a sedative.

Preparations: Lactucarium, dose 0.3–1 g; Extract of Lettuce BPC 1934, dose: 0.3–1 g; Fluid Extract, dose: 0.5–4 ml.

Potter's Products: Anased Tablets, Asthma and Bronchitis Mixture No 80A.

Regulatory Status: GSL.

LIFE EVERLASTING

Antennaria dioica Gaertn.
Fam. Compositae

Synonyms: Catsfoot, Cat's Ear, *Gnaphalium dioicum* L.

Habitat: Northern Europe including Britain, Asia, N. America.

Description: A low creeping perennial, with obovate leaves which are white and cottony on the undersurface. Flowers dioecious, in terminal clusters, rayless, pink or red, with red or white sepal-like bracts. Taste, astringent; odour, aromatic, stronger in the female flowers.

Part Used: Herb.

Constituents: (i) Volatile oil (ii) Flavonoids including luteolin (iii) Triterpenes such as ursolic acid and sterols [2].

Medicinal Use: Astringent; as a gargle or styptic and internally for diarrhoea. An extract stimulates phagocytosis in mice inoculated with *Escherichia coli* [80].

LIFE ROOT

Senecio aureus L.
Fam. Compositae

Synonyms: Squaw Weed, Golden Senecio.

Habitat: Europe, including Britain, N. America.

Description: Rhizome 2–5 cm long, with numerous roots; the root bark being hard and blackish surrounding a ring of whitish woody bundles and a large, dark, central pith. Root leaves up to 15 cm long, reniform; those on the stem shorter, incised and pinnatifid. Flowerheads few, in a loose corymb, up to about 2.5 cm broad, with yellow pistillate ray florets and hermaphrodite central tubular florets. Taste, bitter and astringent; odour, faint, slightly acrid.

Part Used: Rhizome, herb.

Constituents: (i) Pyrrolizidine alkaloids; florosenine, otosenine, floridanine [819] (ii) Eremophilane sesquiterpenes, *trans*-9-oxofuranoeremophilane-8α-ethoxy-10α-*H*-eremophilane, cacalol and others [820].

Medicinal Use: Emmenagogue, diuretic, astringent, pectoral. Has been used as a uterine tonic and for amenorrhoea, and for menopausal symptoms. However only samples with alkaloids absent should be taken internally.

Preparations: Powder, dose: 2–4 g; Liquid Extract, dose: 2–4 ml.

LILY OF THE VALLEY

Convallaria majalis L.
Fam. Liliaceae

Synonyms: May Lily, Muguet.

Habitat: A common garden plant.

Description: Leaves broadly lanceolate, up to 15 cm long and about 5 cm wide, parallel-veined with entire margins. Flower stem carries eight to twelve small, stalked, bell-shaped white flowers with six stamens. Rhizome cylindrical, slender, internodes about 5 cm apart bearing numerous slender rootlets, pale brown. Taste, sweet at first, then bitter; odour, pleasant.

Part Used: Leaves, whole plant.

Constituents: Cardiactive glycosides; the cardenolides convallatoxin, convalloside, convallatoxol, desglucocheirotoxin, lokunjoside, convallamaroside, glycosides of bipindogenin, sarmentologenin, sarmentosigenin A, rhodexin A, rhodexoside and others [821, 822, 823, 824, 825] (ii) Flavonoid glycosides, in the leaves [1].

Medicinal Use: Cardiac tonic. It has a similar action to digitalis (Foxglove, q.v.) but is less cumulative, and is used to treat congestive heart failure. The usual form for use is the isolated glycoside convallatoxin. For further details see [4]. Convallamaroside has antifungal and antibiotic activity but this effect is not therapeutically useful since it forms a complex in the body with cholesterol [824]. Lily of the Valley flowers are used in perfumery.

Preparations: Liquid Extract BPC 1934, dose: 0.3–0.6 ml; Tincture BPC 1934, dose: 0.3–1.2 ml.

Regulatory Status: P.

LIME FLOWERS

Tilia platyphylla Scop.
T. cordata Mill, and others
T. × vulgaris
Fam. Tiliaceae

Synonyms: Lindenflowers, *T. europea.*

Habitat: Europe, including Britain.

Description: The flowerstalk bears about three to six yellowish-white, five-petalled flowers on stalks half-joined to an oblong bract. The leaves are heart-shaped, greyish beneath and downy. The flowers are fragrant.

Part Used: Flowers, with or without the bract.

Constituents: (i) Volatile oil, up to about 0.1%, containing farnesol [50] (ii) Flavonoids; hesperidin, quercetin, astralagin, tiliroside and others [2] (iii) Miscellaneous; mucilage (in the bract), phenolic acids such as chlorogenic and caffeic, tannins [2].

Medicinal Use: Nervine, tonic, hypotensive. They may be used for nervous disorders, catarrh, headaches, indigestion and other disorders as an infusion.

Preparations: Liquid Extract, dose: 2–4 ml.

Potter's Products: Blood Pressure Tablets, Blood Pressure Medicinal Tea Bags, Blood Pressure Mixture.

Regulatory Status: GSL.

171

LIME FRUIT

Citrus aurantifolia Swingle
Fam. Rutaceae

Synonyms: C. *medica var acida* Brandis, C. *acris* Mill., C. *limetta* Risso.
Habitat: Indigenous to southern Asia and cultivated widely in the West Indies, Florida and Central America.
Description: Variable in appearance but usually resembling the lemon, except they are nearly globular, smaller and more greenish in colour.
Part Used: Fruit, juice.
Constituents: (i) Volatile oil, consisting of about 75% limonene, with α-and β-pinenes, sabinene, terpinolene, citral, α-terpineol, linalool, α-bergamotene, β-bisabolene etc [5, 826] (ii) Coumarins; the major one being limettin, with bergamottin, bergapten (= 5-methoxypsoralen), dimethoxy-coumarin, 8-geranoxypsoralen isoimperatoren, isopimpinellin and others [826, 827, 828] (iii) Miscellaneous; vitamin C etc.
Medicinal Use: Antiscorbutic, refrigerant. Limes are used more for flavouring than medicinally, although the juice is a traditional source of vitamin C. The expressed oil is used in perfumery. The coumarins such as bergapten are well-known for causing photosensitization; this effect is sometimes utilized in the formulation of sun-tan preparations, however they should be used with care and may cause allergies in sensitive individuals.

LINSEED

Linum usitatissimum L.
Fam. Linaceae

Synonyms: Flax Seed.
Habitat: Cultivated in many temperate and tropical countries.
Description: The seeds are brown, oval, pointed at one end, polished and about 0.5 cm long although this varies. Taste, mucilaginous, slightly unpleasant; odour, faint.
Part Used: Seeds and the oil expressed from the seed. The pericyclic fibres from the stem are used to prepare flax fibre.
Constituents: (i) Fixed oil, "linseed oil" (30–40%), consisting mainly of glycerides of linoleic and linolenic acids (ii) Mucilage, about 6% (iii) Linamarin and lotaustralin, cyanogenetic glucosides (iii) Protein, about 25% [2,37].
Medicinal Use: Demulcent, emollient, laxative, antitussive, pectoral. It is useful in bronchitis and coughs, and for internal laxative and demulcent use. Externally it may be used as poultice for burns, scalds and boils etc. The oil has a number of uses in the paint and other industries.
Regulatory Status: GSL.

LIPPIA

Lippia dulcis Trev.
Fam. Verbenaceae

Synonyms: Yerba Dulce, Cimarron.
Habitat: Mexico.
Description: Leaves, about 5 cm long, ovate, pointed, serrate above with prominent veins and glandular hairs. Taste and odour, aromatic, agreeable.

Part Used: Leaves.
Constituents: Volatile oil, about 0.3%, containing camphor. Alkaloids and saponins have been found to be absent [829].
Medicinal Use: Demulcent, expectorant.

LIPPIA CITRIODORA

Aloysia triphylla Britt.
Fam. Verbenaceae

Synonyms: Lemon Verbena, Herb Louisa, *Lippia citriodora* (Ort.) HBK, *L. triphylla* L'Her, *Verbena citriodora* Cav.
Habitat: Native to Argentina and Chile, cultivated in Europe and N. Africa and elsewhere.
Description: The leaves occur in whorls of three or four on the stem, lanceolate, about 7–10 cm long with the lateral veins almost at right angles to the midrib. Odour and taste, lemony.
Part Used: Leaves.
Constituents: (i) Volatile oil, about 0.2%, composed of about 35% citral, with cineole, limonene, dipentene, linalool, borneol, nerol and geraniol [50, 829] (ii) Mucilage, tannin, flavonoids etc [830].
Medicinal Use: Antispasmodic, sedative, antipyretic. The oil is reported to be antispasmodic in guineapigs [830].

LIQUORICE

Glycyrrhiza glabra L.
Fam. Leguminosae

Synonyms: Licorice, Spanish or Italian liquorice is *G. glabra* var *typica* Reg. et Herd., Persian or Turkish liquorice is *G. glabra* var *violacea* Boiss, Russian liquorice is *G. glabra* var *glandulifera* Waldst. et Kit. Chinese or Manchurian liquorice is from the closely related *G. uralensis* Fisch.
Habitat: Native to the Mediterranean region and parts of Asia, cultivated worldwide.
Description: Liquorice "root" is well-known. The root and stolons vary in appearance depending on origin. They are usually found cut into lengths of up to 15–20 cm and of variable diameter, stolons normally being narrower than roots. The external surface when unpeeled is dark reddish brown, longitudinally wrinkled with occasional root scars. Internally it is yellowish and fibrous, with a radiate structure; the stolons have a central pith. Liquorice is also imported into this country as extracts or blocks. Taste and odour, sweet, characteristic.
Part Used: Root, underground stem or stolon.
Constituents: (i) Triterpenes of the oleanane type, mainly glycyrrhizin (= glycyrrhizic or glycyrrhizinic acid), and its agylcone glycyrrhetinic acid (= glycyrrhitic acid), liquiritic acid, glycyrrhetol, glabrolide, iso-glabrolide, licoric acid, and phytosterols [1, 2, 5, 48, 284, 830, 831] (ii) Flavonoids and isoflavonoids; liquiritigenin, liquiritin, rhamnoliquiritin, neoliquiritin, licoflavonol, licoisoflavones A and B, licoisoflavanone, formononetin, glabrol, glabrone, glyzarin, kumatakenin and others

173

[5, 832, 833, 834, 836, 837, 838, 839] (iii) Coumarins; liqcoumarin, umbelliferone, herniarin glycyrin [5, 832, 840] (iv) Chalcones; liquiritigenin, isoliquiritigenin, neosoliquiritin, rhamnoisoliquiritin, licuraside, licochalcones A and B, echinatin and others [5,841,837] (v) Polysaccharides, mainly glucans (284) (vi) Volatile oil, containing fenchone, linalool, furfuryl alcohol, benzaldehyde and others (see [5] and references therein) (vi) Miscellaneous; starch, sugars, amino acid etc. [5].

Medicinal Use: Demulcent, antiinflammatory, expectorant, antitussive, spasmolytic. Other important uses are in the treatment of gastric and duodenal ulcers and for adrenocortical insufficiency. Liquorice has been used for thousands of years throughout the world for its medicinal properties, and recent pharmacological work has substantiated many of these and discovered new uses. The major active ingredient is glycyrrhizin, which is responsible for the sweet taste; being 50 times sweeter than sugar [284]. It is the main expectorant ingredient [842], and an 18-β derivative of glycyrrhetinic acid has an antitussive activity comparable to that of codeine [5]. Both glycyrrhizin and glycyrrhetinic acid are antiinflammatory [284, 842, 843] and antiallergic [284], helping to explain their efficacy in asthma. They have been shown to be hepatoprotective, mediating their activity through an antioxidative rather than a corticosteroid-like mechanism [844]. Liquorice is used clinically in China for liver diseases and has produced an improvement in liver function tests in hepatitis, clearing jaundice and alleviating abdominal distension, nausea and vomiting [48]. It is thought that these effects may also be due in part to the ability of glycyrrhizin to induce immune interferon in both mice and humans [845]. Liquorice has antiulcer activity and a derivative of glycyrrhetinic acid, carbenoxolone, is used clinically for ulcers, including aphthous ulcers. However, glycyrrhizin and glycyrrhetinic acid have mineralocorticoid activity [846, 284] which may result in hypokalaemia, hypertension and oedema when large doses are taken over a long period [284, 847] and this limits their use in the long term management of stomach ulcers. Extracts of deglycyrrhizinized liquorice have been prepared and in fact have a similar protective effect against experimentally induced ulcers [848], however they have not yet been clinically proven [849]. Glycyrrhizin has recently been found to have an anticariogenic activity by inhibiting bacterial growth and plaque formation; it has been suggested as a vehicle for topical oral medications [842]. Liquorice has oestrogenic activity in animals [5], this is probably due to the isoflavonoids present. Liquiritigenin and isoliquiritigenin are monoamine oxidase inhibitors *in vitro* [841] and may therefore have antidepressant activity. Liquiritin also has significant antiinflammatory activity in the rat paw oedema test [284]. Liquorice extracts inhibit histamine release in rats and appear to have a centrally-acting muscle relaxant activity [284, 850] and detoxify certain drugs such as strychnine, urethane, cocaine, mercurous chloride and picrotoxin in animals [7]. The polysaccharide fraction has immunostimulating activity [851, 852].

Preparations: Liquorice Liquid Extract BP, dose: 2–5 ml; Liquorice Extract Powder BPC 1973, dose: 0.6–2 g; Liquorice Lozenges BPC 1973; Liquorice Compound Powder BPC 1973, dose: 5–10 g.
Potter's Products: Antibron Tablets, Asthma and Bronchitis Tablets No. 153. Asthma and Bronchitis Medicinal Tea Bags.
Regulatory Status: GSL.

LIVERWORT, AMERICAN

Hepatica nobilis Mill
Fam. Ranunculaceae

Synonyms: Kidneywort, Liverleaf, *H. triloba* Chois, *Anemone hepatica* L.
Habitat: USA, and cultivated as a garden plant elsewhere.
Description: Leaves long-stalked, leathery, smooth, dark green above, rounded with three broad, angular lobes, Taste, slightly astringent and bitter; odourless.
Part Used: Herb.
Constituents: (i) Protoanemonin, which dimerizes on drying to produce anemonin (ii) Miscellaneous; anthocyanins, flavonoids and a glycoside hepatrilobin [2].
Medicinal Use: Pectoral, astringent, tonic. Has been used in disorders of the liver and indigestion. Protoanemonin has antibiotic activity.
Preparations: Liquid Extract, dose: 2–8 ml.

LIVERWORT, ENGLISH

Peltigera canina (L.) Will.
Fam. Peltigeraceae

Synonyms: Liverwort, Lichen Caninus.
Habitat: Moist, shady places in Britain and Europe.
Part Used: Plant.
Constituents: Peltigeroside [2].
Medicinal Use: Mild purgative. Formerly used for liver complaints.
Preparations: Liquid Extract, dose: 2–8 ml.

LOBELIA

Lobelia inflata L.
Fan. Campanulaceae

Synonyms: Indian Tobacco, Pukeweed.
Habitat: Eastern USA, cultivated elsewhere.
Description: Leaves pale green or yellowish, sessile, alternate, ovate-lanceolate, 3–8 cm long, with a toothed margin and pubescent lamina. The fruit consists of an inflated, ovoid or flattened bilocular capsule containing numerous small, brown, reticulate seeds. Taste, acrid; odour, faintly irritant.
Part Used: Herb, collected when the lower fruits are ripe.

175

Constituents: (i) Piperidine alkaloids, mainly lobeline, with lobelanidine, lobelanine, and minor amounts of norlobelanine (= isolobelanine), lelobanidine, lobinine, isolobinine, lobinanidine and others [853, 854, 855] (ii) Chelidonic acid (iii) Miscellaneous; resins, gums, fats etc. [5].

Medicinal Use: Respiratory stimulant, expectorant, emetic, diaphoretic, Lobelia is highly regarded for the treatment of asthma, bronchitis and as a tobacco deterrent; it is the major ingredient in many antismoking mixtures. Lobeline has similar but less potent pharmacological properties to nicotine, which helps to alleviate the withdrawal symptoms associated with stopping smoking. Lobeline stimulates respiration in animals by stimulating the respiratory centre and at high doses stimulates the vomiting centre. It has also been used as a poultice for treating boils and ulcers. In Chinese medicine *L. radicans* Thunb. (= *L. chinensis* Louv. is used for the same purposes and also to treat snake bite (where respiratory depression is involved) and jaundice [7].

Preparations: Powder, dose: 200–600 mg; Ethereal Lobelia Tincture BPC 1973, dose: 0.3–1 ml; Simple Lobelia Tincture BPC 1949, dose; 0.6–2 ml; Liquid Extract, dose: 0.2–0.6 ml.

Potter's Products: Balm of Gilead Cough Mixture, Horehound and Aniseed Cough Mixture, Vegetable Cough Remover, Antismoking Tablets.

Regulatory Status: GSL with restricted dosage.

LOGWOOD

Haematoxylon campechianum L.
Fam. Leguminosae

Synonyms: Peachwood.

Habitat: Central America, naturalized in the West Indies.

Description: The wood is normally sold in chips for dyeing purposes, it has a dark, purplish-brown colour with a greenish iridescence which indicates it has been fermented. For medicinal use the unfermented chips are preferred; these have a bright reddish brown tint.

Part Used: Wood.

Constituents: (i) Haematoxylon, a red-brown pigment, about 10% (ii) Tannin, resin and voltatile oil [4].

Medicinal Use: Astringent. Formerly used for diarrhoea and haemorrhage.

Preparations: Decoction of Logwood BPC 1934, dose: 15–60 ml; Liquid Extract of Logwood BPC 1934, dose: 2–8 ml.

LOOSESTRIFE

Lysimachia vulgaris L.
Fam. Primulaceae

Synonyms: Yellow Loosestrife, Yellow Willowherb.

Habitat: In wet places and by rivers in Britain and Europe.

Description: The herb reaches about 1 m, bearing short-stalked, oval-lanceolate leaves in whorls of two to four. The flowers are yellow, 1.5–2 cm in diameter, in axillary and terminal panicles. Taste, astringent, slightly acid; odourless.

Part Used: Herb.
Constituents: Saponins (unspecified), rutin, tannins [2].
Medicinal Use: Astringent, for nosebleeds, wounds and menorraghia; expectorant.

LOVAGE

Levisticum officinale Koch
Fam. Umbelliferae

Synonyms: Ligusticum levisticum L.

Habitat: Native to the Mediterranean region, cultivated in Britain and the USA.

Description: The plant is a perennial herb reaching 2 m or more. The leaves are divided into wedge-shaped segments, the stems hollow and the flowers are yellow, borne on umbels. The fleshy rhizome has a greyish-brown external surface and bears numerous longitudinally furrowed rootlets. The bark is thick, spongy, often with small cavities, whitish, and separated from the wood by a dark line. The wood is yellowish, radiate and shows glistening oil glands in transverse section. Taste, sweet, then slightly bitter; odour, strongly aromatic, characteristic.

Part Used: Root and rhizome.

Constituents: (i) Volatile oil, containing phthalides (about 70%), including E- and Z-butylidenephthalide, E- and Z-ligustilide, senkyunolide, isosenkyunolide, validene-4,5-dihydrophthalide, butylphthalide and others [856, 857, 858]; and terpenes such as α- and β-pinene, α- and β-phellandrene, carvacrol, etc. [5] (ii) Coumarins; bergapten, coumarin, psoralen, umbelliferone [859, 860] (iii) Miscellaneous; plant acids, e.g. butyric, isovaleric; β-sitosterol, resins, gums etc. [5].

Medicinal Use: Sedative, carminative, spasmolytic, diaphoretic, expectorant, antimicrobial. Lovage is used for dyspepsia, colic, dysmenorrhoa and cystitis, and as a gargle or mouthwash for tonsillitis and aphthous ulcers. The phthalides have sedative and anticonvulsant activity in animals [308, 861] and lovage extracts and oil are reportedly strongly diuretic in mice and rabbits [5]. Lovage is used as a flavouring in food products and alcoholic beverages.

Preparations: Liquid Extract, dose: 0.3–2 ml.

Regulatory Status: GSL.

LUCERNE

Medicago sativa L.
Fam. Leguminosae

Synonyms: Alfalfa, Purple Medick.

Habitat: Native to the Mediterranean region, cultivated widely.

Description: The herb reaches up to about 50 cm. Leaves trifoliate, leaflets obovate, with an acute apex and serrate margin, upper surface glabrous, lower surface with scattered, whitish hairs; stems hollow, ridged. Flowers papilionaceous, blue, in a raceme. Pods loosely spiral, with appressed hairs. Taste and odour, slight.

Part Used: Herb.

Constituents: (i) Isoflavones; biochanin A, daidzein, formononetin, genistein and occasionally pterocarpan phytoalexins [37, 862, 863] (ii) Coumarins; coumestrol, daphnoretin, lucernol, medicagol, sativol and trifoliol [862, 863] (iii) Alkaloids; stachydrine, homostachydrine, and in the seeds, trigonelline [5] (iv) Nutrients, including pro-vitamin A, vitamins of the B group, C, D, E, and K, folic acid, biotin and others [5] (v) Saponins based on hederagenin, medicagenic acid and soyasapogenols A, B, C, D and E [863, 864, 865, 866] (vi) Porphyrins; phaeophorbide A and chlorophyllide A [867] (vii) 4-Aminobutyric acid, in the root [868] (viii) Miscellaneous; sterols and their esters, hydrocarbons such as triacontane and their corresponding alcohols [5].

Medicinal Use: Nutrient, appetite stimulant; used to help patients put on weight during convalescence. The isoflavones are oestrogenic in animals [862, 863] and the porphyrins have been shown to have the potential to affect liver function and biliary secretion in rats, resulting in photosensitization [867]. The saponins have an anticholesterolaemic effect in monkeys [869]. Lucerne is a major animal food crop. The young sprouts are used in salads.

Regulatory Status: GSL.

LUNGMOSS

Lobaria pulmonaria (L.) Hoffm.
Fam. Stictaceae

Synonyms: Oak Lungs, Lungwort, *Sticta pulmonaria* L.

Habitat: Found on old trees and rocks throughout Europe, including Britain.

Description: The lichen is flat, greyish or greenish-brown, leathery, forked, the lobes being about 1.5 cm broad at the widest part. The inner surface is reticulate with small depressions, which are evident on the upper surface as convexities. Taste, mucilaginous bitter, slightly acrid; odour, characteristic.

Part Used: Lichen.

Constituents: (i) Stictic, sticinic, norstictic, gyrophoric, thelophoric and related acids [2, 37, 870] (ii) Fatty acids including palmitic, oleic and linoleic acids [37] (iii) Mucilage [2] (iii) Tannins [2] (iv) Miscellaneous; proteins, ergosterol, fucosterol [37].

Medicinal Use: Astringent, demulcent, expectorant, mucolytic, orexigenic. It may be taken as an infusion for coughs, asthma and bronchitis.

Preparations: Dried lichen, dose: 1–2 g; Liquid Extract, dose 1–2 ml.

LUNGWORT

Pulmonaria officinalis L.
Fam. Boraginaceae

Synonyms: Lungwort Herb.

Habitat: Shady places throughout Europe including Britain, cultivated in gardens.

Description: Leaves lanceolate, up to 60 cm long but usually much smaller, downy, spotted or blotched with white, abruptly narrowing at the base.

Part Used: Leaf.

Constituents: (i) Allantoin (ii) Flavonoids; quercetin and kaempferol (iii) Miscellaneous; tannins, mucilage, vitamin C, saponins (unspecified) [871]. Pyrrolizidine alkaloids, common in other plants of the Boraginaceae, have been shown to be absent from all samples of *Pulmonaria officinalis* tested [193].

Medicinal Use: Emollient, expectorant, antihaemorrhagic, astringent. It is used particularly for bronchitis, laryngitis and catarrh, but can also be used for diarrhoea and haemorrhoids and applied topically as a vulnerary.

Preparations: Liquid Extract, dose; 2–4 ml.

Potter's Products: Balm of Gilead Cough Mixture.

Regulatory Status: GSL.

M

MACE

Myristica fragrans Huott.
Fam. Myristicaceae

Habitat: Native to the Molucca Islands and New Guinea, introduced into Sri Lanka and the West Indies.

Description: Mace is the arillus surrounding the nutmeg; it is a brittle, semi-translucent, net-like, reddish or orange-brown structure. When pressed with the nail it exudes oil. Taste and odour, aromatic, pungent, characteristic.

Part Used: Arillus.

Constituents: Volatile oil, containing myristicin, elemene and safrole, together with monoterpene hydrocarbons such as camphene, α- and β-pinene, sabinene, cymene, α-thujene and the monoterpene alcohols linalool, geraniol, borneol and others (872, 873, 874, 875]. This is rather similar in composition to that of nutmeg (q.v.) but with higher concentrations of myristicin.

Medicinal Use: Stimulant, carminative. High doses cause intoxication and hallucinations, see Nutmeg. Mace is used as a flavouring in cookery.

MADDER

Rubia tinctorum L.
Fam. Rubiaceae

Synonyms: Dyer's Madder.

Habitat: Native to Southern Europe and parts of Asia, cultivated elsewhere.

Description: The root is normally found in commerce as short, cylindrical pieces about 4 mm in diameter, with a thin, easily detached cork, leaving a red-brown, longitudinally furrowed inner bark. The transverse section shows a pinkish-red column marked with concentric striae. Taste, sweetish, then acrid; odour, slight.

Part Used: Root.

Constituents: (i) Anthraquinone derivative, such as ruberythric acid, and its primaveroside, alizarin, and purpurin [1, 218] (ii) Asperuloside, an iridoid [876].

Medicinal Use: Formerly used for menstrual and urinary disorders and for liver diseases. For information on asperuloside see Clivers.

MAGNOLIA

Magnolia glauca L.
Fam. Magnoliaceae

Synonyms: M. virginiana L. M. acuminate, M. tripetata.

Habitat: USA, cultivated as a garden plant elsewhere.

Description: The inner bark occurs in long, fibrous strips, the outer surface rough, almost granular and pitted; the inner surface striated but almost smooth. Fracture short with the inner part tough and fibrous.

Part Used: Bark.
Constituents: Largely unknown. About 0.04% volatile oil [2].
Medicinal Use: Stimulant, tonic, aromatic, diaphoretic, antiinflammatory.
Rarely used now, although the flower buds of *M. biondii* Pamp., *M. denudata* Desr., *M. salicifolia* and other species are used in oriental medicine.
Preparations: Powder, dose: 2–4 g; Liquid Extract, dose: 2–4 ml.

MAIDENHAIR

Adiantum capillus-veneris L.
Fam. Polypodiaceae

Synonyms: Venus Hair, Rock Fern.
Habitat: Southern Europe, occasionally found further north including Britain, and parts of the USA and Canada.
Description: Fronds up to 30 cm long, two or three times pinnate, each leaflet or "pinnule" up to about 1 cm, fan-shaped, with a toothed upper margin, narrowing at the base to a short petiolule. Veins prominent, converging at the base, and spore-cases (sori) visible at the edge of the undersurface. Stems shiny, dark brown. Taste, sweetish and astringent; odour, faint.
Part Used: Fern.
Constituents: (i) Flavonoid glycosides; rutin, isoquercetin, astragalin [37], kaempferol 3,7-diglucoside and kaempferol 3-sulphate [877,878] (ii) Hydroxycinnamic acid sulphate esters, four of which have been isolated [877] (iii) Terpenoids including adiantone [37].
Medicinal Use: Expectorant, antitussive, demulcent. Maidenhair is used as an ingredient of cough and bronchial medicines, and as a hair tonic. It may be used as an infusion. An extract of the plant has diuretic and hypoglycaemic activity in animals [879, 880].
Preparations: Powder, 0.5–2 g.
Regulatory Status: GSL.

MALABAR NUT

Adhatoda vasica Nees.
Fam. Acanthaceae

Synonyms: Arusa, Adulsa, *Justicia adhatoda* L.
Habitat: India.
Description: Leaves up to 15 cm long, 4 cm broad, short-stalked, opposite, lanceolate, tapering to an acute apex with entire margins. Taste, bitter; odour, tea-like.
Part Used: Leaves.
Constituents: (i) Alkaloids; peganine (= vasicine), 6-hydroxypeganine, vasicinone, vasicoline and anisotine [881] (ii) Miscellaneous; essential oil, of undetermined composition, adhatodic acid and vasakin [881, 882].
Medicinal Use: Expectorant, febrifuge, antispasmodic. In India this drug is highly esteemed as a remedy in bronchial, asthmatic and pulmonary diseases. Extracts have been shown to inhibit salivary secretion and block

exogenous and endogenous acetylcholine and adrenaline, and to have local anaesthetic activity in animals. The oil has *in vitro* antitubercular activity [882].

Preparations: Powdered leaves, dose: 1–2 g; Tincture, dose: 2–4 ml; Liquid Extract, dose 1–2 ml.

MALE FERN

Dryopteris filix-mas (L.) Schott.
D. abbreviata (Lam & DC) Newm.
D. borrei Newm.
and hybrids and varieties
Fam. Polypodiaceae

Synonyms: Aspidium, *Aspidium fillix-mas* Sw. American Aspidium or Marginal Fern is *D. marginalis* (L.) Gray.

Habitat: Native to Europe and parts of Asia.

Description: The dried rootstock is reddish brown externally, about 4–6 cm in diameter and up to about 25 cm long, and consists of the rhizome with the bases of the fronds attached but trimmed of rootlets. The transverse section shows six to ten vascular bundles in the rhizome and the frond bases, and should be greenish in colour. Taste, sweetish then astringent, bitter and nauseous; odour, slight but unpleasant.

Part Used: Rhizome.

Constituents: (i) Phloroglucinol derivatives, a mixture known as "filicin" and composed of filicinic acid, filicylbutanone, aspidinol, albaspidin, flavaspidic acids, paraspidin and desaspidin [883, 884] (ii) Triterpenes; 9(11)-fernene, 12-hopene, 11,13(13)-hopadiene [885] (iii) Miscellaneous: n-alkanes, mainly C_{29} and C_{31}, volatile oil, resins etc. [5]. *D. marginalis* contains similar types of compounds [886].

Medicinal Use: Taenifuge, vermifuge. The main active constituents are thought to be flavaspidic acid and desaspidin [884]. Male fern is normally used in conjunction with a saline purgative to expel the parasite; however it should not be used with castor oil as this increases the absorption and toxicity. Symptoms of poisoning include nausea, vomiting, delirium, cardiac and respiratory failure.

Preparations: Powdered rhizome, dose: 1–10 g; Male Fern Extract BPC 1973, dose: 3–6 ml; Male Fern Extract Capsules BP 1958; Male Fern Extract Draught BPC 1973, dose: 50 ml.

Regulatory Status: P

MANACA

Brunfelsia hopeana (Pohl) Benth.
Fam. Solanaceae

Synonyms: Pohl, Vegetable Mercury.

Habitat: S. America, W. Indies.

Description: The root has a papery, pale-brown epidermis, in transverse section showing several concentrc rings of the xylem traversed by slender medullary rays. Taste, sweetish; odour, faintly aromatic.

Part Used: Root.

Constituents: (i) An alkaloid, manacine (ii) Flavonoids; aesculetin, manacein (iii) Gelsemic acid [2].

Medicinal Use: Alterative, diuretic, antirheumatic. May be taken by infusion.

Preparations: Liquid Extract, dose: 0.5–4 ml.

MANDRAKE, AMERICAN

Podophyllum peltatum L.
Fam. Berberidaceae

Synonyms: May Apple, Devil's Apple, Wild Lemon. Indian Podophyllum is *P. hexandrum* Royle (= *P. emodi* Wall.).

Habitat: North America.

Description: The rhizome is a reddish-brown colour and occurs in pieces up to about 20 cm long and 0.5 cm in diameter. The outer surface can be smooth or wrinkled, depending on the time of collection. Nodes, visible as swellings with stem and leaf scars, occur at intervals of 3–5 cm. Fracture, starchy or horny, revealing a whitish interior; odour, unpleasant, acrid.

Part Used: Rhizome and the resin extracted from it.

Constituents: (i) Lignans; the main one being podophyllotoxin, with the β-D-glucoside, dehydropodophyllotoxin, 4-demethylpodophyllotoxin, α- and β-peltatins and their glucosides, picropodophyllin and its β-D-glucoside and others [887, 888, 889, 890, 891] (ii) Miscellaneous; flavonoids, mainly kaempferol and quercetin and their glucosides, resin, starch, gums etc. [5]. *P. hexandrum* contains similar lignans with the exception of α-and β-peltatins, which are reportedly absent; the concentration of podophyllotoxin and its dehydro and demethyl derivatives is very much higher [889, 893, 893].

Medicinal Use: Cathartic, purgative, antineoplastic, antiviral. The resin, known as podophyllin, is used as a topical application, as an ointment or frequently dispersed in alcohol or Compound Benzoin Tincture, for venereal warts, verrucae and similar conditions. It is caustic and irritant and must be used with care. Internal administration is no longer advised, particularly during pregnancy, due to the cytotoxicity. Podophyllin and podophyllotoxin are embryocidal in animals and fatalities in humans have been recorded after ingestion. A derivative of podophyllotoxin, etoposide, is used clinically for the treatment of certain cancers. A considerable research is being carried out into the development of new antitumour drugs based on these lignans, which is beyond the scope of this book; for review see [894].

Preparations: Podophyllum Resin BP; Compound Podophyllum Paint BP; Podophyllum Tincture BPC 1949.

Regulatory Status: POM.

MANNA

Fraxinus ornus L.
Fam. Oleaceae

Habitat: Southern Europe and parts of Asia.
Description: A saccharine exudation from the incised bark of the tree. Pale yellowish or whitish pieces, irregular on one side and smoother and curved on the other. Taste, sweet, honey-like, without bitterness; odour, slight.
Part Used: Exhudation.
Constituents: Mannitol, 40–60% [4].
Medicinal Use: Nutritive, mild laxative.

MAPLE, RED

Acer rubrum L.
Fam. Sapindaceae

Synonyms: Swamp Maple.
Habitat: America.
Description: Long, quilled pieces, externally blackish-brown, slightly polished, with numerous transverse lenticels and scattered, brownish, small warts. Inner bark very tough and fibrous, pale reddish brown or buff. Taste, astringent and slightly bitter.
Part Used: Bark.
Constituents: Unknown.
Medicinal Use: Formerly used by the American Indians as an application for sore eyes, because of its astringency.

MARIGOLD

Calendula officinalis L.
Fam. Compositae

Synonyms: Marybud, Calendula, Gold-bloom, *Caltha officinalis.*
Habitat: A common garden plant.
Description: Flowerheads bright yellow or orange. Ligulate florets, usually detached from the ovary, are used; these are 15–25 mm long and about 3 mm broad, one to three toothed with four or five veins and an entire margin, with a short corolla tube containing the bifid stigma and style. Taste, saline, slightly bitter; odour, faint.
Part Used: Petals, flowerheads.
Constituents: (i) Triterpenes, pentacyclic alcohols such as faradol, brein, arnidiol, erythrodiol, calenduladiol, heliantriol C and F, ursatriol, longispinogenine; the calendulosides A–D (in the root at least); α- and β-amyrin, taraxasterol, τ-taraxasterol and lupeol [895, 896, 897, 898, 899] (ii) Flavonoids; isorhamnetin glycosides including narcissin, and quercetin glycosides including rutin [386] (iii) Volatile oil (iv) Chlorogenic acid [386].
Medicinal Use: Antiinflammatory, spasmolytic, antihaemorrhagic, styptic, vulnerary, antiseptic. Internally it may be taken as an infusion for stomach disorders, gastric and duodenal ulcers and dysmenorrhoea; and externally as a lotion or ointment for cuts and bruises, nappy rash, sore nipples,

burns, scalds etc. An alcoholic extract has been shown to have *in vitro* antitrichomonal activity [900].

Preparations: Liquid Extract, dose 1–4 ml; Tincture BPC 1934, dose: 0.3–1.2 ml.

Potter's Products: Special Formula Stomach Tablets DI.

Regulatory Status: GSL.

MARJORAM

Origanum majorana L.
Fam. Labiatae

Synonyms: Sweet Marjoram, *O. hortensis* Moensch. Wild Marjoram, or Origano, is *O. vulgare* L.

Habitat: Native to the Mediterranean region, cultivated widely in gardens.

Description: The herb grows to about 25 cm high, branched above, with opposite, small, oval leaves up to about 1.5 cm long and 1 cm broad. The flowers are white or pink, small, almost hidden by green bracts, and arranged in small rounded spikes. Taste and odour, pleasant, aromatic, characteristic.

Part Used: Herb.

Constituents: (i) Volatile oil, up to 3%, composed of *cis-* and *trans*-sabinene hydrate, sabinene, linalool, carvacrol, 4-terpineol, α- and γ-terpinene, estrogole, eugenol and others [5] (ii) Flavonoids; luteolin-7-glucoside, diosmetin-7-glucoside and apigenin-7-glucoside (iii) Miscellaneous; rosmarinic acid, caffeic acid, triterpenoids such as ursolic acid, oleanolic acid, sterols; vitamins A and C etc. [5, 901]. *O. vulgare* contains volatile oil with a widely varying composition; major components include thymol, β-bisabolene, caryophyllene, linalool and borneol. Other constituents are similar to those of *O. majorana* [5].

Medicinal Use: Stimulant, antispasmodic, emmenagogue, diaphoretic. Extracts have been shown to have antioxidative and antiviral activity [99, 902]; this is probably due to the flavonoids and rosmarinic acid. Marjoram is almost always used as a culinary flavouring rather than a medicine.

Regulatory Status: GSL.

MARSHMALLOW

Althaea officinalis L.
Fam. Malvaceae

Habitat: Europe including Britain, naturalized in the United States.

Description: A downy perennial reaching up to 2 m. Leaves broadly ovate or cordate, 10–20 cm long and about 10 cm wide, with 3–7 rounded lobes, palmate veins and a crenate margin. The flowers are pink, five petalled, up to 3 cm in diameter. The root as it appears in commerce is dried, fibrous, cream-white when peeled, deeply furrowed longitudinally and with some root scars. Taste, sweet, mucilaginous; odour slight.

Part Used: Leaves, root.

Constituents: In the root: (i) Mucilage, 18–35%; consisting of a number of polysaccharides; one is composed of L-rhamnose, D-galactose, D-galacturonic acid and D-glucuronic acid in the ratio 3:2:3:3 [903], another a highly branched L-arabifuranan [904], another a trisaccharide structural unit [905] and one with a high proportion of uronic acid units [906] (ii) Miscellaneous; about 35% pectin, 1–2% asparagine, tannins [183]. In the leaves: (i) Mucilage; including a low molecular weight D-glucan [907] (ii) Flavanoids such as kaempferol, quercetin and diosmetin glucosides (iii) Scopoletin, a coumarin (v) Polyphenolic acids, including syringic, caffeic, salicyclic, vanillic, *p*-coumaric etc. [908].

Medicinal Use: Demulcent, emollient, expectorant. Both the leaves and root are used for coughs and bronchial complaints and for gastritis, enteritis, peptic ulcer and gastric inflammation in general, and for urinary inflammation and cystitis. They may be used externally as a soothing poultice and vulnerary, usually in the form of an ointment, for boils, ulcers and abscesses. The mucilages have proven biological activity including the stimulation of phagocytosis *in vitro* [903] and hypoglycaemic activity in mice [905]. Extracts of Marshmallow root are used to make confectionery.

Preparations: Liquid Extract (Leaves), dose: 2–5 ml; Liquid Extract (Root), dose: 2–5 ml; Marshmallow Syrup BPC 1949, dose: 2–8 ml.

Potter's Products: Special Formula Stomach Tablets D1, Special Formula Stomach Tablets D4, Tonsillitis Mixture No. 145, Brown Marshmallow Ointment, Mallow and Slippery Elm Drawing Ointment.

Regulatory Status: GSL.

MASTERWORT
Peucedanum ostruthium (L.) Koch
Fam. Umbelliferae

Synonyms: Imperatoria ostruthium L.

Habitat: Parts of Europe but rare in Britain, Australia.

Description: Rhizome cylindrical, compressed, 5–10 cm long and 1–2 cm in thickness, with nodes at intervals of about 1.5 cm and few scattered roots; some pieces terminating in slender, smooth, underground suckers. Fracture short, hard and tough. Taste and odour, aromatic, pungent.

Part Used: Rhizome.

Constituents: (i) Volatile oil, 0.2–1.4%, containing about 95% terpenes, including α-pinene, *d*-phellandrene, *d*-limonene etc. [2] (ii) Furocoumarins; peucedanin, oxypeucadanin, imperatorin, isoimperatorin and osthol [2, 909] (iii) Flavonoids, including hesperidin [2] (iv) Phthalides (unspecified) [910].

Medicinal Use: Stimulant, antispasmodic, carminative. Has been used for asthma, flatulence, dyspepsia and menstrual complaints. The furocoumarins may cause photosensitization [909].

Preparations: Liquid Extract, dose: 4–8 ml.

Regulatory Status: GSL.

MASTIC

Pistacia lentiscus L.
Fam. Anacardiaceae

Habitat: Greece, Cyprus.

Description: The resin occurs in small, rounded or pear-shaped, transparent tears which, when masticated, forms a dough-like mass. Taste and odour, cedar-like.

Part Used: Resin.

Constituents: (i) Resins; α- and β-masticoresins (ii) Volatile oil, about 2%, containing pinene [2].

Medicinal Use: Has been used in dentistry for filling teeth.

MATICO

Piper angustifolia R. and P.
Fam. Piperaceae

Synonyms: Matica, *Artanthe elongata* Miq.

Habitat: S. America.

Description: Leaves usually occur broken in commerce, recognizable by the reticulate surface, convexly on the upper surface due to deeply sunk veins, which are prominent on the lower surface. The under surface is also hairy. Taste and odour, aromatic, tea-like.

Part Used: Leaves.

Constituents: (i) Essential oil containing camphor, borneol, azulene (ii) Tannins, resins etc. [2].

Medicinal Use: Astringent, stimulant, diuretic, styptic. Used for leucorrhoea, haemorrhage, piles etc.

Preparations: Powder, dose: 2–8 g; Tincture BPC 1923, dose: 4–8 ml; Liquid Extract Matico BPC 1923, dose: 2–8 ml.

MAYWEED

Anthemis cotula L.
Fam. Compositae

Synonyms: Stinking Mayweed, Dog Chamomile, *Maruta cotula* DC, *M. foetida* Cass.

Habitat: Europe, including Britain.

Description: The herb resembles Chamomile in appearance, but the flowers have no membranous scales at the base and the outer florets no styles. Taste and odour, unpleasant, acrid.

Part Used: Herb.

Constituents: (i) Sesquiterpene lactones; anthecotulide and several of its dehydro and dihydro derivatives [911].

Medicinal Use: Antispasmodic, emmanagogue, emetic. Has been used for amenorrhoea and sick headaches. Anthecotulide is a potent allergen, and this species, when misidentified as Chamomile, has been responsible for causing allergies in humans [912].

MEADOW LILY

Lilium candidium L.
Fam. Liliaceae

Synonyms: White Lily, Madonna Lily.

Habitat: Native to Southern Europe, cultivated in gardens in Britain and the US.

Description: The bulb consists of free, fleshy scales, lanceolate and curved, about 3 cm long and 1 cm broad in the centre. Taste, mucilaginous, bitter and unpleasant.

Part Used: Bulb.

Constituents: Unknown. The aerial parts contain a flavonoid alkaloid called lilanine [913] and a flavonoid lilyn [914].

Medicinal Use: Demulcent, astringent. Has been used internally for female complaints and dropsy, and externally as a poultice for ulcers, inflammation etc. A total extract stimulates phagocytosis in mice [80].

MEADOWSWEET

Filipendula ulmaria (L.) Maxim
Fam. Rosaceae

Synonyms: Queen-of-the-Meadow, Bridewort, *Spireaea ulmaria* L.

Habitat: A common wild plant in Britain, throughout Europe, parts of Asia and an espacape in N. America.

Description: Leaves long-stalked, pinnate, with 2–5 pairs of toothed leaflets more than 2 cm long, and small leaflets in between. Stipules green above, downy beneath. Flowers in dense clusters, creamy, with 5 or 6 petals, 2–5 mm across. Taste, astringent and slightly aromatic.

Part Used: Herb.

Constituents: (i) Volatile oil; containing salicylaldehyde (ca. 75%), ethylsalicylate, methylsalicylate, methoxybenzaldehyde and others [915] (ii) Phenolic glycosides; spiraein, monotropin, gaultherin [37, 916, 917] (iii) Flavonoids; spiraeoside, rutin, hyperoside, avicularin [386, 421, 917] (iv) Polyphenolics; the major one of which has a molecular weight of 1877, and other tannins, mainly hydrolysable tannides [918, 919] (v) Miscellaneous; chalcones (unspecified), phenylcarboxylic acids, traces of coumarin, ascorbic acid [917, 916].

Medicinal Use: Stomachic, antacid, astringent, antirheumatic. Decoctions of meadowsweet have antiulcer effects against a variety of experimental ulcerogenic procedures, including aspirin and ethanol (but not histamine) induced, in rats [916,920]; obviously the phenolic glycosides and volatile oil are not exerting the same effects as other salicylates in these preparations (see [4] for more information on this). Extracts also have other properties including lowering of motor activity, increasing the tonus of isolated guineapig and rabbit intestine and uterus [915, 921]. The tannins are bactericidal *in vitro* against *Corynebacterium diphtheriae*, *Shigella dysentericae* and *Diplococcus pneumoniae* [922].

Preparations: Liquid Extract, dose: 2–4 ml.

Potter's Products: Acidosis Tablets, Gastritis Mixture No. 112A.

Regulatory Status: GSL.

MELILOT
Melilotus officinalis (L.) Pallas.
Fam. Leguminosae

Synonyms: Ribbed Melilot, Common Melilot, King's Clover, Yellow Sweet Clover, *M. arvensis* Willd.

Habitat: Grows on bare and waste ground throughout Europe.

Description: An erect biennial reaching up to about 1 m. Leaves pinnately trifoliate, the upper ones being longer and narrowed at both ends. The yellow flowers are in axillary racemes, typically papilionaceous with the keel shorter than the wings, 5–6 cm long. The pod is 3–5 mm long, ribbed and hairless. Odour, like new-mown hay, due to the coumarin.

Part Used: Herb.

Constituents: (i) Coumarin derivatives; the glycoside melilotoside, which hydrolyses on drying to produce free coumarin, dihydrocoumarin, melilotin, melilotic acid and melilotol. Dicoumarol (= melitoxin) is produced when melilot has spoiled and fermentation has taken place (386, 339, 923] (ii) Flavonoids; robinin and others [924], tannin etc.

Medicinal Use: Aromatic, carminative, spasmolytic. Flower and leaf extracts have shown analgesic activity, prolongation in pentobarbital induced hypnosis time and smooth muscle relaxant activity in mice; they are also hypotensive and vasodilatory in rabbits [925]. Dicoumarol is a potent anticoagulant and should be present only at very low levels.

MESCAL BUTTONS
Lophophora williamsii (Lemaire) Coult.
Fam. Cactaceae

Synonyms: Peyote, Peyotl, Pellote, Anhalonium. This is the "Sacred Mushroom" of the Aztecs.

Habitat: Mexico, parts of the southern US.

Description: The dried cactus is cut into slices about 2–5 cm in diameter and 0.5–1 cm thick, hence the name. Fracture, short and horny, pale brown. Taste, gritty, mucilaginous, pungent and bitter.

Part Used: Cactus stem.

Constituents: Alkaloids, the main one being mescaline; with N-acetyl mescaline, N-methyl mescaline, anhalamine, anhalidine, lophophorine and many others. See [1, 112, 926, 927] and references therein.

Medicinal Use: Hallucinogen, emetic. Of little medicinal value but is used illicitly as a narcotic and hallucinogen. See [927] for full review.

Regulatory Status: CD. (Misuse of Drugs Act 1973). POM.

MEZEREON
Daphne mezereum L.
D. gnidium L.
D. laureola L.
Fam. Thymeliaceae

Synonyms: Spurge Olive, Spurge Laurel.

Habitat: Native to Europe, cultivated elsewhere as an ornamental.

Description: The root is brownish, very tough, with the outer bark peeling off easily to leave the fibrous inner bark. Taste, acrid and caustic; odour unpleasant when fresh.

Part Used: Root, root bark, bark.

Constituents: Diterpene ortho esters; daphnetoxin, mezerein and other related compounds [928, 929, 440] and references therein.

Medicinal Use: The orthoesters are co-carcinogenic and mezerein has antileukaemic activity [930, 931]; they are currently of great scientific interest. Mezereon can no longer be recommended for medicinal use but was formerly taken as a stimulant, alterative and antirheumatic.

MILK THISTLE

Silybum marianum (L.) Gaertn.
Fam. Compositae

Synonyms: Marian Thistle, Mediterranean Milk Thistle, *Carduus marianus.*

Habitat: Throughout Europe, rare in Britain.

Description: Leaves spiny, dark green with a crenate margin and conspicuous white veins. Flowerheads rayless, purple, solitary with sepal-like bracts ending in sharp yellow spines. Taste and odour, slight.

Part Used: Seeds, aerial parts.

Constituents: (i) Flavolignans; the mixture of these is known as "silymarin" and composed mainly of silybin (= silibinin), with isosilybin, dihydrosilybin, silydianin, silychristin, and in some varieties at least, silandrin, silymonin, silyhermin and neosilyhermin [932, 933, 934, 935, 68] and references therein.

Medicinal Use: Hepatoprotective. Milk thistle was formerly used in this country for nursing mothers, as a bitter tonic, demulcent, as an antidepressant, for liver complaints, and for the same purposes as Holy Thistle (q.v.); in Germany it has been used extensively for liver diseases and jaundice and this is the most important use today. Silymarin has been shown conclusively to exert an antihepatotoxic effect in animals against a variety of toxins, particularly those of the death cap mushroom *Amanita phalloides* [935, 936, 937, 68]. This mushroom is sometimes eaten after mistaken identification, although not normally by the British who are unadventurous with food, and contains some of the most potent liver toxins known. These are the amatoxins and the phallotoxins, both of which cause haemorrhagic necrosis of the liver, with the amatoxins being the most poisonous [937]. Pretreatment of animals with silymarin and silybin gives 100% protection against this type of poisoning [936, 937], and when silybin was given by intravenous injection to human patients up to 48 hours after ingestion of the death cap it was found to be highly effective in preventing fatalities [938]. Silymarin has been used successfully to treat patients with chronic hepatitis and cirrhosis [939, 940]; it is active against hepatitis B virus [941], is hypolipidaemic and lowers fat deposits in the liver in animals [942].

Preparations: Silymarin, dose: 420 mg daily.

MISTLETOE

Viscum album L.

Fam. Loranthaceae

Synonyms: European Mistletoe, Birdlime Mistletoe.

Habitat: A parasite growing on deciduous trees, particularly fruit trees and poplars, throughout Europe.

Description: Woody, regularly branched, with elliptical, yellowish-green, leathery leaves in pairs; monoecious, inconspicuous four-petalled flowers, followed by sticky, white, globular berries in winter.

Part Used: Young leafy twigs.

Constituents: (i) Glycoproteins; the mistletoe lectins I, II and III and viscumin [943, 944, 945] (ii) Polypeptides; the viscotoxins I, II, III and IVB [946] (iii) Flavonoids; usually quercitin-derived and dependent on the host tree to some extent [947] (iv) Phenylcarboxylic acids; e.g. caffeic and gentisic [947] (v) Polysaccharides, in the berries, one of which is viscic acid [948, 949] (vi) Alkaloids, in a Korean variety *V. album coloratum* [950] (vii) Lignans; syringin, syringaresinol 4,4''-diglucoside (= eleutheroside E) and others [951]. For review, see [953], and for protein constituents of other species see [954].

Medicinal Use: Hypotensive, cardiac tonic, immunostimulant, antineo-plastic, sedative, antispasmodic. Mistletoe is used for high blood pressure and tachycardia, as a nervine and for certain cancers. The cardiotonic activity is thought to be due to the lignans, which show significant cAMP-phosphodiesterase inhibitory activity [951]. The polysaccharides stimulate the immune response in mice [949] and a commercial preparation of mistletoe increased antibody production in rats stimulated with antigen after irradiation [954]. The antineoplastic activity of mistletoe is well documented [943, 944, 946, 952, 955]. The viscotoxins bind to DNA and viscumin inhibits protein synthesis [955], and the alkaloids, where present, have antileukaemic activity *in vitro* and in mice [950]. A commercial preparation has been used in Europe to treat several types of cancer. It is a study of 50 patients with malignant pleural effusions, the exudation disappeared in a remarkable 92% of patients after 3–4 treatments [956]; in another study on the prophylactic, postoperative treatment of carcinoma of the bronchial tree, patients showed a significant prolongation of survival time [957]. A group of women with advanced carcinoma of the ovary, treated with a mistletoe preparation, showed much better survival times than a similar group treated with a con-ventional therapy, despite the less favourable prognosis of the group treated with mistletoe. Side effects were said not to be serious [958].

Preparations: Powder, dose: 2–6 g; Liquid Extract, dose: 1–3 ml; Tincture BPC, dose: 0.5 ml.

Potter's Products: Cardivallin Tablets, Mistletoe and Scullcap Nerve Tablets High Blood Pressure Mixture.

Regulatory Status: Berries P.

MONSONIA

Monsonia ovata Cav.
Fam. Geraniaceae

Habitat: S. Africa.

Description: Leaves opposite, very small, stalked, ovate, serrate, with filiform stipules. Flowers white, axillary, geranium-like, either solitary or occasionally in pairs on one peduncle. Stems branched, with slender spreading hairs, up to 30 cm long. Taste, astringent, slightly aromatic.

Part Used: Whole plant.

Constituents: Undetermined.

Medicinal Use: Astringent; formerly used for acute and chronic diarrhoea and ulcerated lower bowel.

MOTHERWORT

Leonurus cardiaca L.
Fam. Labiatae

Synonyms: Lion's Tail.

Habitat: Grows in waste places throughout Europe and occasionally in Britain.

Description: Leaves stalked, palmately 5–7 lobed, serrate, downy on the undersurface with prominent, reticulate veins. Stems unbranched, quadrangular. Flowers downy, pinkish-purple or white, the lower lip spotted purple, about 12 mm long, in axillary whorls. Taste, very bitter; odour, slight.

Part Used: Herb.

Constituents: (i) Iridoids; leonuride and others not yet identified [959, 62] (ii) Diterpenes of the labdane type, such as leocardin, a mixture of two epimers of 8β-acetoxy-9α,13α,15,16-bisepoxy-15-hydroxy-7-oxo-labdan-6β,19-olide [960] (iii) Flavonoids; rutin, quinqueloside, genkwanin, quercetin, quercitrin, isoquercitrin, hyperoside, and apigenin and kaempferol glucosides [961, 962] (iv) Caffeic acid 4-rutinoside [963].

Medicinal Use: Cardiac tonic, sedative, nervine, antispasmodic, emmenagogue. Studies in China have shown that extracts have antiplatelet aggregation actions and decrease the levels of blood lipids [964, 965]; they also have an inhibitory effect on pulsating myocardial cells *in vitro* [966]. These preliminary investigations indicate that the long established use of Motherwort in cardiac conditions may be scientifically valid.

Preparations: Powder, dose: 2–4 g; Liquid Extract, dose: 2–4 ml.

Potter's Products: Cardivallin Tablets, Blood Pressure Tablets No. 400.

Regulatory Status: GSL.

MOUNTAIN ASH

Pyrus aucuparia (L.) Gaertn.
Fam. Rosaceae

Synonyms: Rowan Tree, Witchen, *Sorbus aucuparia* L.

Habitat: Europe and the British Isles, particularly at high altitudes.

Description: A well-known tree. The fruit is scarlet, globular, 6–9 mm in diameter, with calyx teeth at the apex. The bark is greyish, smooth, with a soft, spongy outer layer and a short, granular fracture.

Part Used: Berries, bark.

Constituents: A glycoside of parasorbic acid, an α,β- unsaturated lactone [824].

Medicinal Use: Astringent, antibiotic. Either the glycoside, or the parasorbic acid formed by enzymatic hydrolysis, is the antibiotic principle [824]. The ripe berries have been used as a gargle in sore throats and tonsillitis, and a decoction of the bark for diarrhoea etc.

MOUNTAIN FLAX

Linum catharticum L.
Fam. Linaceae

Synonyms: Purging Flax.

Habitat: A wild British and European plant growing in meadows.

Description: Leaves opposite, small, the lower ones obovate, the upper lanceolate, with entire margins. Flowers small, white, with 5 pointed petals, serrate sepals, arranged in a loose panicle. Taste, bitter and acrid; odourless.

Part Used: Herb.

Constituents: (i) Volatile oil, about 0.15% (ii) Linin, a bitter substance (iii) Tannin [2].

Medicinal Use: Laxative, diuretic, antirheumatic.

Preparations: Liquid Extract, dose: 2–4 ml.

Regulatory Status: GSL.

MOUNTAIN GRAPE

Berberis aquifolium Pursh.
Fam. Berberidaceae

Synonyms: Oregon Grape, Holly-leaved Berberis, *Mahonia aquifolia* Nutt.

Habitat: N. America, cultivated as a garden plant elsewhere.

Description: The plant grows to about 2 m in height, producing bright green, spiny, leathery leaves and small yellow flowers. The root is about 1–4 cm in diameter, with a thin, yellowish or brownish grey bark, longitudinally wrinkled, greenish yellow internally; and a hard, yellowish wood with numerous medullary rays. Taste, bitter; odourless.

Part Used: Root, rhizome.

Constituents: Alkaloids of the isoquinoline type; berberine, berbamine, hydrastine, oxycanthine [112].

Medicinal Use: Alterative, tonic, cholagogue, antidiarrhoeal. Mountain grape is used for gastritis and skin diseases such as psoriasis and eczema as well as for similar purposes to Barberry; it contains similar alkaloids. For pharmacological actions of these, see Barberry.

Preparations: Liquid Extract, dose: 1–2 ml.

MOUNTAIN LAUREL

Kalmia latifolia L.
Fam. Ericaceae

Synonyms: Sheep Laurel, Lambkill, Spoonwood.
Habitat: USA.
Description: An evergreen shrub. Leaves broadly lanceolate, leathery, about 6 cm long and 3 cm broad, with narrowly reflexed margins and a prominent midrib. Taste, astringent and slightly bitter; odour, slight.
Part Used: Leaves.
Constituents: (i) Hydroquinone glycosides including arbutin (ii) Andromedatoxin (iii) Phlorizin [2].
Medicinal Use: Cardiac sedative, astringent. Has been used for febrile conditions, inflammation, diarrhoea and haemorrhage. Large doses are toxic. For information on arbutin see Uva-ursi.

MOUSE EAR

Pilosella officinarum C. H and F. W. Schultz
Fam. Compositae

Synonyms: Mouse Ear Hawkweed, *Hieraceum pilosella* L.
Habitat: A common British and European plant growing in sandy soil.
Description: A small creeping plant giving off leafy runners. The leaves are lanceolate, about 3 cm long, greyish above with scattered slender hairs and whitish underneath due to the dense covering of branched hairs. Flowers solitary, pale yellow, composite, about 2–3 cm diameter, outer florets often reddish underneath. Taste, bitter; odour, faint.
Part Used: Herb.
Constituents: (i) Umbelliferone, a coumarin (ii) Flavonoids including luteolin and its glycosides (iii) Caffeic and chlorogenic acids [967, 968].
Medicinal Use: Expectorant, diuretic, spasmolytic, sialogoge, vulnerary. It is used mainly for whooping cough, bronchitis and asthma as an infusion, and for wounds as a compress. An extract shows weak antifungal activity [969].
Preparations: Liquid Extract, dose: 2–4 ml.
Regulatory Status: GSL.

MUGWORT

Artemisia vulgaris L.
Fam. Compositae

Synonyms: Felon Herb.
Habitat: Grows in waste places throughout Europe.
Description: A downy perennial reaching about 1.5 m in height. Leaves pinnatisect, with five to seven lobes, deeply incised, serrate, dark green and almost hairless on the upper surface and silvery and downy underneath. Flowers yellowish or purplish brown, rayless, in branched spikes. Taste, bitter; odour, aromatic.
Part Used: Herb.

Constituents: (i) Volatile oil, containing linalool, 1,8-cineole, β-thujone, borneol, α- and β-pinene, nerol, neryl acetate, linalyl acetate, myrcene, vulgarole, α-, β- and γ-cadinol, cadinenol, muurolol, spathulenol and others [970, 971, 972] (ii) Vulgarin, a sesquiterpene lactone [37] (iii) Flavonoids; quercetin-3-glucoside, quercetin-3-rhamnoglucoside and 5,3'-dihydroxy-3,7,4'-trimethoxyflavone [973, 974] (iv) Coumarin derivatives; 7,8-methylendioxy-9-methoxycoumarin [974] (v) Triterpenes such as 3β-hydroxurs-12-en-27,28-dionic acid, β-amyrin, β-sitosterol [974, 37].

Medicinal Use: Emmenagogue, diaphoretic, choleretic, anthelmintic, diuretic, stomachic, orexigenic. Mugwort is taken as an infusion for amenorrhoea, anorexia and dyspepsia, and less often for threadworm or roundworm infestation. Used in Chinese medicine for nausea and vomiting. The oil is antimicrobial to some extent [975] but is irritant to the skin [48]. Should not be taken during pregnancy.

Preparations: Liquid Extract, dose: 2–4 ml.

Regulatory Status: GSL.

MUIRA-PUAMA

Liriosma ovata Miers.
Fam. Oleaceae

Habitat: Brazil.

Description: The root in commerce usually occurs as hard, tough fibrous, light brown, woody splinters, 5–8 cm long and about 0.5–1 cm across, without any root bark. Taste, slightly astringent; odourless.

Part Used: Root.

Constituents: Active compounds unknown. Esters of behenic acid, lupeol and phytosterols are present [2].

Medicinal Use: Aphrodisiac, astringent. Used for impotence and diarrhoea.

Preparations: Liquid Extract, dose: 0.5–5 ml.

Regulatory Status: GSL.

MULBERRY

Morus nigra L.
M. alba L.
Fam. Moraceae

Synonyms: Black or Purple Mulberry (= *M. nigra*), White Mulberry, (= *M. alba*).

Habitat: Both are cultivated worldwide in temperate regions.

Description: The fruit of the black mulberry resembles that of the blackberry, except that the remains of the calyx can be seen on each fleshy lobe of the fruit. Taste and odour, pleasant, characteristic.

Part Used: Fruit, leaves, root bark.

Constituents: *M. nigra* fruit: Invert sugar, pectin, fruit acids, vitamin C [2]. *M. alba*, leaves: (i) Flavonoids; rutin, moracetin (ii) Anthocyanins; cyanidin and delphinidin glucosides [33] (iii) Artocarpin, cycloartocarpin and analogues [976], root bark: (i) Flavonoids; including the kuwanons, sangennons, mulberrosides and mulberrofurans [977,978 and references therein].

Medicinal Use: Fruit; nutrient, refrigerant, mild laxative. Leaves and rootbark; diuretic, hypotensive, expectorant. Extracts of *M. alba* are hypoglycaemic, slightly antispasmodic and hypotensive in rats [33, 978]. The kuwanons, mulberrosides and sangennons have differing effects on platelet cyclooxygenase and lipoxygenase, see [978].

Preparations: Fruit; Syrup of Mulberry BPC 1934, dose: 2–5 ml.

Biblical Reference: 2 Samuel 5 : 23–24; 1 Chronicles 14 : 14–15; Luke 17 : 6.

MULLEIN

Verbascum thapsus L.
V. thapsiforme Schrad.
V. phlomoides L.
Fam. Scrophulariaceae

Synonyms: Aarons Rod, Great Mullein (= *V. thapsus*.) Orange Mullein (= *V. phlomoides*).

Habitat: *V. thapsus* is native to Britain, the other spp. to Europe and parts of Asia.

Description: *V. thapsus:* a stout perennial, covered with thick, woolly down, usually unbranched. Leaves broadly lanceolate, crenate, with a decurrent base, stems winged. Flowers yellow, almost flat, 15–30 mm in diameter. Taste, mucilaginous and slightly bitter; odour, faint.

Part Used: Herb.

Constituents: *V. thapsus* has not been well investigated. It contains mucilage, flavonoids such as verbascoside, hesperidin, saponins, volatile oil, tannins [2,37]. *V. thapsiforme:* Iridoid glycosides: aucubin, catalpol, isocatalpol, methylcatalpol, 6-O-β-D-xylopyranosyl catalpol [979] (ii) Flavonoids; rutin, hesperidin and others [386].

Medicinal Use: Expectorant, demulcent, diuretic, emollient, vulnerary. Mullein is used particularly for bronchitis and catarrh and externally for inflammation and to aid wound healing. Gerard has an interesting recipe: "the yellow flowers being steeped in oil and set in warm dung until they be washed into the oil and consumed away, to be a remedy for piles".

Preparations: Liquid Extract, dose: 2–5 ml.

Regulatory Status: GSL.

MUSKSEED

Abelmoschus moschatus Medic.
Fam. Malvaceae

Synonyms: Ambrette Seed, Muskmallow, *Hibiscus abelmoschus* L.

Habitat: Indigenous to India, cultivated elsewhere in the tropics.

Description: The seeds are kidney-shaped, compressed, about 3 mm in diameter, greyish brown, with numerous striations which are concentric around the hilum. Taste, oily; odour, musky.

Part Used: Seed.

Constituents: (i) Oil, containing ambrettolide, ambrettolic acid, (Z)-5-tetradecen-14-olide, (Z)-5-tetradecenyl acetate and (Z)-5-dodecenyl acetate and farnesol [980] (ii) Phospholipids such as α-cephalin, phosphotidylserine and others [981].

Medicinal Use: Stimulant, aromatic, antispasmodic, insecticide. Used more often as a perfume and cosmetic ingredient.

MUSTARD
BLACK MUSTARD
WHITE MUSTARD

Brassica nigra (L.) Koch.
B. juncea (L.) Czern et Coss.
Sinapsis alba L.
Fam. Cruciferae

Synonyms: Black Mustard: Brown Mustard, *S. juncea* (*B. juncea*); White Mustard: *B. alba* L., *B. hirta* Moench.

Habitat: *B. nigra* and *S. alba* are cultivated in Europe and the USA, *B. juncea* in India.

Description: The seeds are globular, 1–2 mm in diameter, with white mustard seeds being up to 2.5 mm diameter. Taste and odour when ground, strong, pungent, characteristic.

Part Used: Seed.

Constituents: (i) Glucosinolates; black mustard contains sinigrin, which on hydrolysis by the enzyme myrosin produces allyisothiocyanate, and white mustard sinalbin, which produces *p*-hydroxybenzyl isothiocyanate (ii) Miscellaneous; sinapine, sinapic acid, fixed oil, protein, mucilage etc. For further information and references see [1,5].

Medicinal Use: Rubefacient, counter-irritant, stimulant, diuretic, emetic. Usually used medicinally as an external application for rheumatic pains, bronchitis etc. It must be used with caution. All types of mustard are used as condiments and flavourings.

Preparations: Volatile Oil of Mustard BPC 1949.

Regulatory Status: Volatile Oil: GSL for external use only (at restricted strength).

Biblical Reference: Matthew 13:31 and 17:20; Mark 4:31; Luke 13:19 and 17:6.

MYROBALANS

Terminalia chebula Retz.
Fam. Combretaceae

Synonyms: Black Chebulic.

Habitat: India.

Description: The immature fruits of a large tree, roundish or ovate in shape and about the size of a hazel nut, larger and pointed when ripe.

Part Used: Fruit.

Constituents: (i) Sennoside A, and anthraquinone glycoside [982] (ii) Tannins, ellagic and gallic acids (iii) Chebulic acid (iv) Fixed oil [2].

Medicinal Use: Astringent, laxative; like Rhubarb (q.v.) it has both cathartic and astringent properties. This has been known for centuries, it is now explained by the constituents, the well-known laxative sennoside A (for actions, see Senna) and the astringent tannins.

MYRRH

Commiphora molmol Engl.
C. abyssinica (Berg.) Engl.
and possibly other *Commiphora* spp.
Fam. Burseraceae

Synonyms: *Balsamodendron myrrha* Nees. Guggal Gum or Resin, "Guggulu" is from *C. mukul* Hook ex Stocks.

Habitat: North east Africa and Arabia. *C. mukul* is of Indian origin.

Description: The oleo-gum resin exudes from fissures or incisions in the bark and is collected as irregular masses or tears, varying in colour from yellowish to reddish brown, often with white patches. The surface may be oily or covered with fine dust. Taste, bitter and acrid; odour aromatic.

Part Used: Oleo-gum Resin.

Constituents: (i) Volatile oil, containing heerabolene, cadinene, elemol, eugenol, cuminaldehyde, numerous furanosesquiterpenes including furanodiene, furanodienone, curzerenone, lindestrene, 2-methoxy furanodiene and other derivatives [983, 984, 985, 986, 987] (ii) Resins including α-, β- and γ-commiphoric acids, commiphorinic acid, heeraboresene, α- and β-heerabomyrrhols and commiferin [988] (iii) Gums, composed of arabinose, galactose, xylose and 4-O-methylglucuronic acid [983, 988] (iv) Sterols etc. [988].

Guggul resin contains steroids such as *E*- and *Z*-guggulsterone, the *Z*-guggulsterols [989, 990] and volatile oil containing cembrene A and numerous other constituents similar to *C. molmol* [991, 992].

Medicinal Use: Stimulant, expectorant, antiseptic, antiinflammatory, antispasmodic, carminative. Myrrh is used internally for stomach complaints, tonsillitis, pharyngitis and gingivitis, and externally for ulcers, boils and wounds. It is reportedly antimicrobial *in vitro* [5]. Extracts of *C. abyssinica* stimulate phagocytosis in mice inoculated with *E. coli* [80].

Guggul resin is hypolipidaemic and hypocholesteraemic in humans and in animals [993, 994]; it increases catecholamine biosynthesis and activity in cholesterol-fed rabbits [994], inhibits platelet aggregation [990], has antiinflammatory effects in rats [995] and appears to activate the thyroid gland in rats and chickens [996].

Preparations: Myrrh Tincture BPC 1973, dose: 2.5–5 ml.

Potter's Products: Antispasmodic Tincture, Vegetable Cough Remover, Natural Herb Tablet, Hydrastis Compound Digestive Tablet No. 24.

Regulatory Status: GSL.

Biblical References: Exodus 30:23; Esther 2:12; Psalm 45:8; Proverbs 7:17; Song 1:13, 3:6, 4:6 and 14; 5:1 and 13; Matthew 2:11; John 19:39.

MYRTLE

Myrtus communis L.
Fam. Myrtaceae

Habitat: Indigenous to Southern Europe, cultivated elsewhere.

Description: An evergreen shrug with ovate, smooth, glossy leaves.

Part Used: Leaves.

Constituents: (i) Tannins, pyrogallol derivatives [183] (ii) Flavonoids such as myricetin (about 90%) with kaempferol and quercetin glycosides [997] (iii) Volatile oil, containing α-pinene, cineole, myrtenol, nerol, geraniol and dipentene [183].

Medicinal Use: Antiseptic, antiparasitic. Used for urinary infections as a substitute for Buchu (q.v.). Leaf extracts show antimicrobial activity *in vitro* [183], probably due to the tannins. It is used as an infusion.

Biblical References: Nehemiah 8:15; Isaiah 41:9 and 55:13; Zechariah 1:8 and 11.

N

NETTLE

Urtica dioica L.
Fam. Urticaceae,

Synonyms: Stinging Nettle.
Habitat: Nettles grow in waste places everywhere.
Description:

> "Tender-handed, grasp the nettle
> And it stings you for your pains
> Grasp it like a man of mettle
> And it soft as silk remains"

Stems up to 1.5 m, quadrangular, with opposite, stalked, cordate or lanceolate leaves, serrated at the margin. Flowers green with yellow stamens, in panicles; the male and female flowers on separate plants.
Part Used: Herb.
Constituents: (i) Chlorophyll in high yields (ii) Indoles such as histamine and serotonin (iii) Acetylcholine (iv) Vitamin C and other vitamins, protein and dietary fibre [998, 2].
Medicinal Use: Diuretic, astringent, tonic, antihaemorrhagic. Nettles are used for haemorrhage and skin complaints, including eczema and skin eruptions, usually as an infusion. Extracts are reported to be mildly hypoglycaemic. Massive exposure to nettle plants has caused severe symptoms of shock in animals [999].

Nettles are used as a source of chlorophyll.
Preparations: Liquid Extract, dose: 2.5–5 ml.
Potter's Products: Curophyll Tea.
Regulatory Status: GSL.
Biblical References: Job 30:7; Proverbs 24:31; Isaiah 34:13; Hosea 9:6; Zephaniah 2:9.

NIGHT-BLOOMING CEREUS

Selenicereus grandiflorus Britt. and Rose
Fam. Cactaceae

Synonyms: Sweet-scented Cactus *Cereus grandiflorus* Mill.
Habitat: West Indies.
Description: The stems and flowers are often preserved in spirit. Stems fleshy, five- to seven-angled, about 1–2 cm in diameter. The flowers are large, 10–13 cm in diameter, with oblong-lanceolate white petals and linear, orange, hairy calyx segments; numerous stamens and a many-rayed stigma.
Part Used: Fresh or preserved plant.
Constituents: (i) Alkaloids, including cactine [1000] (ii) Flavonoids, based on isorhamnetin [2].
Medicinal Use: Cardiac stimulant, diuretic, tonic. Used for palpitations, angina etc. cactine is reported to have a digitalis-like activity on the heart.

Preparations: Liquid Extract BPC 1949, dose: 0.05–0.5 ml; Tincture BPC 1934, dose: 0.1–2 ml.

NIKKAR NUTS

Caesalpinia bonducella Flem.
Fam. Leguminosae

Synonyms: Nichol Seeds, *Guilandia bondue* G. Bonducella.
Habitat: The Savannas, grown in the W. Indies and India.
Description: The pods are covered with prickles and contain the hard, polished, yellow seeds, which are about the size of an acorn.
Part Used: Seeds.
Constituents: (i) Caesalpinine, an alkaloid (ii) Bitter principles such as bonducin (iii) Fixed oil, saponins etc. [2].
Medicinal Use: Febrifuge, tonic. The seeds have been roasted and used to make an antidiabetic preparation.

NUTMEG

Myristica fragrans Houtt.
Fam. Myristicaceae

Synonyms: *Myristica fragrans* L.
Habitat: Native to the Molucca Islands and New Guinea, introduced into Sri Lanka and the W. Indies.
Description: The seed is ovoid, about 3 cm long and 2 cm broad, with a pale brown surface reticulately patterned with grooves, lines and specks. The internal structure is variegated brown and white, due to the infolding of the darker perisperm into the endosperm. Odour, aromatic, characteristic; taste, bitter, aromatic.
Part Used: Seed.
Constituents: (i) Volatile oil, about 10% but variable, containing camphene and pinene as the major constituents, with cymene, α-thujene, γ-terpinene, linalool, terpineol, myristicin (about 4–8% of the oil), safrole, elemicin, copaene, eugenol, isoeugenol, methyleugenol and others [1001, 1002, 1003, 1004] (ii) Miscellaneous; diarylpropanoids, sclareol, fixed oils and protein [5, 1001, 1005, 1006].
Medicinal Use: Carminative, spasmolytic, antimetic, orexigenic, topical antiinflammatory. Nutmeg is used medicinally for nausea and vomiting, flatulence, indigestion and diarrhoea. Extracts of nutmeg decrease kidney prostaglandin levels in rats [1007], inhibit contractions of rat stomach strips produced by prostaglandin E_2 and decrease levels of prostaglandin-like material produced by isolated human colon [1008]. They also inhibit platelet aggregation; this activity was found to be due to eugenol and isoeugenol [1004]. Nutmeg has been used successfully in the treatment of Crohn's disease [1009]. However nutmeg oil decreases fertility in rats [1010] and some constituents are carcinogenic [1011]. Large doses cause intoxication, hypnosis and tachycardia; these actions are thought to be due to the hallucinogenic myristicin, but some of the other constituents have

hypnotic activity at least [1012,1013]. Nutmeg is a popular domestic culinary spice.

Preparations: Powder, dose: 0.3–1 g; Nutmeg Oil BPC, dose: 0.05–0.2 ml.

Regulatory Status: GSL.

NUX VOMICA

Strychnos nux vomica L.
Fam. Loganiaceae

Synonyms: Poison Nut.

Habitat: India to Northern Australia.

Description: The seeds are disc-shaped, up to about 2 cm in diameter and about 0.5 cm thick, usually flattened, often with a keeled margin, greyish-green with a satiny sheen due to the closely appressed hairs. On the convex side the raphe is visible as a line going from the central hilum to the micropyle. Fracture, extremely hard and horny, showing the white cotyledons, straight radicle and small embryo. Taste, very bitter; odourless.

Part Used: Seeds.

Constituents: Indole alkaloids, the main one being strychnine, accounting for approximately 50% of the alkaloids, with strychnine N-oxide, brucine and its N-oxide, α- and β-colubrine, condylocarpine, diaboline, geisso-schizine, icajine, isostrychnine, normacusine, novacine, pseudobrucine, pseudo-α-colubrine, pseudo-β-colubrine, pseudostrychnine, vomicine and others [1, 732] (ii) Miscellaneous; loganin, chlorogenic acid, fixed oil [1].

Medicinal Use: Stimulant, bitter, tonic. The action is mainly due to strychnine, which is a potent CNS stimulant. Nux vomica has been used as a tonic and analeptic but this cannot really be justified; its therapeutic properties are limited and recorded fatalities from deliberate or accidental ingestion are numerous. Poisoning causes muscle stiffness and spasm, resulting in the fixed grinning expression known as "risus sardonicus" due to clamping of the jaw; contraction of the abdominals and the diaphragm arrests respiration and death may easily result.

Preparations: Nux Vomica Elixir BPC 1973, dose: 5 ml; Nux Vomica Liquid Extract BP, dose: 0.05–0.2 ml; Nux Vomica Tincture BP, dose: 0.5–2 ml.

Regulatory Status: POM.

O

OAK

Quercus robur L.
and other species of *Quercus*.
Fam. Fagaceae

Synonyms: Tanner's Bark.

Habitat: Throughout Europe, planted elsewhere.

Description: The bark has a greyish external surface with occasional brown lenticels, a reddish brown inner surface with longitudinal striations. Fracture fibrous, showing projecting medullary rays. Taste, astringent; odour, slightly aromatic.

Part Used: Bark.

Constituents: Tannins 15–20%, consisting of phlobatannin, ellagitannins and gallic acid [1, 4].

Medicinal Use: Astringent, haemostatic, antiseptic. it is used as a decoction in frequent small doses for diarrhoea, and as an enema for haemorrhoids and gargle for throat problems.

Preparations: Liquid Extract, dose: 0.5–5 ml.

Potter's Products: Peerless Composition Essence.

Regulatory Status: GSL.

Biblical References: Genesis 35:4, 8; Joshua 24:26; Judges 6:11, 19; 2 Samuel 18:9–14; Kings 13:14; 1 Chronicles 10:12; Isaiah 1:29–30, 2:13, 6:13, 44:14; Ezekiel 6:13, 27:6; Hosea 4:13; Amos 2:9; Zechariah 11:2.

OATS

Avena sativa L.
Fam. Graminae

Synonyms: Groats.

Habitat: Widely distributed as a cereal crop.

Description: The seeds with the husks removed are found crushed, as a coarse powder of flakes, creamy white and buff coloured with a mealy taste.

Part Used: Seeds.

Constituents: (i) Proteins, prolamines known as avenins [1012] (ii) C-glycosyl flavones [1013] (iii) Avenacosides, which are spirostanol glycosides [1014] (iv) Fixed oil, vitamin E, starch etc.

Medicinal Use: Antidepressant, thymoleptic, cardiac tonic. Used for debility, menopausal symptoms and depression. Reports that extracts counteract dependence on cigarettes and morphine have been disputed [1015, 1016, 1017]. Oats are externally emollient and the colloidal fraction is used in bath preparations for eczema and dry skin.

Preparations: Liquid Extrract, dose: 0.6–2 ml.

Potter's Products: Compound Elixir of Avena with Helonias, Mixture No 108A Tonic No 1.

Regulatory Status: GSL.

OLIVE

Olea europea L.
Fam. Oleaceae

Habitat: Native to the Mediterranean region.

Description: An evergreen shrub, from the fruit of which is expressed the oil. Virgin, or cold expressed oil has a greenish tinge and is used as a food, refined oil is yellowish. Both have a characteristic odour.

Part Used: Oil.

Constituents: Glycerides of oleic acid, about 70–80%, with smaller amounts of linoleic, palmitic and stearic acid glycerides [2, 4].

Medicinal Use: Nutritive, emollient, mild aperient. It may be used externally as an emollient in liniments and embrocations, as an enema in chronic constipation, to soften ear wax and for numerous other purposes. The leaves have a hypotensive action in rats [556].

Preparations: Olive Oil BP, dose (as a laxative) 15–60 ml.

Regulatory Status: GSL.

Biblical References: Genesis 8 : 11; Exodus 27 : 20 and 30 : 24; Leviticus 24 : 2; Kings 18 : 32; Job 15 : 33, Psalm 52 : 8 and 128 : 3; Micah 6 : 15 and others.

OLIVER BARK

Cinnamomum oliveri Baill.
Fam. Lauraceae

Synonyms: Australian Cinnamon, Black Sassafras.

Habitat: New South Wales and Queensland.

Description: The bark occurs in flat strips, with a coarsely granular, brown outer surface with white cork patches. Odour of sassafras and cinnamon.

Part Used: Bark.

Constituents: Volatile oil, containing about 40–45% methyleugenol, 25% safrole, 20% camphor and 15% α-pinene [2].

Medicinal Use: Stimulant. In view of the carcinogenicity of both safrole and methyleugenol [1011] it would be best avoided.

Preparations: Tincture, dose: 2–4 ml.

ONION

Allium cepa L.
Fam. Liliaceae

Habitat: Widely cultivated throughout the world.

Description: Such a common vegetable hardly requires description.

Part Used: Bulb.

Constituents: (i) Volatile oil, containing allylpropyldisulphide, dimethyl-sulphide, methylpropyldisulphide, thiopropanal-S-oxide [580, 1018, 1019, 1020] (ii) Sulphur-containing compounds; allicin, alliin, methylalliin, cycloalliin, *trans*-S-(1-propenyl)cysteine sulphoxide, S-methylcysteine [580, 1018, 1020] (iii) Flavonoids; kaempferol, quercetin, cyanidin and paeonidin glycosides [5, 33] (iv) Miscellaneous; phenolic acids, sterols, sugars, vitamins etc. [5].

Medicinal Use: Expectorant, diuretic, carminative, antispasmodic. Like garlic (q.v.) onion is the subject of intensive modern research. Extracts of onion are hypoglycaemic in humans when taken orally [584]; this is attributable to the allylpropyldisulphide and allicin [1018, 586]. More recently onion extracts have been shown to have antiasthmatic effects, acting at least in part by antagonizing platelet-activating factor [1021, 1022]. Alliin and allicin have an inhibitory effect on platelet aggregation [1023]. Onions have well-known antibiotic activity, due mainly to allicin [583]. For more information on these types of compounds see garlic.
Biblical References: Numbers 11 : 5.

ORANGE
BITTER ORANGE
SWEET ORANGE

Citrus aurantium var *amara* L.
C. aurantium var *sinensis* L.
Fam. Rutaceae

Synonyms: Bitter Orange: Seville Orange, Bigarde Orange; Sweet Orange: China Orange, *C. sinensis* (L.) Osbeck, *C. dulcis* Pers.
Habitat: Bitter orange: Southern Spain, Sicily, W. Indies; sweet orange: cultivated worldwide in warm countries.
Description: The orange is too well-known to require description.
Part Used: Peel, oil, juice, fruit.
Constituents: (i) Volatile oil, both types of fairly similar composition, containing about 90% limonene with aldehydes such as octanal and decanal. Sweet orange oil contains more aldehydes [5, 1024, 1025] (ii) Flavonoids; hesperidin, neohesperidin, naringin, tangeretin, nobiletin and others [5, 1026, 1027] (iii) Coumarins; umbelliferone, 6,7-dimethoxy-coumarin and bergapten [5, 1028] (iv) Miscellaneous; triterpenes such as limonin, vitamin C (in the juice), carotenoids, pectin etc. The bitterness is attributed to the triterpenes and flavonoids [1, 5].
Medicinal Use: Carminative, aromatic, stomachic. The flavonoids are antiinflammatory, antibacterial and antifungal. Orange peel and oils are used more as a flavouring in foods, drinks and medicine. The juice is a well-known source of vitamin C.
Preparations: Bitter Orange: Orange Tincture BP; Orange Syrup BP; Concentrated Orange Peel Infusion BP. Sweet Orange: Orange Oil BP; Compound Spirit BP.

ORRIS

Iris florentina L.
I. germanica
I pallida Lam.
Fam. Iridaceae

Synonyms: Florentine Orris, Orris Root.
Habitat: Cultivated Italy and Morocco and grown in many countries, including Britain, as ornamentals.

Description: The rhizome may be peeled or unpeeled. The better quality rhizome is peeled, creamy-white, irregular in shape, often flattened or constricted in places and bearing small marks where the rootlets have been removed. Fracture very hard; odour, characteristic, like violets.

Part Used: Rhizome.

Constituents: (i) Essential oil, about 0.1–2%, known as "orris butter", consisting of about 85% myristic acid, with irone, ionone, methyl myristate [1, 4, 37] (ii) Isoflavones; irilone (in *I. germanica* and *I. florentina*, irilone-4'-glucoside, irisolone-4'bioside, irigenin, iristecto-genin-B, irisflorentin, irifloside and iridin (in *I. florentina* [1029, 1030, 1031] (iii) Triterpines; β-sitosterol, α- and β-amyrin [1031].

Medicinal Use: Demulcent, aromatic, expectorant, antidiarrhoeal. It has been taken for coughs and diarrhoea as an infusion. Orris is used in dental preparations, in cachous and in perfumery.

Preparations: Powder, dose: 0.2–1 g.

Regulatory Status: GSL (for external use only).

OSIER, RED, AMERICAN

Cornus sericea L.
Fam. Cornaceae

Synonyms: Rose Willow, Red Willow, Silky Cornel.

Habitat: USA.

Description: Bark in thin, irregular pieces or short quills, purplish externally, somewhat warty; inner surface brown and finely striated. Fracture short. Taste, atringent and bitter; odour, slight.

Part Used: Bark, root-bark.

Constituents: Unknown.

Medicinal Use: Astringent, bitter, tonic. Has been used for diarrhoea, dyspepsia and vomiting.

OX-EYE DAISY

Chrysanthemum leucanthemum L.
Fam. Compositae

Synonyms: Moon Daisy, Marguerite, *Leucanthemum vulgare* Lam.

Habitat: Europe, including Britain, and parts of Asia and Russia.

Description: The leaf stem is angular, up to about 60 cm, bearing dark green, serrate, spatulate leaves. The white, yellow-centred solitary flowers are 25–50 mm in diameter, with an involucre of green bracts with membranous black edges. Taste, bitter and tingling; odour, faintly valerianic.

Part Used: Herb.

Constituents: No information available.

Medicinal Use: Antispasmodic, diuretic, tonic. It has been used as an infusion in a similar way to chamomile (q.v.) but is emetic in large doses.

P

PAPAYA

Carica papaya L.
Fam. Caricaceae

Synonyms: Pawpaw, Papaw.

Habitat: Cultivated in most tropical countries.

Description: The fruit is the size of a small melon, and when ripe is a greenish yellow or orange colour. The flesh is a yellow sweet pulp with numerous black seeds.

Part Used: Papain an enzyme mixture prepared from the fruit, seeds and leaf.

Constituents: (i) Proteolytic enzymes, chiefly papain and chymopapain [4] (ii) Carpaine, an alkaloid (traces in the fruit, more in the seeds and leaf) [33] (ii) In the seeds: carpasemine, benzylsenevol [33].

Medicinal Use: Digestive. The enzymes hydrolyse polypeptides, amides and esters, particularly when used in an alkaline environment, and are used to aid digestion and in digestive disorders. These enzymes have also found other uses, for their action on scar tissue and help in wound healing, in disorders of the eye and spinal disorders. Inhalation of the enzyme powder has caused allergies but otherwise it is non-toxic when taken orally. Papain is used to tenderize meat and for other dubious purposes in the food industry. The leaves and seeds of the papaya are used in native medicine as an anthelmintic, and the roots and leaves as a diuretic.

Preparations: Elixir of Papain BPC 1949, dose: 2.5–5 ml; Glycerin of Papain BPC 1934, dose: 2.5–5 ml.

Potter's Products: Pegina Indigestion Remedy.

Regulatory Status: GSL.

PARAGUAY TEA

Ilex paraguariensis St. Hil.
Fam. Aquifoliaceae

Synonyms: Mate, Yerba Mate, Jesuit's Brazil Tea.

Habitat: Brazil and Argentina.

Description: The leaves appear in commerce either broken or as coarse powder. They are ovate, up to 15 cm long, with a crenate or serrate margin and a leathery texture. Taste astringent, bitter; odour, characteristic, aromatic.

Part Used: Leaves.

Constituents: (i) Xanthine derivatives; caffeine, 0.2–2%, theobromine, 0.3–0.5%. Theophylline was found to be absent [1032, 25] (ii) Volatile oil (ii) Polyphenolics, tannins and chlorogenic acid, about 16% [1, 25] (iii) Miscellaneous; vanillin vitamin C [50].

Medicinal Use: Stimulant, diuretic, mild analgesic. Used for mild depression and rheumatic pains in combination with other remedies. In South

America this is used frequently in place of ordinary tea. The beneficial effects are due mainly to the caffeine and theobromine content.

Preparations: Liquid Extract, dose: 2.5–5 ml.

Potter's Products: Blood Pressure Medicinal Tea Bags, Lion Cleansing Herbs.

Regulatory Status: GSL.

PAREIRA
Chondrodendron tomentosum R. and P.
Fam. Menispermaceae

Synonym: Pareira brava

Habitat: South America.

Description: The root is about 2–5 cm in diameter, tortuous, black, longitudinally furrowed with transverse ridges and some constrictions. Internally it is greyish-brown, and the transverse section shows three or four concentric rings, traversed by wide medullary rays. The stem pieces are similar but the external surface is greyish and marked with numerous round, warty lenticels. Taste, bitter then slightly sweet; odourless.

Part Used: Root, stem.

Constituents: Alkaloids, *d*-tubocurarine, *l*-curarine, *l*-beebirine, chondrocurine and others [926, 1033].

Medicinal Use: Formerly used as a tonic, diuretic and aperient. Pareira is mainly used as a source of tubocurarine, a potent muscle relaxant used to paralyse muscles during surgical operations. Tubocurarine is unstable when taken orally [4]. Species of *Chondrodendron* were used to prepare "curare", the famous South American arrow poisons.

Preparations: Liquid Extract, dose: 2.5–10 ml.

PARSLEY
Petroselinum crispum (Mill) Nym.
Fam. Umbelliferae

Synonyms: *P. sativum* Hoffm., *Carum petroselinum* Benth. and Hook., *Apium petroselinum* L.

Habitat: Native to the Eastern Mediterranean, cultivated worldwide.

Description: Parsley is a well-known plant, easily distinguished by its dissected leaves and distinctive taste. The root is yellowish white, up to 10 cm long and 2 cm wide, usually found chopped in commerce, longitudinally wrinkled with occasional root scars. Taste and odour, characteristic, aromatic.

Part Used: Root, seeds, leaf.

Constituents: (i) Volatile oil, containing apiole, myristicin, β-phellandrene, *p*-mentha-1,3,8-triene, 4-isopropyl-1-methylbenzene, 2-(*p*-toluyl)propan-2-ol, limonene, eugenol, α-thujene, α- and β-pinene, camphene, γ-terpinene, osthole and others [1034, 1035] (ii) Coumarins; bergapten, xanthotoxin, isopimpinellin, psoralen, 8- and 5-methoxypsoralen and imperatorin [1036, 1037] (iii) Flavonoids; apiin, luteolin, apigenin-7-glucoside, luteolin-7-glucoside and others [452]. (iv) Phthalides; Z-ligustilide and senkyunolide [910] (iv) Proteins, fats, vitamins etc. [5].

Medicinal Use: Diuretic, spasmolytic, carminative, aperient, antiseptic, expectorant, antirheumatic, sedative. The flavonoids, particularly apigenin, have been shown to be antiinflammatory, to inhibit histamine release and to act as a free radical scavenger [436, 437]. Apiole is reportedly antipyretic [25] and the phthalides are sedative in mice [308]. The leaves are a common culinary herb.

Preparations: Liquid Extract, dose: 2.5–5 ml; Liquid Extract (Seed), dose: 2.5–5 ml.

Regulatory Status: GSL.

PARSLEY PIERT

Aphanes arvensis L.
Fam. Rosaceae

Synonyms: *Alchemilla arvensis* Scop.

Habitat: Native to Europe, including Britain.

Description: A more or less prostrate, hairy annual, with 3-lobed, fan-shaped, serrate leaves and small, insignificant green flowers with no petals, found in axillary clusters, surrounded by toothed, leaf-like stipules. Taste, astringent; odourless.

Part Used: Herb.

Constituents: Largely unknown. Tannins are present.

Medicinal Use: Diuretic, demulcent. Used particularly for kidney and bladder complaints, often taken as an infusion.

Preparations: Liquid Extract, dose: 2.5–5 ml.

Potter's Products: Diuretab No 116.

Regulatory Status: GSL.

PASSION FLOWER

Passiflora incarnata L.
Fam. Passifloraceae

Synonyms: Maypop.

Habitat: Native to the USA, cultivated elsewhere.

Description: The plant is a climber, reaching up to about 9 m in length, bearing ovate or cordate leaves, palmately 3-lobed, coiled tendrils and white, cross-shaped flowers.

Part Used: Leaves, whole plant.

Constituents: (i) Alkaloids, harman, harmine, harmaline, harmol and harmalol. The presence of the latter four has been disputed [1038, 1039, 1040, 1041, 1042] (ii) Flavonoids; apigenin and various glycosides, homoorientin, isovitexin, kaempferol, luteolin, orientin, quercetin, rutin, saponaretin, saponarin and vitexin [1043, 1044) (iv) Miscellaneous; an 8-pyrone derivative, sterols, sugars, gums etc. [1045, 5].

Medicinal Use: Sedative, hypnotic, antispasmodic, hypotensive, anodyne. Passiflora extracts have CNS depressant activities and are hypotensive [25]; they are used for their sedative and soothing properties, to lower

209

blood pressure, prevent tachycardia and for insomnia. The alkaloids and the flavonoids are both reported to have sedative activity in animals [1046], as is the 8-pyrone derivative [1045]. Apigenin is well-known for its pharmacological activity, particularly its antispasmodic and antiinflammatory activity [436, 437].

Preparations: Liquid Extract, dose: 0.5–1 ml.

Potter's Products: Passiflora Tablets, Passiflora Elixir, Cardivallin Tablets, Anased Tablets.

Regulatory Status: GSL.

PATCHOULI

Pogostemon cablin (Blanco) Benth.
Fam. Labiatae

Synonyms: Patchouly, *P. patchouli* Pell., *P. heyneanus* Benth.
Habitat: Tropical Asia.
Description: A perennial herb with ovate leaves which give a strong, characteristic odour when rubbed.
Part Used: Leaves.
Constituents: Volatile oil, containing sesquiterpenes, mainly patchouli alcohol, with pogostol, norpatchulenol, β-patchoulene, α-guaiene and others [5].
Medicinal Use: None. The oil is used in perfumery.

PAWPAW, AMERICAN

Asimina triloba (L.) Dur.
Fam. Annonaceae

Synonyms: Custard Apple.
Habitat: USA.
Description: Seeds flat, brown, slightly polished with darker brown lines on the surface, oblong-oval, with a greyish hilum at one end. Taste and odour, resinous.
Part Used: Seeds. The fruit is edible.
Constituents: Asimine, an alkaloid [33].

PEACH

Prunus persica Stokes
Fam. Rosaceae

Synonyms: Persica vulgaris Nutt., *Amygdalus persica* L.
Habitat: Cultivated in many parts of the world.
Description: The peach tree and its fruit are well known.
Part Used: Bark, leaves, oil expressed from the seeds. Peaches are normally grown for the fruit.
Constituents: Oil: mainly glycerides of oleic acid, with some palmitic and stearic acid glycerides, some benzaldehyde and cyanhydrin. Leaves: cyanogenetic glycosides [2].
Medicinal Use: Sedative, diuretic, expectorant. The bark and leaves have been used as an infusion. The oil may be used as an emollient and in toilet preparations.
Regulatory Status: GSL.

PELLITORY *Anacyclus pyrethrum* (L.) Link.
Fam. Compositae
Synonyms: Anthemis pyrethrum L. *Matricaria pyrethrum* Baill.
Habitat: Spain and other Mediterranean countries.
Description: The root occurs in dark brown, cylindrical pieces, longitudinally furrowed, often with a tuft of soft, woolly hairs at the crown. Taste, acrid, pungent, causing a flow of saliva; odour, characteristic.
Part Used: Root.
Constituents: Anacycline, isobutylamide, inulin, a trace of essential oil [2].
Medicinal Use: Rubifacient, counter-irritant, used externally for toothache.
Regulatory Status: GSL.

PELLITORY-OF-THE-WALL *Parietaria officinalis* L.
and other spp.
Fam. Urticaceae
Synonyms: P. diffusa Mert. and Koch.
Habitat: Native to Europe, including Britain.
Description: A perennial herb with slender, lanceolate-ovate leaves and brittle, reddish, ridged stalks. The flowers are unisexual, green with yellow stamens, the female flowers terminal and the male flowers in axillary clusters. Taste and odour, slight.
Part Used: Herb.
Constituents: (i) Flavonoids; 3-glucosides and 3-rhamnosides of quercetin, kaempferol and isorhamnetin; 3-sophorosides of quercetin and kaempferol and 3-neohesperidosides of kaempferol and isorhamnetin [1047] (ii) Glucoproteins (allergens) [1048].
Medicinal Use: Diuretic, demulcent. It is used to treat cystitis, pyelitis and dysuria as well as kidney stones.
Preparations: Liquid Extract, dose: 2.5–5 ml.
Regulatory Status: GSL.

PENNYROYAL *Mentha-pulegium* L.
Fam. Labiatae
Synonyms: European Pennyroyal.
Habitat: A common wild or garden plant, in Britain, France and Germany. American Pennyroyal is *Hedeoma pulegioides* (L.) Pers.
Description: A prostrate, or sometimes erect perennial, with ovate leaves up to about 2–3 cm long and only slightly serrate; lilac flowers in axillary clusters with a hairy, ribbed calyx tube. Taste and odour, mint-like but characteristic.
Part Used: Herb.
Constituents: (i) Volatile oil, consisting mainly of pulegone (about 85%), isopulegone, menthol, isomenthone, limonene, piperitone, neomenthol [4, 25, 124] (ii) Miscellaneous; bitters and tannins [124]. American Pennyroyal contains similar constituents [124].

Medicinal Use: Carminative, diaphoretic, stimulant, emmenagogue. it has been principally used for delayed menses, however in effective doses it is abortifacient and toxic. In small doses and as an infusion it is used for colds, colic and dyspesia. Topically it may be used for skin eruptions, itching and gout. The oil is an insect repellant. Not to be used during pregnancy.

Preparations: Liquid Extract, dose: 0.5–5 ml; Pennyroyal Oil BPC 1934, dose: 0.05–2 ml; Spirit of Pulegium, dose: 0.6–1.2 ml.

Regulatory Status: GSL.

PEONY

Paeonia officinalis L.
Fam. Ranunculaceae

Synonyms: Common Peony. The botanical name of this plant is in some doubt. Species such as *P. lactiflora* Pallas (*P. albiflora* Pallas), which is used in China, may in fact be the same plant.

Habitat: A common garden plant.

Description: The root is spindle-shaped, furrowed, and pinkish grey or whitish externally when scraped. Taste, sweet then bitter; odourless.

Part Used: Root.

Constituents: No information available for *P. officinalis.* However *P. lactiflora*, which is used in Oriental medicine, has been investigated: (i) Monoterpenoid glycosides; paeoniflorin, albiflorin, oxypaeoniflorin, benzoylpaeoniflorin (ii) Benzoic acid (iii) Pentagalloyl glucose [284 and references therein).

Medicinal Use: Antispasmodic, tonic. Again no information available. *P. lactiflora* is used for the same purposes, and as an astringent and analgesic. Paeoniflorin has a smooth muscle relaxant activity, is vasodilatory, has some CNS depressant effects, is antiinflammatory and immunostimulating in animals. Pentagalloyl glucose is antiviral *in vitro* against *Herpes simplex*. For review see [284].

PEPPER

Piper nigrum L.
Fam. Piperaceae

Synonyms: Black Pepper, White Pepper.

Habitat: Cultivated widely in the tropics, especially in India, Indonesia and South America.

Description: Black pepper consists of the unripe fruit, which is globular, about 3–6 mm in diameter, with a wrinkled, reticulated dark brown or greyish-black surface. White pepper is prepared from riper fruit with the outer pericarp removed; it has therefore a slightly smaller diameter and the vascular bundles are visible as longitudinal lines on the yellowish-white surface. Taste and odour, pungent, characteristic; white pepper is more pungent than black but less aromatic.

Part Used: Fruit.

Constituents: (i) Volatile oil, about 2–4% in black pepper but very little in white pepper, containing β-bisabolene, camphene, β-caryophyllene, α-cubebene, β-farnesene, hydrocarveol, limonene, myrcene, myristicin, α- and β-pinene, sabinene, safrole, α- and β-selinene, α-thujene, and others [5, 50, 1049, 1050] (ii) Alkaloids, in both types, the major pungent principle being piperine, up to 11%, with piperanine, piperettine, piperolein A and B, piperidine and traces of others [1049, 1051, 1052] (iii) Miscellaneous; fixed oil, protein etc. [5].

Medicinal Use: Carminative, stimulant. Pepper has been used for indigestion and flatulence. It is used throughout the world as a condiment.

PEPPERMINT
Mentha × *piperita* L.

(a hybrid between *M. spicata* L. and *M. viridis*) Fam. Labiatae

Synonyms: Black Mint is *M. piperita* var *vulgaris* Sole; White Mint is *M. piperita* var *officinalis* Sole.

Habitat: Cultivated widely, particularly in Europe and America.

Description: Stems quadrangular, those of black mint are purplish. Leaves up to 9 cm long, 3 cm broad, petiolate, with a serrated margin. Those of the black mint are tinged with purple. The flowers are small, lilac or reddish-purple, in tight whorls at the base of the leaves. Taste and odour, characteristic.

Part Used: Herb, distilled oil.

Constituents: (i) Essential oil, up to 1.5%, containing menthol, menthone and menthyl acetate as the major components, with isomenthone, menthofuran, isomenthol, neomenthol, piperitone, α- and β-pinene, limonene, cineole, pulegone, viridiflorol, ledol and others [1, 5, 50, 1053, 1054] (ii) Flavonoids; menthoside, rutin and others (iii) Miscellaneous; rosmarinic acid, azulenes, choline, carotenes etc. [5, and other references therein].

Medicinal Use: Spasmolytic, carminative, antiemetic, diaphoretic, antiseptic. The herb is used in herbal teas and peppermint oil is used in many indigestion and colic mixtures. It is an ingredient of some cough and cold remedies; menthol is used in similar ways for oral ingestion and inhalation. The spasmolytic and carminative effects have been shown experimentally *in vivo* and *in vitro* [269, 1055], thus confirming what has been common knowledge for centuries. Peppermint extracts also have antiviral effects [99]. Peppermint is a popular flavouring for confectionery, ice cream, sauces and liqueurs, as well as for toothpastes, mouthwashes and medicines.

Preparations: Powdered Herb, dose: 2–4 g; Peppermint Oil BP, dose: 0.05–2 ml; Peppermint Spirit BPC, dose: 0.3–2 ml; Concentrated Peppermint Water BPC 1973, dose: 0.25–1 ml.

Potter's Products: Elder Flowers and Peppermint with Composition Essence.

Regulatory Status: GSL.

PERIWINKLE

Vinca major (L.) Pich.
Fam. Apocynaceae

Synonyms: Greater Periwinkle, *V. pubescens* Urv.

Habitat: Indigenous to Southern Europe, grown widely elsewhere as an ornamental.

Description: A semi-procumbent shrub with stems up to about 1 m; leaves dark green, broadly lanceolate, up to about 8 cm long and 5 cm broad, with entire margins. Flowers blue, solitary, with five joined petals, up to 5 cm in diameter. Taste, slightly bitter and acrid; odourless.

Part Used: Herb.

Constituents: (i) Indole alkaloids; majdine, isomajdine, majoridine, akuammine, akuammicine, carpanaubine, ervine, reserpinine, serpentine, sarpagine, tetrahydroalstonine, vincamajine and vincamajoreine [1056, 1057, 1058, 1059] (ii) Tannins.

The cytotoxic dimeric alkaloids present in the Madagascar Periwinkle, *Cantharanthus roseus* (L.) Don., (= *Vinca rosea* L.), which are used to treat certain types of cancer, have not been found in *V. major.*

Medicinal Use: Astringent, antihaemorrhagic. It is used particularly to treat menorrhagia and leucorrhoea, and for nose bleeds, mouth ulcers and sore throats.

Preparations: Powder, dose; 2–4 g; Liquid Extract, dose: 2.5–5 ml.

Potter's Products: Vinca Major Compound Mixture.

Regulatory Status: GSL.

PERUVIAN BALSAM

Myroxylon pereirae Klotsch.
Fam. Leguminosae

Synonyms: Balsam of Peru.

Habitat: Central America.

Description: The balsam is a dark brown to black, oily fluid which exudes from the tree after the bark has been beaten and scorched. It is soaked up with rags and boiled with water to separate the balsam, which sinks to the bottom. Taste, acrid and bitter; odour, sweet, balsamic, vanilla-like.

Part Used: Balsam.

Constituents: (i) Essential oil, about 50–65%, comprised mainly of benzyl benzoate, benzyl cinnamate (= cinnamein), cinnnamyl cinnamate (= styracin), free benzoic and cinnamic acids, vanillin, farnesol, styrene, nerolidol and coumarin (1, 5, 183] (ii) Resins, about 25–30%, consisting of peruresinotannol combined with cinnamic and benzoic acids [1].

Medicinal Use: Stimulant, expectorant, antiseptic. It is used to treat catarrh and diarrhoea and externally for wounds, ulcers, pruritis, nappy rash, eczema and ringworm. It is an ingredient of some soaps and cosmetics and used as a perfume fixative. Peruvian balsam is known to cause allergies in sensitive individuals [1060].

Regulatory Status: GSL.

PICHI

Fabiana imbricata Ruiz et Pav.
Fam. Solanaceae

Habitat: South America.

Description: Stem irregularly branched, the twigs covered with closely overlapping heath-like leaves, which are fleshy, obtuse, and keeled with a prominent midrib beneath. Flowers, if present, white, tubular, constricted at the throat. Taste, bitter; odour, faint, agreeable.

Part Used: Leaves, twigs.

Constituents: (i) Fabianine, an alkaloid (ii) Coumarins; scopoletin and β-methylaesculetin and their glycosides (iii) Essential oil (iv) Tannins, choline, acetovanillin [2].

Medicinal Use: Diuretic, tonic, hepatic, stimulant. It has been used particularly for dyspepsia and jaundice, and for kidney complaints.

Preparations: Liquid Extract, dose: 2.5–5 ml.

Regulatory Status: GSL.

PILEWORT

Ficaria ranunculoides Moench.
Fam. Ranunculaceae

Synonyms: Lesser Celandine, *Ranunculus ficaria* L.

Habitat: Common in Europe, including Britain, and Western Asia.

Description: Leaves mostly radical, the petioles up to about 15 cm long, the lamina up to 4 cm long and 5 cm broad, ovate, cordate or reniform. Flowers solitary, on long peduncles, bright yellow with three sepals and 8–12 lanceolate petals each with a nectary at the base. Roots fleshy, oblong or club-shaped, up to about 3 cm long. Taste, slightly bitter; odour, faint.

Part Used: Herb.

Constituents: (i) Saponins based on hederagenin and oleanolic acid; the most abundant being hederagenin glucoside, and others with rhamnose, arabinose and glucose as the sugar moieties [1061, 1062, 1063, 1064] (ii) Protoanemonin and anemonin [37, 1065] (iii) Tannins [1065].

Medicinal Use: Antihaemorrhoidal, astringent. As the name denotes, it is used chiefly for piles, taken internally and also applied externally in the form of an ointment or suppository. The saponins have a local antihaemorrhoidal effect [1062] which is increased by the astringency of the tannins. The saponins are also fungicidal [1064]. Protoanemonin has antibiotic activity, however it easily dimerizes to anemonin which is inactive [1014].

Preparations: Liquid Extract, dose: 2.5–5 ml; Pilewort Ointment BPC 1934.

Potter's Products: Piletabs; Pile Compound Herb; Green Pilewort Ointment; Pilewort Compound Tablets No 375.

Regulatory Status: GSL.

PIMPERNEL, SCARLET

Anagallis arvensis L.
Fam. Primulaceae

Synonyms: Poor Man's Weatherglass.

Habitat: Europe including Britain, parts of Asia and Russia.

Description: A prostrate annual; leaves opposite, about 1–2 cm long and 1 cm broad, ovate, sessile, with black dots on the undersurface. Flowers small, scarlet, star-like, finely toothed at the tip with hairs along the margins. The flowers open in sunshine and close when humid, hence the synonym. Taste, mucilaginous, acrid; odourless.

Part Used: Herb.

Constituents: (i) Saponins based on derivatives of oleanolic acid, including anagalline, its aglycone anagalligenone B and other glycosides of protoprimulagenin A [1066, 1067, 1068] (ii) Cucurbitacins B, D, E, I, L and R, and the related arvenins I, II, III and IV [1069].

Medicinal Use: Diuretic, diaphoretic, expectorant. The saponins are antiviral [1067, 1068]. The cucurbitacins are cytotoxic (see Bryony, White). This herb is poisonous and cannot be recommended.

Preparations: Powder, dose: 1–4 g.

Regulatory Status: GSL.

PINE OILS
PUMILIO PINE
SCOTCH PINE

Pinus spp.
P. mugo Turra, and varieties
P. sylvestris L.
Fam. Pinaceae

Synonyms: Swiss Mountain Pine, Dwarf Pine (*P. mugo*).

Habitat: *P. mugo* is native to central and southern Europe, *P. sylvestris* to Europe and Asia, and cultivated in the USA.

Part Used: Oil distilled from the needles.

Constituents: *P. mugo:* α- and β-pinene, *d*-limonene, dipentene, camphene, myrcene, bornyl acetate, hexanal, cuminaldehyde, cadinene and others [5, 445]. *P. sylvestris:* α-pinene (the major constituent), with β-pinene, *d*-limonene, α- and γ-terpinene, β-ocimene, myrcene, camphene, sabinene, terpinolene, bornyl acetate, borneol, cineole, caryophyllene, chamazulene, 3β-oxy*trans*-biformene and its acetate, and others [5, 445, 1070].

Medicinal Use: Antiseptic, decongestant, expectorant. The pine oils are commonly used in cough and cold remedies, particularly inhalations, and in rubefacients for use in muscle stiffness and rheumatism. They are also used as flavour and fragrance ingredients in toiletries, detergents and disinfectants.

Regulatory Status: GSL (External use only).

PINE, WHITE

Pinus strobus L.
Fam. Pinaceae

Synonyms: Eastern White Pine, Deal Pine.

Habitat: Native to N. America, found widely in the northern hemisphere.

Description: The inner bark occurs in pieces about 2–3 mm thick, bright buff coloured on the inner surface, smooth and finely striated; on the outer surface there are numerous scattered, small oil glands. Fracture, tough, shortly fibrous. Taste, mucilaginous, astringent; odour, slight.

Part Used: Inner bark.

Constituents: (i) Coniferin, coniferyl alcohol (ii) Diterpenes; strobol, strobal, abienol (iii) Triterpenes, e.g. 3β-methoxyserrat-14-en-21-one (iv) Essential oil, mucilage [5, 1071].

Medicinal Use: Expectorant, demulcent, diuretic. Mainly used in the form of a syrup for coughs and colds.

Preparations: Liquid Extract of White Pine BPC 1934, dose: 1–5 ml; Compound Syrup of White Pine BPC 1934, dose: 5–10 ml.

Regulatory Status: GSL.

PINK ROOT
Spigelia marilandica L.
Fam. Loganiaceae

Synonyms: Indian Pinkroot, Wormgrass, Maryland Pink.

Habitat: USA.

Description: It is a perennial herb growing to about 45 cm, bearing bright red flowers.

Part Used: Herb, rhizome.

Constituents: (i) Spigeleine, an alkaloid (ii) Essential oil (iii) Tannin [2].

Medicinal Use: Vermifuge, taken as an infusion morning and evening with a purgative such as Senna (q.v.).

Preparations: Powdered Herb or Root, dose: children over 4 years, 0.5–4 g, adults, 2–5 g; Liquid Extract, dose: 2.5–5 ml.

PINUS BARK
Tsuga canadensis Carr.
Fam. Pinaceae

Synonyms: Hemlock Spruce, Hemlock bark, *Pinus canadensis* L., *Abies canadensis* Michx.

Habitat: North America.

Description: The bark occurs in pieces of very variable size and up to 2 cm thick. Outer surface of older pieces with rhytidome, deeply fissured; younger bark with exfoliating cork, reddish coloured. Inner surface light yellowish brown, longitudinally striated. Fracture short, fibrous. Taste, astringent; odour, faintly terebinthinate.

Part Used: Bark.

Constituents: Little information available. (i) Essential oil, containing α-pinene, bornyl acetate, cadinene (ii) Tannins, 10–14% (iii) Resin [2, 37].

Medicinal Use: Astringent, tonic, diuretic, diaphoretic, antiseptic. Used for diarrhoea, cystitis, colitis, leucorrhoea; and for gingivitis and laryngitis as a gargle or mouthwash.

Preparations: Liquid Extract Hemlock Spruce BPC 1934, dose: 1–5 ml.

Potter's Products: Peerless Composition Essence.

Regulatory Status: GSL.

PIPSISSEWA

Chimaphila umbellata Nutt.
Fam. Pyrolaceae

Synonyms: Prince's Pine, Ground Holly, Umbellate Wintergreen.
Habitat: Parts of Europe (not including Britain) and northern N. America.
Description: A short perennial. Leaves leathery, oblanceolate, about 3 cm long and 1 cm across, with a serrate margin and rounded apex.
Part Used: Leaves.
Constituents: (i) Quinones; including the hydroquinones arbutin and isohomoarbutin, and the naphthaquinones renifolin and chimaphilin [5, 218] (ii) Flavonoids; hyperoside, avicularin, kaempferol etc. [5, 1072] (iii) Triterpenes; ursolic acid, taraxasterol, β-sitosterol etc [5] (iv) Miscellaneous; methyl salicylate, epicatechin gallate, tannins etc [5].
Medicinal Use: Astringent, alterative, tonic. Used for kidney disorders in a similar manner to Uva-Ursi (q.v.), which also contains hydroquinones. These, and the chimaphilin, are responsible for the urinary antiseptic properties. It is also used for rheumatism, and extracts have been reported to have hypoglycaemic activity in animals [1073].
Preparations: Liquid Extract, dose: 2.5–5 ml.
Regulatory Status: GSL.

PITCHER PLANT

Sarracenia purpurea L.
Fam. Sarraceniaceae

Habitat: North America.
Description: A carnivorous plant with "pitchers" 15–20 cm or more long, formed from the leafstalks and stipules, the latter forming a sharp wing on the inner side, the leaf blade forming a rounded, heart-shaped hood. Taste, bitter and astringent; odourless.
Part Used: Root, leaves.
Constituents: Not well investigated. Glycosides; sarracenin and sarracenic acid, of unknown structure [2]. The closely related *S. flava* contains the poisonous alkaloid coniine [1074].
Medicinal Use: Stomachic, diuretic, laxative, usually as an infusion. At one time this plant had a great but obviously undeserved reputation as a prophylactic against smallpox.
Preparations: Powdered Root, dose: 0.5–2 g; Liquid Extract, dose: 2.5–5 ml.

PLANTAIN

Plantago major L.
Fam. Plantaginaceae

Synonyms: Greater Plantain.
Habitat: A common weed in Britain and many other parts of the world.
Description: Leaves strongly veined, in a basal rosette, broadly oval, with a blunt apex, abruptly narrowing at the base into a long petiole. Flowers tiny, yellowish-green with purple then yellowish anthers, in a long, dense, spike. Taste, astringent; odourless.

Part Used: Leaves.
Constituents: (i) Iridoids; aucubin, 3,4-dihydroaucubin, 6'-O-β-gluco-sylaucubin, catalpol [1075, 1076] (ii) Flavonoids; apigenin and its 7-glucoside, luteolin, scutellarin, baicalein, nepetin, hispidulin and plantago-side [1075, 1077, 1078] (iii) Miscellaneous; tannin, oleanolic acid, plant acids such as chlorogenic, neochlorogenic, fumaric, hydroxycinnamic and benzoic acids and their esters [1079].
Medicinal Use: Antiinflammatory, diuretic, antihaemorrhagic. Aucubin is a mild aperient, it also stimuates the secretion of uric acid by the kidneys [196, 197]. Apigenin is an antiinflammatory agent [436, 437] and baicalein is antiinflammatory and antiallergic (see Scullcap). Plantain is used widely in Chinese medicine to treat urinary diseases, tuberculous ulcers, bacillary dysentery, hepatitis and other conditions. Extracts have been shown there to be antimicrobial, and have complex effects on the cardiovascular system in animals [7].
Preparations: Liquid Extract, dose: 2.5–5 ml.
Regulatory Status: GSL.

PLEURISY ROOT
Aslepias tuberosa L.
Fam. Asclepiadaceae
Synonyms: Butterfly Weed.
Habitat: USA.
Description: The rootstock is slightly annulate, with a knotty crown. Roots longitudinally wrinkled, greyish-brown externally, whitish internally, composed of concentric cylinders of tissue which can easily be separated. Fracture uneven, tough, short, starch. Taste, nutty, bitter; odour, faint.
Part Used: Root.
Constituents: (i) Cardenolides, including asclepiadin [1080] (ii) Flavonoids; rutin, kaempferol, quercetin and isorhamnetin [1081] (iii) Miscellaneous; friedalin, α- and β-amyrin, lupeol, viburnitol, choline sugars and amino acids [1081].
Medicinal Use: Expectorant, tonic, diaphoretic, antispasmodic. It is also reputed to be mildly aperient and carminative. The main use is in the treatment of pleurisy, as the name implies, to relieve the pain and ease breathing. It has also been used for certain uterine disorders, and oestrogenic activity has been demonstrated in rats [1082].
Preparations: Liquid Extracts, dose: 2.5–5 ml.
Potter's Products: Pleurisy Mixture No. 115, Vegetable Cough Remover.
Regulatory Status: GSL.

POISON OAK
POISON IVY
Toxicodendrom diversilobium (L.) Kuntz
T. radicans (L.) Kuntz
Fam. Anacardiaceae
Synonyms: *Rhus toxicodendron* L.
Habitat: USA.

Description: Leaves trifoliate, about 10 cm long with a downy undersurface. Taste, acrid and astringent; odourless.

Part Used: Leaves.

Constituents: Urushiols, a series of alkyl catechols of varying chain length and double bond position. Poison ivy contains mainly pentadecylcatechols with some heptadecylcatechols, poison oak *vice versa* [1083, 1084]. For review see [1085].

Medicinal Use: The only medicinal use is as a homoeopathic remedy. *Toxicodendron* species are contact allergens, causing sensitization on intitial exposure and dermatitis of varying severity on subsequent exposure. It is possible to build up some sort of immune tolerance using usual techniques in highly sensitive individuals [1085 (review)]. Urushiols induce blastogenesis in peritoneal blood lymphocytes and may therefore stimulate the immune system in a non-specific way [1086]; they also inhibit cyclooxygenase and lipoxygenase *in vitro* [1086].

Preparations: Tincture 1 in 10, dose: 0.05–1 ml.

Regulatory Status: P.

POKE ROOT

Phytolacca americana L.
Fam. Phytolaccaeae

Synonyms: Pokeweed, *P. decandra* L.

Habitat: North America.

Description: The root is usually sold in transverse slices or split lengthways. The outer surface is yellowish to brownish grey, wrinkled longtidinally and marked with transverse bars of cork. The inner surface is whitish or buff, very hard, and shows characteristic concentric rings of vascular tissue separated by parenchyma. The berries are subglobular, purplish black, fleshy, about 8 mm in diameter and composed of 10 carpels, each containing one lens-shaped seed. The powder is strongly sternutatory; taste, slight.

Part Used: Root, berries.

Constituents: Research is continuing, so far the following have been found: (i) Triterpenoid saponins; the phytolaccosides A, B, C, D and E, based on the aglycones phytolaccagenin and phytolaccic acid [1087, 1088, 1089] (ii) Lectins; the mixture known as pokeweed mitogen, consisting of a series of glycoproteins termed Pa^{-1} to Pa^{-5} [1090] (iii) Proteins of undetermined structure [1091, 1092, 1093). Seeds: (iv) polyphenols [1094].

Medicinal Use: Antirheumatic, antiinflammatory, alterative, emetic, cathartic. The phytolaccosides are potent antiinflammatory agents in the rat paw oedema test [1089], and a saponin extract has a comparable antiexudative and antigranulomatous activity to that of hydrocortisone in mice. It had no effect on the adrenal gland but high doses caused thymolysis [1087]. Phytolaccosides B and E inhibited exudate formation after sponge pellet and carrageenan-induced oedema in rats, with antiinflammatory and toxic effects less than those of aescin (see Horsechestnut) [1088]. The proteins are antiviral; they inhibit the replication of the influenza and HSV-1 viruses and poliovirus [1091, 1093, 1094]. The lectins are mitogenic [1090]. Poke root has caused toxic, particularly gastrointestinal, symptoms when accidently eaten by mistake for parsnip or horseradish, and as a freshly made herbal tea [1095]. No toxic effects have been observed from other types of products. The berries are milder in action.

Preparations: Powdered root, dose: 0.06–0.3 g; Liquid Extract, dose: 0.1–0.5 ml; Tincture of Poke Root BPC 1923, dose: 0.2–0.6 ml.

Potter's Products: Tabritis Remedy for Arthritis, Alterative Tablets No. 34, Compound Elixir of Trifolium.

Regulatory Status: GSL.

POLYPODY ROOT

Polypodium vulgare L.
Fam. Polypodiaceae

Habitat: Grows on old walls, trunks of trees etc. in Britain and Europe.

Description: The rhizome is slender, about 3 mm in diameter, striated longitudinally, knotty, with cup-shaped leaf base scars on the upper side at intervals of about 1 cm and rootlet scars on the undersurface. Transverse section horny, greenish-brown, with an irregular circle of vascular bundles near the circumference. Taste, very sweet, faintly acrid; odourless.

Part Used: Rhizome.

Constituents: (i) Saponin glycosides, based on polypodosapogenin, including osladin [1096] (ii) Ecdysteroids; polypodins A and B [2] (iii) Phloroglucin derivatives [1097] (iv) Miscellaneous; essential oil, fixed oil, tannin etc. [2].

Medicinal Use: Expectorant, pectoral, alterative. It has been used in coughs and chest disorders, as a tonic in dyspepsia and loss of appetite, and as an alterative in skin diseases. The sweet taste is due to osladin [1096]. It occasionally produces a rash after ingestion, the reason for this is unknown and it appears to be harmless.

Preparations: Liquid Extract, dose: 1–4 ml.

POMEGRANATE

Punica granatum L.
Fam. Punicaeae

Habitat: Indigenous to NW India and the Middle East, cultivated.in the Mediterranean region and elsewhere.

Description: The tree is very beautiful with scarlet flowers; it is said to have flourished in the garden of Eden. The fruit is well-known. The rind of the fruit occurs in concave fragments, brownish-red externally and yellowish internally with depressions left by the seeds. The bark, mainly stem bark, occurs in flat or quilled pieces, externally yellowish grey, furrowed, occasionally with patches of lichen; internally finely striated. Taste, astringent; odourless.

Part Used: Bark, rind of fruit.

Constituents: (i) Alkaloids known as pelletierenes; pelletierine, isopelletierine, methylisopelletierine and pseudopelletierine [1074] (ii) Ellagitannins; punicacorteins A, B, C and D, punicalin, punicalagin, punigluconin, casuariin and casuarinin [1098].

Medicinal Use: Taenifuge, astringent. This is a very old remedy, being mentioned in the papyrus Ebers (Egypt, *circa* 1550 BC). It is taken by decoction, followed by a purgative. The alkaloids are anthelmintic; pelletierine in particular causes the tapeworm to relax its grip on the wall of the intestine so it can be expelled by the cathartic. If systemic absorption of pelletierine occurs it may give rise to toxic symptoms such as muscle cramps and dizziness. The ellagitannins are responsible for the astringency.

Preparations: Powdered Fruit Rind, dose: 3.5–7 g; Liquid Extract of Root Bark, dose: 1–7 ml.

Biblical References: Exodus 39 : 24–24; Numbers 13 : 23 and 20 : 5; Deuteronomy 8 : 8; 1 Samuel 14 : 2; Song of Solomon 4 : 3 & 13, 6 : 7 & 11, 7 : 12, 8 : 2 and others.

Regulatory Status: P.

POPLAR

Populus alba L.
P. tremuloides Michx.
P. nigra L. and other spp.
Fam. Salicaceae

Synonyms: White Poplar (= *P. alba*), Quaking Aspen, American Aspen (= *P. tremuloides*), Black Poplar (= *P. nigra*).

Habitat: *P. alba* and *P. nigra* are European species, *P. tremuloides* is N. American.

Description: The bark occurs as curved or flattened pieces or may be shredded. The outer layer is usually removed, leaving a dull brown surface. The inner surface is smooth and varies in colour from nearly white to brown. Taste, bitter; odourless.

Part Used: Bark.

Constituents: (i) Phenolic glycosides; salicin and populin (salicin benzoate), in all the above species [25] (ii) Tannins [37]. (iii) *P. nigra* at least contains the lignan (+)-*iso*lariciresinol mono-β-D-glucopyranoside [1099].

Medicinal Use: Antiinflammatory, anodyne, astringent, diuretic, stimulant. The salicylates are well known for their antiinflammatory activity [4]. Poplar has also been used to treat urinary complaints, such as cystitis, stomach, and liver disorder, debility and anorexia.

Preparations: Powdered Bark, dose: 1–5 g; Liquid Extract, dose: 1–5 ml.

Potter's Products: Tabritis Remedy for Arthritis, Rheumatism Compound Herb, Herbprin.

Regulatory Status: GSL.

Biblical References: Genesis 30 : 37; Hosea 4 : 13.

POPPY

Papaver somniferum L.
Fam. Papaveraceae

Synonyms: Opium Poppy.

Habitat: Native to Asia, cultivated widely elsewhere for food and medicinal purposes and as a garden ornamental.

Description: The flowers vary in colour from white to reddish purple, but are usually pale lilac with a purple base spot. The capsules are sub-spherical, depressed at the top with the radiating stigma in the centre, below which are the valves through which the seeds are dispersed. There is a swollen ring just above where the capsule joins the stem. The seeds are small, greyish, reniform and attached to the internal projections or placentae.

Part Used: Capsule, latex exuded from the unripe capsule (Opium).

Constituents: (i) Alkaloids; the major one is morphine, with codeine and thebaine and lesser amounts of very many others including narceine, narcotine, papaverine, salutaridine and sanguinarine [1, 4, 174] (ii) Meconic acid [1].

Medicinal Use: Narcotic, analgesic, antispasmodic, antidiarrhoeal, antitussive, diaphoretic. The total alkaloidal extract is known as papaveretum and is used routinely for preoperative analgesia and relaxation. Morphine is a very potent analgesic, however due to its potential for inducing dependence is used only under particular circumstances such as for terminal illness. Synthetic derivatives are normally used in its place. Papaverine is spasmolytic and is used in cough mixtures for this purpose. Opium is the starting material for the production of heroin. For further details see [1, 4]. Poppy seeds are used in the food industry to produce oil, on bread, and as bird seed. They do not contain alkaloids.

Preparations: Papaveretum BPC, Opium BP and many others, see [4].

Regulatory Status: Depending on strength, P, POM, or CD (Misuse of Drugs Act 1973).

POPPY, RED

Papaver rhoeas L.
Fam. Papaveraceae

Synonyms: Corn Poppy.

Habitat: Common throughout Europe and Britain, especially in fields and disturbed ground.

Description: Flowers solitary, with four, silky, bright red petals often with a dark centre. The stamens are numerous with blue-black anthers, and the stigma is radiate. The two sepals, which fall off soon after opening, and the stalk are covered with bristly hairs.

Part Used: Flowers.

Constituents: (i) Alkaloids, the papaverrubines, rhoeadine, isorhoeadine, stylopine, protopine and many others, variable in composition due to the existence of chemical races [112, 1100] (ii) Meconic acid [1101] (iii) Mekocyanin, a red pigment [1] (iv) Mucilage, tannin.

Medicinal Use: Anodyne, expectorant. Red poppy is also used as a colouring, it is used as an infusion and in the form of a syrup.
Preparations: Syrup of Red Poppy BPC 1949, dose: 2.5–5 ml.
Regulatory Status: GSL.

PRICKLY ASH

Zanthoxylum americanum Mill
Z. clava-herculis L.
Fam. Rutaceae

Synonyms: Toothache Tree, Yellow Wood. Northern Prickly Ash is *Z. americanum*; Southern Prickly Ash is *Z. clava-herculis*.
Habitat: Canada and the USA.
Description: Northern prickly ash bark occurs in curved or quilled fragments, about 1 mm thick, externally brownish grey, faintly furrowed with whitish patches and flattened spines about 5 mm long. Southern prickly ash is about 2 mm thick, with conical, corky spines up to 2 cm long. Fracture short, green in the outer and yellow in the inner part. Taste, bitter and pungent, causing salivation.
Part Used: Bark, berries.
Constituents: Bark: (i) Alkaloids, in both species; γ-fagarine, β-fagarine (= skimmianine), magnoflorine, laurifoline, nitidine, chelerythrine, tambetarine and candicine [1102, 1103] (ii) Coumarins, in *Z. americanum*; xanthyletin, xanthoxyletin, alloxanthyletin [5, 1102] (iii) Amides, in *Z. clava-herculis*; herculin, neoherculin [2, 1102, 1103] (iv) Asarinin, a lignan, in *Z. clava-herculis* [5] (v) Resin, tannin, volatile oil.
Medicinal Use: Antirheumatic, analgesic, diaphoretic, carminative, antipyretic, antidiarrhoeal. It is used both internally and externally to treat rheumatism and toothache, for fevers and as a tonic, and for circulatory insufficiency. Chelerythrine is antimicrobial. A West African species *Z. zanthoxyloides* (Lam.) Watson, used for similar purposes, has been extensively investigated chemically and pharmacologically. It has related but different constituents and contains fagaramide, a potent prostaglandin inhibitor in animal tests. For review see [33].
Preparations: Liquid Extract of Bark, dose: 1–3 ml; Liquid Extract of Berries, dose: 0.5–1.5 ml.
Potter's Products: Tabritis Remedy for Arthritis, Compound Elixir Trifolium, Eczema and All Skin Diseases Mixtures No 83 and No 83A, Acne Mixture No 128.
Regulatory Status: GSL.

PRIMROSE

Primula vulgaris Huds.
Fam. Primulaceae

Habitat: A well known wild flower growing in woods and grassy banks in Britain and parts of Europe, Asia and N. Africa.
Description: The leaves are up to about 12 cm long and 3 cm broad, oblanceolate, with a rounded apex and tapering to a decurrent base. The

margin is irregular and the lamina shows a characteristic, reticulate venation, depressed above and prominent and hairy beneath. Rootstock knotty, with successive leaf base scars and cylindrical, branched rootlets. Taste, insipid; odourless.

Part Used: Root, herb.

Constituents: (i) Saponins, including primulaveroside (ii) Phenolic glycosides (iii) Flavonoids [1104].

Medicinal Use: Antiinflammatory, antispasmodic, vermifuge, emetic, vulnerary. Seldom used today but formerly used for rheumatism, gout, insomnia and as a poultice to heal wounds.

PRUNE

Prunus domestica L.
Fam. Rosaceae

Synonyms: Plum tree.

Habitat: Widely cultivated.

Description: The prune, or dried plum, is too well known to require description.

Part Used: Fruit.

Constituents: Pulp: sugars, about 44%, malic acid. Kernel: fixed oil, about 45%, amygdalin and benzoic acid [1].

Medicinal Use: Laxative, refrigerant, nutritive. Prunes are either eaten as a food or added to other preparations for their laxative effect.

Preparations: Confection of Senna BPC 1959, dose: 4–8 g.

Regulatory Status: GSL.

PSYLLIUM

Plantago ovata Forsk.
P. indica L.
P. psyllium L.
Fam. Plantaginaceae

Synonyms: *P. ovata:* blond psyllium, ispaghula, spogel, Indian plantago, *P. decumbens* Forsk., *P. ispaghula* Roxb. *P. psyllium:* dark psyllium, Spanish or French psyllium, brown psyllium. *P. indica:* black psyllium, *P. arenaria* Waldst et Kit. The seeds of *P. major* have been used as a substitute, and *P. asiatica* L. is used in the Far East.

Habitat: Native to the Mediterranean region, cultivated widely throughout the world, including Russia and China. *P. ovata* is cultivated in India and Pakistan, *P. indica* in Europe and Egypt, and *P. psyllium* in France, Spain and Cuba.

Description: *P. ovata* seeds are pinkish or greyish brown, boat shaped, 1.8–3.3 mm long; *P. indica* seeds are blackish brown and slightly smaller; *P. psyllium* seeds are deep brown and glossy.

Part Used: Seeds. The whole plant, as well as the seeds, of *P. asiatica* is used in Oriental medicine.

Constituents: (i) Mucilage, 10–30%, consisting of a mixture of polysaccharides composed of mainly of D-xylose units, with smaller amounts of L-arabinose and aldobiouronic acid [1105] (ii) Monoterpene alkaloids; (+)-boschniakine (= indicaine) and (+)-boschniakinic acid (= plantagonine) [1106] (iii) Miscellaneous; triterpenes such as stigmasterol, β-sitosterol, campesterol, α- and β-amyrin; sugars, fixed oil rich in polyunsaturated fatty acids etc. [5]. The herb of *P. psyllium* and *P. indica* contains the iridoid plantarenaloside [1107]. *P. asiatica* contains 3'4 dihydroaucubin and other iridoids [1108].

Medicinal Use: Bulk laxative. The seeds swell when moistened into a gelatinous mass, promoting peristaslis and hydrating the faeces. The bulk thus formed also has a beneficial effect in diarrhoea. *P. ovata* has also been shown to absorb a mixture of food additives including cyclamate, preventing harmful effects, in rats [1109], and an alcoholic extract is reported to lower blood pressure, slow heart rate, have anticholinergic activity and stimulate peristalsis in animals [1110]. The mucilage of *P. asiatica* is hypoglycaemic in mice [1111] and the seeds show a liver protective effect on carbon tetrachloride induced hepatotoxicity in mice, this is due to the aucubin content [48]. The fresh plant is used clinically in China to treat certain types of hepatitis with apparently great success [7].

Potter's Products: Lion Cleansing Herbs (*P. ovata*).

Regulatory Status: GSL.

PUFF BALL

Lycoperdon spp.
Calvatia spp.
Fam. Lycoperdaceae

Habitat: Europe including Britain.

Description: The fungus forms a globose or depressed ball, varying in size from 10 cm to 30 cm in diameter, sometimes furrowed at the base. Whitish when young, with a white internal mass containing yellow spores, darkening with age and when ripe, discharging brownish or blackish spores by rupturing the skin.

Part Used: Fungus.

Constituents: *L. bovista* L. contains a glycoside lycoperdin, xanthine derivatives and amino acids [2]. *C. lilacina* (Berk) Henn. contains *p*-carboxyphenylazoxycyanide [1112].

Medicinal Use: Haemostatic.

PULSATILLA

Anemone pulsatilla L.
and other spp.
Fam. Ranunculaceae

Synonyms: Pasque Flower, Wind Flower, Meadow Anemone, *Pulsatilla vulgaris* Mill.

Habitat: Europe and parts of Russia.

Description: Leaves feathery, hairy, stalked, up to about 15 cm long, 8 cm broad, bipinnate, the leaflets opposite, each segment trifid, narrow, with acute points. Leafstalks cylindrical, channelled on the upper surface, purplish at the base. Flowers large, solitary, purple, with numerous stamens with bright yellow anthers. Sepals hairy, purplish. Taste when fresh, acrid and burning; odourless.

Part Used: Herb.

Constituents: (i) Lactones; protoanemonin, which dimerizes on drying to anemonin, ranunculin [1113, 1014] (ii) Triterpenoid saponins, unspecified [2,7] (iii) Miscellaneous; anemone camphor, tannins, volatile oil [25].

Medicinal Use: Nervine, antispasmodic, alterative. Used for nervous exhaustion and amenorrhoea in women, as a sedative and for catarrh. Protoanemonin is antibacterial and irritant [1014, 1113], however it is not found in dried plant material so the irritancy does not constitute a practical problem [1014].

Preparations: Liquid Extract of Pulsatilla BPC 1934, dose: 0.12–0.3 ml; Tincture of Pulsatilla BPC 1934, dose 0.3–2 ml; Solution of Caulophyllum and Pulsatilla BPC 1934, dose 5–10 ml; Elixir of Euonymus and Pulsatilla BPC 1934, dose: 5–15 ml.

Potter's Products: Blood Pressure Tablets No 400, Uterine Sedative Tablets No 444.

Regulatory Status: GSL.

PUMPKIN

Cucurbita maxima Duchesne.
and other spp.
Fam. Cucurbitaceae

Habitat: Cultivated widely.

Description: The seeds are broadly ovate, about 2 cm long, whitish, with a shallow groove and flat ridge round the margin. The hilum is near the pointed end. Taste, nutty; odourless.

Part Used: Seeds.

Constituents: (i) Oil, the main component of which is linoleic acid, with oleic, palmitic and to a lesser extent stearic acids [1115] (ii) Cucurbitacins, to a variable extent depending on variety etc [1116, 33].

Medicinal Use: Taenicide, diuretic, demulcent. It has been taken for tapeworm with a saline purgative. The cucurbitacins are toxic, see Bryony.

Regulatory Status: P.

PYRETHRUM

Chryanthemum cinerariaefolium Visiana
and other spp.
Fam. Compositae

Synonyms: Insect Flowers, Dalmation Insect Flowers, *Pyrethrum cinerariaefolium* Trev.

Habitat: Indigenous to the Balkans but widely cultivated elsewhere.

Description: The unopened flowerheads are preferred; they are about 6–9 mm in diameter, with two or three rows of lanceolate greenish-yellow, hairy bracts. The receptacle is nearly flat, without paleae; the ligulate florets are creamy-white and the tubular florets yellow. Taste, slightly acrid; odourless.

Part Used: Flowers.

Constituents: (i) Pyrethrins; esters of chrysanthemic and pyrethric acids, known as pyrethrin I and II, cinerin I and II, jasmolin I and II etc. (ii) Sesquiterpene lactones (iii) Pyrethrol, a triterpenoid [1].

Medicinal Use: Insecticide. It is harmless to humans and may be used as a spray, lotion or powder, or for fumigation.

Q

QUASSIA

Picrasma excelsa (Sw.) Planch
Quassia amara L.
Fam. Simaroubaceae

Synonyms: Bitter Wood. Jamaica Quassia, *Picraenia excelsa* Lindl., (= *P. excelsa*); Surinam Quassia (= *Q. amara*). Japanese Quassia is *Picrasma ailanthoides* Planch., (= *P. quassinoides* Bennett).

Habitat: *P. excelsa* is native to the West Indies, *Q. amara* to South America and *P. ailanthoides* to the Far East.

Description: Quassia occurs in commerce as logs, chips or shredded. The wood is whitish, becoming yellow on exposure to the air. Cork may be present, with blackish or greyish markings due to fungus, in inferior samples. Taste, intensely bitter; odourless.

Part Used: Wood.

Constituents: (i) Quassinoids; quassin, isoquassin (= picrasmin), neoquassin and 18-hydroxyquassin, in *P. excelsa* [1, 306, 1117]; quassin, quassinol, 18-hydroxyquassin, neoquassin, quassimarin and similikalactone in *Q. amara* [306, 1118]. *P. ailanthoides* also contains quassinoids, the nigakilactones A–N and the nigakihemiacetals A–F [1119, 1120] (ii) Alkaloids, of the β-carboline type, including canthin-6-one, 5-methoxycanthin-6-one, 4-methoxy-5-hydroxycanthin-6-one and N-methyl-1-*vinyl*-β-carboline [1121], in *P. excelsa*; and similar alkaloids in *P. ailanthoides* [1122] (iii) Miscellaneous; scopoletin, β-sitosterol etc. [1, 5].

Medicinal Use: Tonic, bitter, anthelmintic, febrifuge, antimalarial. The quassinoids are responsible for the bitterness and pharmacological activity; many of them are amoebicidal *in vitro* and *in vivo* [306, 1123, 1124]. The alkaloids do not appear to contribute to the antimalarial activity [1125]. Quassimarin has been reported to have antileukaemic properties [1118]. Quassia extracts have been used to expel threadworms, administered as an enema. Quassia has long been used as a bitter flavouring in alcoholic and soft drinks.

Preparations: Powdered Wood, dose: 0.3–0.6 g; Concentrated Quassia Infusion BPC 1959, dose: 2.5–5 ml; Quassia Enema BPC 1949, dose: 600 ml; Quassia Tincture BP 1948, dose: 2.5–5 ml.

Potter's Products: Tonsillitis Mixture No. 145.

Regulatory Status: GSL.

QUEBRACHO

Aspidosperma quebracho-blanco Schlecht.
Fam. Apocynaceae

Synonyms: White Quebracho. Red Quebracho is *Schinopsis quebracho-colorado* (Schlecht) Barkl. et T Meyer.

Habitat: Argentina.

Description: The bark occurs in curved or flat pieces up to about 2.5 cm thick, greyish and deeply fissured externally. The inner surface is yellowish brown, often with a reddish tint, and striated. The transverse fracture shows a coarsely granular outer layer and a fibrous or splintery, darker inner layer. Taste, bitter; odourless.

Part Used: Bark.

Constituents: (i) Indole alkaloids; aspidospermine, aspidospermatine, akuammicine, yohimbine (= quebrachine), eburnaminine, quebrachamine, pyrifolidine and others [5, 29, 112, 1126] (ii) Miscellaneous; rhazinilam, tannins, sugars, sterols etc [5, 1126].

Medicinal Use: Antiasthmatic, tonic, febrifuge. The alkaloids are hypotensive, but arterial hypertensive, spasmolytic and diuretic, with respiratory stimulant and peripheral vasoconstricting actions. For actions of yohimbine see Yohimbe. Large doses have toxic effects, including nausea and vomiting [4].

Preparations: Liquid Extract, dose: 0.5–1.5 ml.

Regulatory Status: POM.

QUEEN'S DELIGHT

Stillingia sylvatica L.
Fam. Euphorbiaceae

Synonyms: Queen's Root, Yaw Root.

Habitat: USA.

Description: The root usually occurs in tapering, tough, fibrous pieces. It is greyish brown externally with a pinkish-white wood, showing numerous small resin glands. Taste, bitter and acrid; odour, characteristic and unpleasant.

Part Used: Root.

Constituents: (i) Diterpene esters of the daphnane and tigliane type, including prostatin and gnidilatin [1127] (ii) Fixed oil, volatile oil and resins [37].

Medicinal Use: Alterative, laxative, tonic, diuretic. It is generally given as a tonic and "blood purifier" in combination with other remedies. The diterpene esters are irritant [1127], however they are unstable and unlikely to be present in most extracts and preparations.

Preparations: Liquid Extract, dose: 0.5–2 ml; Tincture, dose: 1–4 ml.

Potter's Products: Compound Elixir of Trifolium, Alterative Tablet No. 34.

Regulatory Status: GSL.

QUINCE

Cydonia oblongata Mill.
Fam. Rosaceae

Habitat: Native to the Middle East but cultivated elsewhere for its fruit.

Description: The seeds are usually clumped in a double row by the dried mucilage contained in the testa. In appearance and size they resemble apple pips but have been pressed into a more angular shape.

Part Used: Seeds.

Constituents: Mucilage, about 20%; amygdalin, about 0.4%; fixed oil; tannins [2].

Medicinal Use: Demulcent. The seeds have been used in diarrhoea and in the form of a lotion to soothe the eyes. The fruit is used to make jam.

R

RAGWORT

Senecio jacobaea L.
Fam. Compositae

Synonyms: Common Ragwort, Tansy Ragwort.

Habitat: Grows as a common weed in many parts of the world, including Britain.

Description: A medium or tall perennial, usually hairless. Leaves alternate, pinnately lobed, with the end lobe small and blunt, the segments deeply and irregularly toothed. Flowers rayed, 15–25 mm in diameter, daisy-like bright golden yellow, in dense, flat-topped clusters.

Part Used: Herb.

Constituents: (i) Volatile oil, containing germacrene D and 1-undecene as the major components, with 1-nonene, myrcene, *trans*-ocimene and β-caryophyllene [653] (ii) Pyrrolizidine alkaloids; seneciphylline, senecionine, jacoline, jaconine, jacobine, jacozine and others [1128, 1129].

Medicinal Use: Formerly used as a diaphoretic, in coughs and colds and for rheumatism and gout. The alkaloids are hepatotoxic [1130] and ragwort should not be taken internally or applied to broken skin. It is occasionally used externally as an ointment or lotion for rheumatic pains, myalgia and other similar conditions.

RASPBERRY

Rubus idaeus L.
Fam. Rosaceae

Habitat: Cultivated in most temperate countries.

Description: Leaves stalked, pinnate with 3–5 leaflets, up to 12 cm in length, the terminal leaflet being longer than the others. Leaflets ovate, acuminate, rounded at the base, with an irregularly dentate, mucronate, toothed margin, green on the upper surface, white and densely tomentose on the lower. Taste, astringent; odourless.

Part Used: Leaves.

Constituents: Largely unknown (i) Polypeptides (unspecified) [37, 1131] (ii) Flavonoids, mainly glycosides of kaempferol and quercetin [160] (iii) Tannins [37].

Medicinal Use: Raspberry leaf tea has been used for centuries to facilitate childbirth. It is recommended that it be drunk freely before and during confinement for maximum benefit. Uterine relaxant effects have been demonstrated in animals on many occasions [1132, 1133, 1134), however despite attempts to fractionate the extract [1134], no further progress has been made. The extract appears to affect only the pregnant uterus from both rats and humans, with no activity on the non-pregnant uterus; evaluation is not easy since obviously only pathological human uterus can be used [1133]. If polypeptides are the active constituents this would explain the problems since they are notoriously difficult to isolate.

Preparations: Liquid Extract, dose: 2–10 ml.
Potter's Products: Raspberry Leaf Tablets, Tonsillitis Mixture No. 145, Motherhood Tea.
Regulatory Status: GSL.

RED CLOVER

Trifolium pratense L.
Fam. Leguminosae

Habitat: Widely distributed throughout Europe including Britain, naturalized in N. America and many other parts of the world.
Description: The flowerheads are globular or egg-shaped, sometimes paired, usually unstalked, reddish purple, about 2–3 cm long and 2 cm broad, composed of numerous individual, typically papilionaceous keeled flowers. Leaflets trefoil, often with a whitish crescent; stipules triangular, bristly.
Part Used: Flowerheads.
Constituents: (i) Isoflavones; biochanin A, daidzein, formononetin, genistein, pratensein and trifoside [1136, 1137, 1138, 1139] (ii) Other flavonoids, including pectolinarin and trifoliin (= isoquercitrin) [5] (iii) Volatile oil, containing furfural [50] (iv) Clovamides; L-Dopa-caffeic acid conjugates [1140] (v) Coumarins; coumestrol, medicagol and coumarin [1137, 1138, 1139] (vi) Miscellaneous; a galactomannan, resins, minerals, vitamins, phytoalexins etc. [1138, 5].
Medicinal Use: Alterative, antispasmodic, expectorant, sedative dermatological agent. Its main use is as an alterative and for skin complaints such as psoriasis and eczema, and as an expectorant in coughs and bronchial conditions. The isoflavones are oestrogenic in animals, which may ingest large quantities as forage [1136, 1138]. Red clover is also reported to have antispasmodic and expectorant properties [25].
Preparations: Liquid Extract, dose: 2.5–10 ml.
Potter's Products: Compound Elixir of Trifolium.
Regulatory Status: GSL.

RED ROOT

Ceanothus americanus L.
Fam. Rhamnaceae

Synonyms: Jersey Tea Root.
Habitat: USA.
Description: Root tough, woody, dark brown, striated or finely wrinkled longitudinally. Bark thin, brittle, deep brown; wood, reddish, with obscure concentric rings. Taste, astringent; odourless.
Part Used: Root.
Constituents: Little information available. Ceanothic acid and emmolic acid [25]. *C. interregmus* and *C. sanguineus* contain cyclopeptide alkaloids [1141].
Medicinal Use: Astringent, expectorant, antispasmodic.
Preparations: Liquid Extract, dose: 0.05–1.5 ml.

REST HARROW

Ononis spinosa L.
Fam. Leguminosae

Synonyms: Cammock, Spiny Rest Harrow.

Habitat: Common on arable and waste land in Europe and Russia.

Description: A woody perennial, with roundish leaves, oval or trefoil, spines, flowers in leafy spikes, pink, papilionaceous, with the wings equalling the keel. The root is more or less flattened, twisted and branched, deeply wrinkled and brown in colour. Taste, sweet and mucilaginous at first, then rather bitter; odour, resembling that of liquorice.

Part Used: Root.

Constituents: (i) Volatile oil, containing *trans*-anethole as the major component, with menthone, isomenthone, camphor, linalool, menthol, estragole, borneol, carvone and *cis*-anethole [1142] (ii) Phenolics; trifo-lirfizin and other pterocarpans, tannins etc [1143, 1144] (iii) Lectins and phytohaemaglutinins [1145] (iv) Triterpenes; α-onocerin, β-sitosterol etc. [1142]. In the aerial parts at least: Flavonoids and isoflavones: rutin, hyperoside, cosmosiin, myricetrin, and apigenin, vitexin, luteolin, kaemp-ferol, quercetin, faceidin, penduletin, formononetin, tectorigenin, and biochanin A glycosides [1146, 1147].

Medicinal Use: Diuretic, antilithic, antiinflammatory, expectorant. Rest harrow is used mainly for its effects on the urinary system, as an infusion.

RHATANY

Krameria triandra Ruiz et Pavon
Fam. Krameriaceae

Synonyms: Peruvian Rhatany. Para Rhatany is *K. argentea* Mart.

Habitat: Peru, Bolivia.

Description: Root woody, cylindrical, deep reddish-brown and rough externally, with a coarsely fibrous bark and hard, tough, woody centre. Taste, very astringent; odourless.

Part Used: Root.

Constituents: Tannins, exclusively condensed tannins composed of pro-cyanidins and propelargonidins with a ratio of from 37 : 63 to 24 : 76 as determined by acid hydrolysis. The astringency is due to polymers with a degree of polymerization of more than 5 [1148, 1149].

Medicinal Use: Astringent. Rhatany is used as an antidiarrhoeal, styptic, antihaemorrhagic and vulnerary. It may be used as an infusion or decoction internally for diarrhoea or haemorrhage, including menorrhagia, as an ointment or suppository for haemorrhoids, topically for chilblains and wounds, as a lozenge, gargle or mouthwash for gingivitis and pharyngitis.

Preparations: Krameria Dry Extract BPC 1954, dose: 0.3–1 g; Krameria Tincture BPC 1949, dose: 2–4 ml.

Regulatory Status: GSL.

RHUBARB
CHINESE RHUBARB

Rheum officinale Baill.
R. palmatum L.
and other varieties and hybrids.

INDIAN RHUBARB
JAPANESE RHUBARB
ENGLISH RHUBARB

R. emodi Wall.
R. palmatum × *R. coreanum*
R. rhaponticum Willd.
Fam. Polygonaceae

Synonyms: Chinese Rhubarb; Dahuang; Indian Rhubarb; Himalayan Rhubarb; English Rhubarb; Rhapontic Rhubarb; Garden Rhubarb.

Habitat: Most rhubarb is cultivated, the origin being shown by the name.

Description: Chinese rhubarb comes in different grades and sizes; the older rhizome is larger and occurs in peeled flats or rounds, often with circular holes made for hanging by a string during the drying process. The cut surface has a bright yellow, marbled or reticulate appearance due to the reddish-brown medullary rays; when freshly cut it is pinkish. Poorer quality grades are paler and less carefully peeled. English rhubarb, not normally found in commerce, is unpeeled, in smaller pieces and has red veins. Taste, bitter; odour, aromatic and characteristic.

Part Used: Rhizome. The young leaf stalks of English rhubarb are used for food.

Constituents: (i) Anthraquinone derivatives: Chinese rhubarb contains chrysophanic acid (= chrysophanol), emodin (= rheum emodin), aloe-emodin, rhein and physcion, with their O-glycosides (mainly mono-glucosides) such as glucorhein, chrysophanein, glucoemodin; lesser amounts of the sennosides A–E, reidin C and others [1, 5, 1150, 1151, 1152, 1153] Both Indian and Japanese rhubarbs contain similar anthraquinones [1, 5, 1154], but English rhubarb contains only chrysophanic acid and some of its glycosides [1150] (ii) Tannins; in Chinese rhubarb: *d*-catechin and epicatechin gallate, with various cinnamoyl and coumaroyl galloyl glucosides and fructoses [1150, 1156, 1157] (iii) Stilbene derivatives; in English rhubarb rhaponticin (= rhapontin) is present, with related stilbene glycosides present in other types [5, 1156] (iii) Miscellaneous; volatile oil, containing diisobutyl phthalate, cinnamic and ferulic acids; rutin, fatty acids, calcium oxalate etc. [5].

Medicinal Use: Astringent, aperient, tonic, stomachic. In large doses rhubarb is a laxative. English rhubarb is similar but milder in action. It has been shown to have both astringent and cathartic properties [1158]; the anthraquinones are laxative and the tannins astringent. In Chinese medicine rhubarb is also very highly regarded; it is used for jaundice, abdominal pains, indigestion, amenorrhoea, carbuncles, scalds and burns. It was shown to have cholinergic action in rodents, to enhance peristalsis and increase the water content of stools. In low doses it increased gastric secretion and therefore acted as an appetite stimulant, and increased the secretion of bile. Emodin was shown to be a powerful antispasmodic in isolated rat intestine. The antiinflammatory and antiseptic action was also demonstrated [7].

Preparations: Chinese Rhubarb: Rhubarb Dry Extract BPC 1954, dose: 120–500 mg; Compound Rhubarb Pills BPC 1963, dose 1 or 2 pills; Compound Rhubarb Powder BPC, dose: 0.5–5 g; Compound Rhubarb Tincture BP, dose: up to 15 ml daily in divided doses.

Potter's Products: Hydrastis Compound Digestive Tablet No. 24, Gout and Rheumatism Tablet No. 31, Bile and Liver Tablet No. 167, Rhubarb and Myrrh Compound Tablet No. 254, Acidosis Tablet, Eczema and All Skin Diseases Mixture No. 83, Stomach and Liver Mixture No. 93, Flatulence Mixture No. 99, Constipation Mixture No. 105.

Regulatory Status: GSL.

RICE
Oryza sativa L.
Fam. Gramineae

Habitat: Widely cultivated in wet, tropical areas.
Description: The grains hardly require description.
Part Used: Seeds.
Constituents: Starch, fixed oil, vitamins etc.
Medicinal Use: Nutritive, demulcent. Boiled rice is easily digested in gastric upsets and rice-water, similar to barley water, can be made.

ROSE
Rosa gallica L.
R. damascena Mill.
R. centifolia L.
and other spp.
Fam. Rosaceae

Habitat: Cultivated throughout the world.
Description: A common, thorny, garden shrub needing no description.
Part Used: Flowers.
Constituents: Oil, containing geraniol, nerol, citronellol, geranic acid, eugenol, myrcene, β-phenethyl alcohol and many other constituents [5].
Medicinal Use: Rarely used medicinally. An important ingredient of many cosmetics and a flavouring agent. The fruits of the Dog Rose (q.v.) are used as an astringent and source of vitamin C.
Preparations: Concentrated Rose Water BPC 1949, Rose Oil BPC 1949.
Regulatory Status: GSL.

ROSEMARY
Rosmarinus officinalis L.
Fam. Labiatae

Habitat: Native to the Mediterranean region, cultivated widely elsewhere.
Description: Stem woody, quadrangular, branched; bearing linear leaves about 1.5–3.5 cm long, green above and whitish beneath, with strongly revolute margins. Flowers if present, bluish-lilac, two-lipped, with two stamens only. Taste and odour, aromatic, characteristic.
Part Used: Herb.

Constituents: (i) Volatile oil, composed of borneol, camphene, camphor, cineole, limonene, linalool, isobutyl acetate, 3-octanone, terpineol, verbenol etc. [5, 50, 1159] (ii) Flavonoids; apigenin, diosmetin, diosmin, genkwanin, 6-methoxygenkwanin, hispidulin, sinensetin, luteolin and derivatives [386, 1160, 1161] (iii) Rosmarinic acid and other phenolic acids [1160] (iv) Diterpenes such as picrosalvin (= carnosol), carnosolic acid and rosmariquinone [386, 1162] (v) Miscellaneous; rosmaricine, the triterpenes ursolic acid, oleanolic acid and derivatives [5, 1163, 1164].

Medicinal Use: Antiinflammatory, tonic, astringent, diaphoretic, stomachic, nervine, anodyne, antiseptic. Rosmarinic acid has been suggested as a possible potential treatment for septic shock, since it suppresses the endotoxin-induced activation of complement, the formation of prostacyclin, both hypotensive phases, thrombocytopaenia and the concomitant release of thromboxane Az [1165]. The antiinflammatory effect of Rosemary extracts [403] may be due to the rosmarinic acid, ursolic acid and apigenin, all of which have this effect. Diosmin is reported to be more effective in decreasing capillary fragility than rutin (see Rue) [5]. A rosmaricine derivative has stimulant and mild analgesic activity [5]. Rosemary has long been a popular ingredient of hair preparations, shampoos and tonics. It is a well-known culinary herb.

Preparations: Rosemary Oil BPC 1973, Rosemary Spirit BPC 1949, dose: 0.3–1.2 ml.

Potter's Products: Medicated Extract of Rosemary, Herbal Shampoo.

Regulatory Status: GSL.

ROSINWEED

Silphium laciniatum L.
Fam. Compositae

Synonyms: Compass Weed.

Habitat: Northern Europe.

Description: Fragments of leaves stiff, papery, brittle, hairless, with a faintly reticulate surface. Root up to about 5 cm long, 2–3 cm in diameter, laterally branched at the base, dark greyish brown, striated longitudinally; the transverse section showing concentric lines and a radiate structure, variegated dark grey and white with a small central pith. Taste, bitter then acrid; odourless.

Part Used: Herb, root.

Constituents: Inulin, in the root; terpenes, resin acids [2].

Medicinal Use: Antispasmodic, diuretic, expectorant, emetic.

Preparations: Liquid Extract, dose: 2–4 ml

RUE

Ruta graveolens L.
Fam. Rutaceae

Synonyms: Garden Rue, Herb of Grace, Herbygrass.

Habitat: Native to Southern Europe, cultivated in Britain and elsewhere as an ornamental.

237

Description: Leaves blue green, alternate, bipinnate, with oblanceolate segments, wedge-shaped below, with numerous translucent, small, punctate oil glands. Flowers yellow with five concave petals incurved at the tip, stem cylindrical, smooth and branched. Taste, pungent; odour, strong and characteristic.

Part Used: Herb.

Constituents: (i) Volatile oil, with 2-undecanone as the major component (50–90%), with 2-haptanol, 2-nonanol, 2-nonanone, limonene, pinene, anisic acid, phenol, guiacol and others [50, 45, 1166] (ii) Rutin and other flavonoids such as quercetin [5,50,386] (iii) Coumarins; bergapten, daphnoretin, isoimperatorin, naphthoherniarin, psoralen, pangelin, rutamarin, rutarin, scopoletin and umbelliferone [386, 1167, 1168, 1169] (iv) Alkaloids; arborinine, γ-fagarine, graveoline, graveolinine, kokusaginine, rutacridine, 1-hydroxy-3-methoxy-N-methylacridone etc [1170, 1171, 1172] (v) Lignans, in the root; savinin and helioxanthin [1173].

Medicinal Use: Stimulant, antispasmodic, emmenagogue. Rue is usually used as a uterine stimulant; it should only be taken in small doses and not by pregnant women. The volatile oil is reportedly anthelmintic. The furocoumarins can cause phototoxicity; this property is utilized in the treatment of psoriasis by psoralen derivatives [4, 45]. Rutin has been extensively investigated for its ability to reduce capillary fragility and is often taken as a food supplement, the so-called "vitamin P". Its other properties include anti-oedema effects [5] and it may be responsible for the antiinflammatory effect of the herb observed in animal tests [403]. It has also been shown to inhibit tumour formation on mouse skin induced by benzo(*a*)pyrene [1174] and increase survival times of rats fed a thrombogenic diet [1175].

Preparations: Powdered Herb, dose 1–2 g; Liquid Extract, dose: 2–4 ml.

Regulatory Status: GSL.

Biblical References: Luke 11 : 42.

RUPTUREWORT

Herniaria glabra L.
Fam. Caryophyllaceae

Synonyms: Smooth Rupturewort, Herniary.

Habitat: Grows throughout Europe but is rare in Britain.

Description: A prostrate, bright green, more or less hairless plant. Flowers green, sessile, in clusters at the base of the small, oval, opposite leaves. Taste, insipid; odourless.

Part Used: Herb.

Constituents: (i) Coumarins; herniarin, scopoletin, umbelliferone (ii) Flavonoids; isorhamnetin and quercetin glycosides (iii) Phenolic acids; salicylic, ferulic, vanillic, *p*-coumaric, caffeic and protocatechiuc [1176, 1177, 1178] (iv) Saponins [1179].

Medicinal Use: Astringent, diuretic. Used principally for bladder complaints in the form of an infusion, and, as the name suggests, for ruptures. Gerard writes: "it is singular good for Ruptures and that very many that have been bursten were restored to health by the use of this herbe also the powder thereof taken with wine . . . wasteth away the stone in the kidney and expelleth them".

S

SABADILLA

Schoenocaulon officinale A. Gray
Fam. Liliaceae

Synonyms: Cevadilla.

Habitat: Mexico and parts of South America.

Description: The seeds are linear, about 6 mm long, pointed, brownish-black, shiny and wrinkled.

Part Used: Seeds.

Constituents: (i) Alkaloids, of the ceveratrum type, including veracevine, sabadilline, sabadine, cevine, cevagenine, germidine and neogermidine [669] (ii) Fixed oil, containing tiglic and angelic acids and their esters [2].

Medicinal Use: Insecticide. The seeds have been used in the form of an ointment for topical use as parasiticide but the alkaloids are too toxic to recommend for this use (see Hellebore, American). They are also toxic to houseflies.

Regulatory Status: POM.

SAFFLOWER

Carthamus tinctorius L.
Fam. Compositae

Synonyms: False Saffron, Dyer's Saffron, Honghua (Chinese).

Habitat: Indigenous to parts of Asia, cultivated elsewhere.

Description: The florets are usually separated from the flowerheads, either loose or compressed into circular masses. The florets are cylindrical, slender, orange, about 1 cm long, with five teeth. Taste, slightly bitter; odour faint.

Part Used: Flowers

Constituents: (i) Carthamone, a benzoquinone pigment, together with carthamin and neocarthamin, both of which are also dihydroflavones [7, 218] (ii) Lignans; tracheloside, matairesinoside and 2-hydroxyarctiin [1180] (iii) A polysaccharide composed of xylose, fructose, galactose, glucose, arabinose, rhamnose and uronic acid residues [1181].

Medicinal Use: Laxative, diuretic. Safflowers were formerly used as an infusion for childrens complaints such as measles, fevers and eruptive skin conditions. The polysaccharide induces antibody formation in mice following peritoneal injection; these antibodies cross react with antisera specific for *Streptococcus pneumoniae* type III and type VIII [1181]. Safflower is used widely in Chinese medicine for injuries, contusions and strains and for amenorrhoea, and has been shown to have antiinflammatory activity [7, 1182]. Extracts have also been tested there on blood coagulation, where a prolongation of clotting time was observed and platelet aggregation inhibited. Other properties included an increase in the tolerance of mice to hypoxia and a stimulant effect on the uterus, particularly the pregnant uterus, in animals. Clinically Safflower is used in China to treat coronary disease, thrombotic disorders and menstrual disturbances, and alcoholic extracts are applied topically to ulcers and wounds [7].

Regulatory Status: GSL.

SAFFRON
Crocus sativus L.
Fam. Iridaceae

Synonyms: Hay Saffron.

Habitat: Native to the Mediterranean region, cultivated in Spain, France, Italy and the Middle East.

Description: Saffron consists of the three filiform, deep orange-red stigmas attached to the upper part of the style. These give the appearance of a loose mass of threads, about 2.5 cm long. Each stigma is tubular, slit at the end and toothed at the apex. Taste, characteristic and bitter; odour, aromatic, characteristic.

Part Used: Flower pistils gathered in the autumn.

Constituents: (i) Volatile oil, containing 2-butenoic acid lactone, cineole, isophorone, oxysafranal, safranal, 3,5,5-trimethyl-4-hydroxy-1-cyclo-hexanone-2-ene and others (ii) Crocins; bitter glycosides including picro-crocin, which decomposes to safranal, crocins -1, -2, -3 and -4 which are glucose and gentiobiose esters of crocetin (= α-crocin) and methylcrocetin (= β-crocetin) and other related compounds (iii) Vitamins B_1 and B_2 (iv) Fixed oil (v) Carotenoid pigments [5, 50, 1183, 1184].

Medicinal Use: Formerly used as a carminative, diaphoretic and emmena-gogue. In Chinese medicine it is used for depression, shock and menstrual difficulties. It is used mainly as a colouring and flavouring for food. The spicy, warm odour is due to the safranal, and the bright yellow colour imparted to food is due to the crocin [50].

Preparations: Powder, dose: 0.5–2.5 g.

Regulatory Status: GSL.

Biblical References: Song of Solomon 4 : 14.

SAGE
Salvia officinalis L.
Fam. Labiatae

Synonyms: Garden Sage, Red Sage. Spanish Sage is *S. officinalis* subspp. *lavadulifolia* (Vahl) Gams, and Greek Sage is *S. triloba* L. fil.

Habitat: Native to the Mediterranean region, cultivated worldwide.

Description: Leaves stalked, 3–5 cm long and 1–2.5 cm broad, oblong lanceolate and rounded at the base and at the apex, crenulate at the margin. The venation is finely but distinctly reticulated, depressed on the upper surface, prominent on the lower. Taste, pungent; odour, strong, character-istic, aromatic.

Part Used: Leaves.

Constituents: (i) Volatile oil, containing α- and β-thujone as the major components, usually about 50%, with cineole, borneol, camphor, 2-methyl-3-methylene-5-heptene and others [5, 50, 386]. Spanish sage does not contain thujone, and Greek sage contains only small amounts [5, 386]. (ii) Diterpene bitters; picrosalvin (= carnosol), carnosolic acid and others [386] (iii) Flavonoids; salvigenin, genkwanin, 6-methoxygenkwanin, his-pidulin, luteolin and derivatives [1185, 368] (iv) Phenolic acids; rosmarinic, caffeic, labiatic etc. [5, 386] (v) Salviatannin, a condensed catechin [1186].

Medicinal Use: Aromatic, astringent, antiseptic, spasmolytic. It may be used as an infusion to reduce perspiration, and also as a gargle or mouthwash for pharyngitis, tonsillitis, sore gums, mouth ulcers and other similar disorders. Rosmarinic acid is antiinflammatory (see Rosemary). Sage oil has been reported to be antimicrobial [25] and antispasmodic in animals [286] and to be non-toxic [25]. Sage is a popular and widely used culinary herb.
Preparations: Liquid Extract, dose: 1–4 ml.
Potter's Products: Catarrh Compound Herb.
Regulatory Status: GSL.

SAGO

Metroxylon rumphii Mart.
Fam. Palmae

Synonyms: Pearl Sago.
Habitat: Cultivated in the tropics.
Description: The starch grains are shortly cylindrical, with one flat end and the opposite end rounded.
Part Used: Prepared pith-starch.
Medicinal Use: Demulcent, nutritive. Used as an easily digested food for convalescents.

SALEP

Orchis spp.
Fam. Orchidaceae

Habitat: Central and Southern Europe.
Description: Salep is the dried tuberous root of many species of *Orchis*, imported from Europe. Tubers whitish or pale brownish yellow, about 2–3 cm long and 8–15 mm in diameter, oblong-oval or elliptical, sometimes compressed, with a stem scar at one end and tapering at the other.
Part Used: Root.
Constituents: Mucilage, about 50%, starch etc. [2].
Medicinal Use: Demulcent, nutritive. Has been used similarly to Arrowroot.

SAMPHIRE

Crithmum maritimum L.
Fam. Umbelliferae

Synonyms: Sea Fennel.
Habitat: Grows on rocks on the coast of East Anglia and other parts of Britain.
Description: A succulent plant, reaching about 25 cm, with glaucous, twice-ternate leaves.
Part Used: Herb.
Constituents: Ascorbic acid, dehydroascorbic acid [1187].
Medicinal Use: Antiobesity agent, antiscorbutic, diuretic. It is an effective protection agains scurvy. It may be taken as an infusion and an item of food, often pickled.

SANDALWOOD
Santalum album L.
Fam. Santalaceae

Synonyms: Santalwood, Australian Sandalwood is *Eucarya spicata*.
Habitat: Native to, and cultivated in, tropical Asia.
Description: The wood is sold for medicinal purposes as fine raspings, yellowish in colour, and with a characteristic fragrant odour.
Part Used: Heartwood and the oil distilled from it.
Constituents: Volatile oil, containing at least 90% of the sesquiterpene alcohols α- and β-santalol; with the sesquiterpene hydrocarbons α- and β-santalene, α- and β-curcumene; santene, borneol, santalol etc [1188, 1189, 1190].
Medicinal Use: Rarely used medicinally. The oil is reportedly diuretic and antiseptic and used to treat urinary disorders. It is a common ingredient of perfumes and cosmetics.
Preparations: Liquid Extract, dose: 2–4 ml; Sandalwood Oil BPC 1949, dose: 0.3–1 ml.
Regulatory Status: GSL.

SANDERSWOOD, RED
Pterocarpus santalus L.
Fam. Leguminosae

Synonyms: Red Sandalwood, Rubywood.
Habitat: Southern India and the Philippines.
Description: Usually met with in commerce as raspings, with a deep purplish red tint. Taste and odour very slight.
Part Used: Wood.
Constituents: (i) Isoflavones; the pterocarpans pterocarpin and isoptero-carpin, and santal (ii) Stilbenes such as pterostilbene (iii) Terpenoids such as pterocarpol [794].
Medicinal Use: Little used medicinally here but in India it is occasionally used for diabetes; the antidiabetic constituent is pterostilbene, which also has insecticidal activity [794]. It is used as a colouring agent, for example in Compound Lavender Tincture.
Regulatory Status: GSL.

SANICLE
Sanicula europea L.
Fam. Umbelliferae

Habitat: Grows in shady places throughout Europe, including Britain.
Description: Leaves long-stalked, green above and paler below, rounded in outline, 5–8 cm in diameter, deeply divided into five irregularly trifid and serrate lobes which are broadly wedge-shaped below. Flowers white, small, in simple umbels. Taste bitter, then acrid; odourless.
Part Used: Herb.
Constituents: (i) Saponins, based on saniculogenins (ii) Allantoin (iii) Essential oil (iv) Chlorogenic and rosmarinic acid (v) Vitamin C [2].

Medicinal Use: Astringent, alterative, vulnerary. It has been taken as an infusion and applied topically.
Preparations: Liquid Extract, dose: 2–4 ml.
Regulatory Status: GSL.

SARSAPARILLA

Smilax aristolochiaefolia Mill
S. regelii Killip et Morton
S. febrifuga Kunth
S. officinalis Kunth
Fam. Liliaceae

Synonyms: S. aristolochiaefolia: American, Mexican, Vera Cruz or Grey Sarsaparilla *S. medica* Schlecht; *S. regelii:* Jamaican, Honduras or Brown Sarsaparilla; *S. febrifuga:* Ecuadorian or Guayaquil Sarsaparilla. Indian Sarsaparilla is *Hemidesmus indicus* Brown (Aristolochiaceae) and is no longer used medicinally.
Habitat: The origins are not always easy to determine but some indication is apparent from the names. The plants are climbing vines native to tropical America and the West Indies.
Description: The roots are narrow, very long, cylindrical, up to about 6 mm in diameter and usually found in commerce folded and bound into bundles. Pieces of rhizome, if present, are much thicker and are cut. The external surface varies from greyish to yellowish or reddish brown; ridges, furrows and scars may or may not be present. The transverse section also shows highly variable features. Taste, sweetish and acrid; odourless.
Part Used: Roots, rhizome.
Constituents: (i) Saponins, based on the aglycones sarsapogenin and smilagenin; the major one being parillin (= sarsaponin), with smilasaponin (= smilacin) and sarsaparilloside (ii) β-sitosterol, stigmasterol and their glucosides [1014, 1191, 1192].
Medicinal Use: Alterative, antiinflammatory, antipruritic, antiseptic. Sarsaparilla was first introduced by the Spanish in 1563 as a sure cure for syphilis. It has been used for many years as a treatment for skin diseases, including psoriasis. In a study many years ago patients with psoriasis were treated over a two-year period with "sarsaponin" tablets prepared from sarsaparilla; and improvement was noted in 62% of cases [1193]. Parillin has antibiotic activity [1014]. The therapeutic actions of sarsaparilla are unknown and little recent work has been carried out. In China, other species of *Smilax* are used for similar purposes, for rheumatism, skin diseases, dysentery and even syphilis with apparent success [5]. Sarsaparilla is an ingredient of soft drinks.
Preparations: Powdered Root, dose: 1–4 g; Concentrated Compound Sarsaparilla Decoction BPC 1949, dose: 8–30 ml; Sarsaparilla Liquid Extract BP 1898, dose: 8–15 ml.
Potter's Products: Jamaican Sarsaparilla Liquid, Alterative Tablet No. 34, Compound Elixir of Trifolium.
Regulatory Status: GSL.

SASSAFRAS
Sassafras albidum (Nutt.) Nees.
Fam. Lauraceae

Synonyms: *S. varifolium* (Salisb.) Kuntze, *S. officinale* Nees and Eberm.

Habitat: Eastern USA and Canada.

Description: The rootbark is a bright, rust brown colour, in irregular pieces, soft and brittle. The fracture is short and corky, in definite layers, showing numerous oil glands. The root itself is sometimes found as chips; it is brownish white, showing distinctive concentric rings traversed by narrow medullary rays. Taste, sweetish and slightly astringent; odour, pleasant, aromatic.

Part Used: Root bark, root.

Constituents: (i) Volatile oil, containing safrole 80–90%, with 5-methoxy-eugenol, asarone, eugenol, A- and β-phellandrene, α-pinene, myristicin, thujone, caryophyllene, anethole and others [1194, 1195] (ii) Alkaloids, boldine, norboldine, isoboldine, norcinnamolaurine, reticuline and others [1196] (iii) Lignans: sesamin desmethoxyaschantin [1196] (iv) Tannin and phlobaphene, resin [37].

Medicinal Use: Carminative, diaphoretic, diuretic, antiseptic, anti-rheumatic. Safrole is carcinogenic in animals [1011, 1197] and should not be taken internally. It is possible to prepare safrole-free extracts but since safrole is responsible for much of the effectiveness of sassafras, and also for its odour and flavour, this is not of much use.

Preparations: Liquid Extract of Root Bark, dose: 2–4 ml; Oil of Sassafras BPC 1954.

Regulatory Status: Root Bark GSL. Oil: for external use only.

SASSY BARK
Erythrophloeum guineense G. Don
Fam. Leguminosae

Synonyms: Mancona Bark.

Habitat: Parts of Africa.

Description: In flat or curved pieces, about 5 mm thick, externally warty, greyish, furrowed longitudinally, with a red-brown inner surface, smooth, sometimes with black stains. Fracture coarsely granular, very hard. Taste, astringent, bitter and acrid; odourless.

Part Used: Bark.

Constituents: Undetermined.

Medicinal Use: Narcotic, astringent, laxative. Very poisonous.

SAVIN
Juniperus sabina L.
Fam. Cupressaceae

Synonyms: Savin Tops.

Habitat: Mountainous regions of Switzerland, Italy and Spain.

Description: The shoots bear imbricated, sessile, opposite leaves, the younger of which are oval or hexagonal, becoming rhomboidal or lanceolate with age and less appressed to the stem. An oil gland is visible on the dorsal surface of each leaf. Taste, bitter and resinous; odour terebinthinate, characteristic.

Part Used: Young shoots.

Constituents: (i) Volatile oil, containing sabinol and sabinol acetate [1] (ii) Lignans including savinin and podophyllotoxin [1198].

Medicinal Use: Emmanagogue, diuretic, anthelmintic. Savin is toxic and should not be used internally. For actions of podophyllotoxin see Mandrake, American.

Regulatory Status: P.

SAVORY, SUMMER
SAVORY, WINTER

Satureja hortensis L.
S. montana L.
Fam. Labiatae

Synonyms: Garden Savory, *Calamintha hortensis* Hort, (= Summer Savory); *S. obovata* Lag., *C. montana* Lam. (= Winter Savory).

Habitat: Both species are native to Southern Europe and N. Africa and cultivated elsewhere.

Description: Summer savory is a herbaceous annual; winter savory a perennial, woody shrub; both have oblong or linear leaves and blue flowers.

Part Used: Herb.

Constituents: Volatile oil; in *S. hortensis* consisting mainly of carvacrol with *p*-cymene, β-pinene. β-phellandrene, limonene, borneol and others [26, 323]; in *S. montana* consisting of carvacrol, *p*-cymene and thymol, with α- and β-pinenes, cineole, borneol and others [5].

Medicinal Use: Rarely used medicinally, reputed to be carminative, expectorant and astringent. Both are used as culinary herbs, summer savory particularly. Summer savory oil is reported to be antimicrobial and spasmolytic [26].

SAW PALMETTO

Sabal serrulata (Michx.) Benth. and Hook
and possibly other spp.
Fam. Palmae

Synonyms: Sabal, *Seronoa serrulata* Hook.

Habitat: Eastern N. America.

Description: The fruits are oval or globular, from 2–2.5 cm long and up to 3 cm broad, externally black, with a thin, hard, but fragile pericarp covering a pale-brown, spongy pulp and a thin papery endocarp. The seed is pale brown, oval or globular, with a hilum near the base. Taste, soapy; odour, nutty, reminiscent of vanilla.

Part Used: Fruit.

Constituents: (i) Essential oil about 1–2% (ii) Fixed oil, consisting of about 25% fatty acids; caproic, lauric, palmitic etc., and 75% neutral fats (iii) Sterols [2, 1199] (iv) Polysaccharides, one in particular being composed of galactose, arabinose and uronic acid units with an average molecular weight of 100,000 [1200].

Medicinal Use: Tonic, diuretic, sedative, endocrine agent, anabolic agent. It is used for debility and wasting diseases, cystitis, prostate enlargement and similar conditions. Very little pharmacological work on these aspects has been carried out. The polysaccharide described above has antiphlogistic effects as measured by the rat paw oedema test [1200] and a polysaccharide fraction stimulated phagocytosis in mice [1201].

Preparations: Powdered Berries, dose: 0.5–1 g; Liquid Extract Saw Palmetto BPC 1934, dose: 0.6–1.5 ml.

Potter's Products: Compound Elixir of Damiana and Saw Palmetto, Strength Tablets, Antiglan Tablets.

Regulatory Status: GSL.

SCAMMONY ROOT, MEXICAN

Ipomoea orizabensis (Pell.) Led.
Fam. Convolvulaceae

Synonyms: Ipomoea, Orizaba Jalap.

Habitat: Mexico.

Description: The root occurs in large transverse or oblique slices, up to 10 cm in diameter and 4 cm thick. It is greyish brown and wrinkled externally, internally the section shows irregular concentric rings and scattered resin glands, resembling jalap (q.v.). Taste, acrid and resinous; odour, slight.

Part Used: Root, and resin extracted from it.

Constituents: (i) Resins, known as scammonin and α-scammonin, which hydrolyse to jalapinolic acid and convolvulenic acids [1, 2]. See Jalap also. (ii) Phytosterols [1].

Medicinal Use: Drastic purgative. Used in a similar way to Jalap (q.v.).

Preparations: Scammony Resin BPC 1963, dose: 30–200 mg.

SCOPOLIA

Scopolia carniolica Jacq.
and other spp.
Fam. Solanaceae

Habitat: Central and Eastern Europe.

Description: Rhizome knotty, about 1–2 cm in diameter, nearly black in colour, with numerous depressed stem scars, Fracture short.

Part Used: Rhizome.

Constituents: Tropane alkaloids, including hyoscine and hyoscyamine, with cuscohygrine, tropine and pseudotropine [1].

Medicinal Use: Narcotic, mydriatic. Used in a similar way to Belladonna and Henbane (q.v.), which it resembles in action. It has been suggested as a source of hyoscine [1].

Regulatory Status: P.

SCULLCAP

Scutellaria lateriflora L.
and possibly other spp.
Fam. Labiatae

Synonyms: Skullcap, Hoodwort, Quaker Bonnet, Helmet Flower. European or Greater Skullcap is *S. galericulata* L. In Oriental Medicine Skullcap refers to *S. baicalensis* Georgi.

Habitat: USA.

Description: Leaves opposite, cordate-lanceolate, shortly stalked with a tapering apex. Flowers blue, with a helmet-shaped upper lip, in axillary racemes. Hybridization with other species readily occurs and substitution may occur in commerce. Taste, bitterish; odour, slight.

Part Used: Herb.

Constituents: (i) Scutellarin, a flavonoid glycoside [2]. *S. baicalensis* contains the flavonoids baicalin, baicalein, wogonin, skullcapflavones I and II, and many other flavones [1202, 1203, 1204, 1205]. *S. galericulata* contains wogonin, baicalin, baicalein, apigenin, scutellarein, eriodictyol and luteolin glycosides among others [648], and *S. ovata* also contains flavones [1206] so it is likely that *S. lateriflora* contains similar compounds; little work has been carried out on this species. (ii) Iridoids; catalpol is present in both *S. lateriflora* and *S. galericulata* [62] (iii) Volatile oil and waxes, mainly C_{31}, C_{33} and C_{35} hydrocarbons [1207] (iv) Tannins [2].

Medicinal Use: Sedative, nervine, antispasmodic, anticonvulsant. Scullcap is highly regarded for hysteria, nervous tension and as an antispasmodic, however experimental work is not yet available to support this, in contrast to the extensive research carried out on *S. baicalensis*. Effects of baicalin include antiinflammatory and antiallergic properties [1204]; it inhibits calcium ionophore-induced leukotriene synthesis in human lymphocytes [1208], the formation of lipoxygenase products and to a lesser extent cyclooxygenase products in leukocytes [1202]. *S. baicalensis* also inhibits lipid peroxidation in rat liver [1203] and has been clinically tested in China and patients with chronic hepatitis, where it improved symptoms in over 70% of patients, increasing appetite, relieving abdominal distension and improving the results of liver function tests [48].

Preparations: Powdered Herb, dose: 1–2 g; Liquid Extract, dose: 2–4 ml.

Potter's Products: Valerian and Scullcap Compound Tablets No. 337, Nervine Medicinal Tea Bags, Mistletoe and Scullcap Nerve Tablets No. 216, Neurelax Tablets, Antispasmodic Drops.

Regulatory Status: GSL.

SCURVY-GRASS

Cochlearia officinalis L.
Fam. Cruciferae

Synonyms: Spoonwort.

Habitat: Grows wild on dry banks, particularly near the coast, throughout Europe.

Description: The basal leaves are long-stalked, kidney-shaped, nearly entire; the stem leaves ovate, becoming sessile upwards, with a few angular teeth. Flowers white and cruciform, in terminal racemes. Taste, pungent and cress-like, less so when dried.

Part Used: Herb.

Constituents: Glucosinolates, e.g. glucoputranjivin [1].

Medicinal Use: Formerly used as an antiscorbutic and diuretic; as a gargle or mouthwash for ulcers and sores in the mouth, and topically for spots and blemishes.

SELF-HEAL

Prunella vulgaris L.
Fam. Labiatae

Synonyms: Siclewort, Heal-all.

Habitat: A common European and British wild plant.

Description: A low, creeping herb, branched, with quadrangular stems, oblong-ovate leaves, about 2–3 cm long and 1 cm broad, with entire margins. Flowers purplish blue, in a dense terminal spike, with two kidney-shaped bracts under each whorl. Taste, saline, faintly bitter; odourless.

Part Used: Herb.

Constituents: (i) Pentacyclic triterpenes based on ursolic, betulinic and oleanolic acids [1209].

Medicinal Use: Astringent, vulnerary. Has been taken internally as a haemostatic and for sore throats, and applied externally to wounds.

SENEGA

Polygala senega L.
Fam. Polygalaceae

Synonyms: Snake Root, Rattlesnake Root. In Chinese medicine Senega refers to *P. tenuifolia* Willd.

Habitat: USA.

Description: The root has a knotty crown, from which slender stems arise, with the remains of rudimentary leaves and buds at the base. The root is light yellowish grey in colour, up to about 1 cm thick, often with a keel-shaped ridge running along the main root on the concave side. Fracture short and brittle, showing a cleft central column. Taste, acrid; odour, rather wintergreen-like. The powder is sternutatory.

Part Used: Root.

Constituents: (i) Triterpenoid saponins. Both *P. senega* and *P. tenuifolia* contain almost identical compounds [1210], based on the aglycones presenegenin, senegenin, hydroxysenegin, polygalacic acid and senegenic acid; *P. senega* contains the senegins II, III and IV [1211]; the latter two of which were found to be identical to onjisaponin B and onjisaponin A respectively from *P. tenuifolia* [1212]. For review see [1210] (ii) Phenolic acids; *p*-coumaric, ferulic, sinapic, *p*-methoxycinnamic and others [1213] (iii) Polygalitol, a sorbitol derivative (iv) Miscellaneous; methyl salicylate, sterols, fats etc [1].

Medicinal Use: Expectorant, diaphoretic, emetic. Senega is used especially for chronic bronchitis, catarrh, asthma and croup. It may be taken as an infusion.

Preparations: Powdered Root, dose: 0.5–1 g; Concentrated Senega Infusion BP, dose: 2.5–5 ml; Senega Liquid Extract BPC, dose: 0.3–1 ml; Senega Tincture BPC 1973, dose: 2.5–5 ml.

Potter's Products: Antibron Tablets, Asthma and Chest Mixture No. 80.

Regulatory Status: GSL.

SENNA

Cassia senna L.
C. angustifolia Vahl.
Fam. Leguminosae

Synonyms: *C. senna:* Alexandrian Senna, *C. acutifolia* Del.; *C. angustifolia:* Tinnevelly Senna.

Habitat: *C. senna* is native to tropical Africa and cultivated in Egypt and the Sudan and elsewhere; *C. angustifolia* is native to India and cultivated mainly in India and Pakistan.

Description: Leaves: the leaflets are greyish to yellowish green, lanceolate, unequal at the base (*C. senna* being more so), petiolate, varying from 1 to 5 cm long and 0.5 to 1 cm broad. Those of *C. senna* are in general smaller. Pods: kidney-shaped, flat, showing the imprint of the seeds through the pod. *C. senna* pods are shorter and broader and green in colour, without the remains of the style visible; those of *C. angustifolia* are longer and narrower, brown, with stylar remains. Taste, sweetish then rather unpleasant; odour, tea-like, characteristic.

Part Used: Leaves, pods.

Constituents: (i) Anthraquinone glycosides; in the leaf; sennosides A and B based on the aglycones sennidin A and sennidin B, sennosides C and D which are glycosides of heterodianthrones of aloe-emodin and rhein. Others include palmidin A, rhein anthrone and aloe-emodin glycosides, some free anthraquinones and some potent, novel compounds of as yet undetermined structure [1153, 1158, 1214, 1215, 1216]. *C. senna* usually contains greater amounts of the sennosides. In the fruit: sennosides A and B and a closely related glycoside sennoside A1 [1217] (ii) Naphthalene glycosides; tinnevellin glycoside and 6-hydroxymusizin glycoside, in both leaves and pods [1218] (iii) Miscellaneous; mucilage, flavonoids, volatile oil, sugars, resins etc [5].

Medicinal Use: Stimulant laxative. The glycosides are absorbed from the intestinal tract and the active anthraquinones excreted into the colon where they exert their stimulant effect. Senna is a safe and effective laxative and used widely throughout the world. The fruits are usually taken as an infusion.

Preparations: Powdered Leaves, dose: 0.5–2 g. From leaf: Senna Confection BPC 1959, dose: 4–8 g; Compound Senna Tincture BPC 1949, dose: 2–4 ml; Compound Liquorice Powder BPC 1973, dose: 5–10 g. From fruit: Senna Liquid Extract BP, dose: 0.5–2 ml; Senna Tablets BP;

249

Compound Senna Mixture BPC 1949, dose: 30–60 ml; Senna Syrup BPC 1959, dose: 2–8 ml.

Potter's Products: Lion Cleansing Herbs, Senna Tablets Standardized, Natural Herb Tablets.

Regulatory Status: GSL.

SHEEP'S SORREL

Rumex acetosella L.
Fam. Polygonaceae

Habitat: Common on dry places throughout Europe.

Description: A slender, short perennial. Leaves arrow-shaped, narrow, often with a reddish tint. Flowers small, green, often turning red, in spikes, typically dock-like. Taste, acid and astringent; odourless.

Part Used: Herb.

Constituents: Anthraquinones; chrysophanol, emodin and physcion [1219].

Medicinal Use: Diuretic. The fresh plant juice is used for urinary conditions.

SHEPHERD'S PURSE

Capsella bursa-pastoris (L.) Medic.
Fam. Cruciferae

Habitat: A common plant growing in many parts of the world.

Description: A very variable annual or biennial. Leaves lanceolate, pinnately lobed, sometimes toothed, sometimes hairy, mainly in a basal rosette with a few on the peduncle. Flowers white, 2–3 mm, cruciferous; pod, an inverted, notched triangle, containing the small seeds, its appearance giving rise to the common name. Taste, pungent; odourless.

Part Used: Herb.

Constituents: (i) Flavonoids; luteolin-7-rutinoside and quercetin-3-rutinoside [421] (ii) Polypeptides of undetermined structure [1220] (iii) Plant acids; fumaric and bursic acids [1221] (iv) Bases; choline, acetylcholine, histamine, tyramine [1221, 1222].

Medicinal Use: Antihaemorrhagic, urinary antiseptic, antipyretic. The polypeptide described above was shown to have contractile activity on rat uterus similar to that of oxytocin [1220]. Other experiments showed that extracts produced a transient decrease in blood pressure and haemostatic activity in animals, however whether this was due to the acetylcholine, choline and tyramine was not clear [1221]. Other properties demonstrated included antiinflammatory, diuretic and anti-ulcer activity [1223]. An inhibitory effect of extracts of shepherd's purse on Ehrlich solid tumour in mice was found to be due to the fumaric acid [1224], a disappointing result as fumaric acid is a ubiquitous compound. Despite the interesting pharmacological effects described for this plant, the active constituents of shepherd's purse have not been satisfactorily ascertained, possibly because they may be labile, which would be the case if polypeptides are involved. The flavonoids may of course contribute to the antiinflammatory action. Unfortunately it does not seem that research is continuing into this problem.

Preparations: Liquid Extract, dose: 1–4 ml.

Potter's Products: Sciargo Medicinal Tea Bags, Sciargo Tablets, Motherhood Tea.

Regulatory Status: GSL.

SILVERWEED

Potentilla anserina L.
Fam. Rosaceae

Habitat: A common European wild plant.

Description: Leaves often silvery, especially below, pinnate, with 12–15 toothed leaflets. Flowers bright yellow, buttercup-like, solitary, with the petals twice as long as the sepals. Taste, astringent; odourless.

Part Used: Herb.

Constituents: (i) Ellagitannins, 2–10% (ii) Flavonoids, including quercetin (iii) Choline, bitters etc. [2].

Regulatory Status: Astringent, tonic.

SIMARUBA

Simaruba amara Aubl.
Fam. Simaroubaceae

Habitat: S. America, Florida, West Indies.

Description: The bark occurs in thin, flat, yellowish or greyish-yellow tough, fibrous, pieces, almost impossible to break, usually folded. Taste, very bitter; odourless.

Part Used: Bark.

Constituents: (i) Quassinoids, including simarubolide, simarolide, 2′acetylglaucarubine, 13,18-dehydroglaucarubine and 2′acetylglaucarubinone [1125] (ii) Alkaloids; 5-hydroxycanthin-6-one [1226] (iii) Limonoids: e.g. melianone and derivatives [1226].

Medicinal Use: Tonic, febrifuge. Simaruba was formerly taken as an infusion for fevers and dysentery and then fell out of use, however recent research has shown that the quassinoids are in fact amoebicidal [1123] and antimalarial *in vivo* in animals and *in vitro* [1224].

Preparations: Liquid Extract, dose: 2–4 ml.

SKUNK CABBAGE

Symplocarpus foetidus Nutt.
Fam. Araceae

Synonyms: Skunkweed, *Dracontium foetidum* L.

Habitat: USA.

Description: Rhizome obconical, truncate at both ends, dark brown, up to about 4 cm in diameter, knotted and woody, bearing numerous roots and root scars. Roots up to 8 cm long, 0.5 cm in diameter, transversely wrinkled; fracture short, showing a white cross section with a small central stele. Taste, acrid; odour, unpleasant.

Part Used: Rhizome and root.

Constituents: Active constituents unknown. (i) Essential oil (ii) 5-hydroxytryptamine [1227] (iii) Resins etc.

Medicinal Use: Antispasmodic, diaphoretic, expectorant, sedative. Used mainly for bronchitis and asthma.

Preparations: Liquid Extract, dose: 2–4 ml.

Potter's Products: Antispasmodic Drops, Horehound and Aniseed Balsam, Vegetable Cough Remover.

Regulatory Status: GSL.

SLIPPERY ELM
Ulmus rubra Muhl.
Fam. Ulmaceae

Synonyms: Red Elm, *U. fulva* Mich.

Habitat: Central and Northern USA.

Description: The inner bark occurs in flat oblong pieces, about 2–4 mm thick, sometimes folded. The outer surface is light yellowish to reddish brown, longitudinally wrinkled or striated, with occasional pieces of dark brown rhytidome. The inner surface is paler and finely ridged. Fracture, fibrous. Taste, mucilaginous; odour, slight but characteristic.

Part Used: Inner bark.

Constituents: Mucilage, composed of galactose, 3-methyl galactose, rhamnose and galacturonic acid residues [1, 2].

Medicinal Use: Demulcent, emollient, nutrient, antitussive. It is used to make a gruel for convalescents and for patients with gastric or duodenal ulcers, by adding boiling water to a small quantity of the powder and flavouring with sugar and cinnamon etc. The mucilage is made by digesting the powder in water, heating gently for an hour and straining. The coarsely powdered bark is also made into poultices for wounds, burns, boils and other skin disorders, where it soothes and draws.

Preparations: See above.

Potter's Products: Slippery Elm Tablets.

Regulatory Status: GSL in powder form only.

SMARTWEED
Polygonum hydropiper L.
Fam. Polygonaceae

Synonyms: Arsesmart, Water Pepper.

Habitat: Found in damp places throughout Europe, including Britain.

Description: Leaves narrow, lanceolate, sheathed at the base. Flowers white, tinged with pink or green, on a narrow, drooping spike. Taste, pungent and biting; odourless.

Part Used: Herb.

Constituents: (i) Sesquiterpenes; polygodial in the leaves and polygonal, isodrimeninol, isopolygodial and confertifolin in the seeds [1228, 1229] (ii) Flavonoids; quercetin, kaempferol, isorhamnetin and rhamnesin [1230] (iii) Polygonolide, an isocoumarin [1231].

Medicinal Use: Stimulant, diuretic, emmenagogue. It is taken mainly for amenorrhoea as an infusion. Culpeper states that "the juice destroys worms in the ears, being dropped into them". Presumably worms in the ears were commoner in those days.

Preparations: Liquid Extract, dose: 4–8 ml.

SNAKE ROOT
Aristolochia reticulata Nutt.
Fam. Aristolochiaceae

Synonyms: Texan Snake Root, Serpentary.

Habitat: USA.

Description: Rhizome small, about 2–3 cm long and 3 mm thick, with numerous filiform, branching, longitudinally furrowed roots below and the remains of stem bases on the upper side. Taste, bitter; odour, camphoraceous, aromatic.

Part Used: Rhizome.

Constituents: Aristolochic acid and aristored [142].

Medicinal Use: Stimulant, diaphoretic, anodyne, antispasmodic, nervine. These properties are due mainly to the aristolochic acid; for details, see Birthwort.

Preparations: Powdered root, dose: 50–100 mg; Liquid Extract, dose: 2–4 ml; Tincture of Serpentary BPC 1949, dose: 2–4 ml.

Regulatory Status: GSL.

SOAP BARK
Quillaja saponaria Mol.
Fam. Rosaceae

Synonyms: Quillaia, Soap Tree, Panama Bark.

Habitat: Native to Chile and Peru, cultivated in California and India.

Description: The bark occurs in flat strips up to about 1 cm thick, externally pale yellowish-white with occasional reddish or brownish black patches of imperfectly removed rhytidome. The inner surface is pale and smooth. Fracture, splintery and laminate. Large crystals of calcium oxalate may be seen glistening with the naked eye. Taste, acrid and astringent; odourless, but the powder is strongly sternutatory.

Part Used: Inner bark.

Constituents: (i) Saponins, the mixture known as quillajasaponin, and consisting of glycosides of quillaic acid and derivatives with complex arrangements of sugar moieties [1232, 1233 and references therein] (ii) Calcium oxalate (iii) Tannins.

Medicinal Use: Expectorant, antiinflammatory, detergent. Formerly used to loosen cough in chronic bronchitis and pulmonary complaints. The saponins have been shown to have antiinflammatory and anti-hypercholesterolaemic activity in animals [1234, 1235] but also to cause irritation, inflammation of the intestines, cytotoxicity and other untoward effects, especially in large doses [4, 5]. Quillaia is now used externally for dandruff shampoos and as a cleansing and sloughing agent.

Preparations: Quillaia Liquid Extract BPC, Quillaia Tincture BPC.

Regulatory Status: GSL.

SOAPWORT

Saponaria officinalis L.
Fam. Caryophyllaceae

Habitat: Grows wild throughout Europe and cultivated as a garden plant.

Description: A rather straggling, hairless perennial. Leaves opposite, entire, lanceolate. Flowers soft pink, five-petalled, with a long calyx tube. Taste, bitter, acrid; odourless.

Part Used: Herb, root.

Constituents: Saponins, about 5% [1].

Medicinal Use: Alterative, detergent. Used medicinally for skin diseases, and domestically in the past, as a soap substitute and to produce a head on beers.

SOLOMON'S SEAL

Polygonatum multiflorum (L.) All.
Fam. Liliaceae

Habitat: Largely found as a cultivated plant and garden escape.

Description: A well-known plant, reaching about 0.5 m; the arched stalks bearing alternate elliptical leaves, underneath which hang the bell-shaped white flowers in small clusters. The rhizome is cylindrical, flattened, about 1 cm in diameter, with circular stem scars at intervals and transverse ridges. Fracture short, waxy, yellowish. Taste, mucilaginous, sweet, then acrid and bitter; odourless.

Part Used: Rhizome.

Constituents: Saponins, based on diosgenin, known as saponosides A and B [1236].

Medicinal Use: Astringent, demulcent, tonic. Formerly used as an infusion for pulmonary complaints and as a poultice for bruises and piles.

SORREL

Rumex acetosa L.
Fam. Polygonaceae

Habitat: Common in moist meadows in Europe, including Britain.

Description: Leaves oblong, arrow-shaped, often with a reddish tinge, with a broad-toothed, membranous, stipular sheath round the stem at the base. Taste, acid and astringent; odourless.

Part Used: Leaves.

Constituents: (i) Flavonoids, e.g. hyperoside (ii) Potassium oxalate and oxalic acid (iii) Vitamin C [2]. In the roots at least: anthraquinones; chrysophanol, physcion and emodin anthrones [1237].
Medicinal Use: Refrigerant, diuretic. The leaves are sometimes eaten in salads and in place of spinach.

SPEARMINT

Mentha spicata L.
Mentha × *cardiaca.*
Fam. Labiatae

Synonyms: Garden Mint, *M. viridis* L.
Habitat: Britain, Europe, Asia, N. Africa, USA.
Description: Leaves bright green, almost sessile, opposite, ovate-lanceolate, up to about 7 cm long, with an acute apex and a serrate margin. The lamina has a more or less crumpled appearance. Taste and odour, pleasant, characteristic.
Part Used: Herb, essential oil.
Constituents: (i) Essential oil, of variable composition, containing carvone, about 50–70%, with dihydrocarvone, limonene, and phellandrene, and to a lesser extent; menthone, menthol, pulegone, menthofuran and many others [5, 1054, 1242] (ii) Flavonoids; diosmin and diosmetin [1243].
Medicinal Use: Stimulant, antispasmodic, carminative. Spearmint is used as a flavouring and culinary herb.
Preparations: Spearmint Oil BPC, dose: 0.5–2 ml; Concentrated Spearmint Water BPC 1954, dose: 0.3–1 ml.
Regulatory Status: GSL.
Biblical References: Matthew 23 : 23; Luke 11 : 42 (Mint).

SPEEDWELL

Veronica officinalis L.
Fam. Scrophulariaceae

Habitat: A common wild plant in Europe, including Britain.
Description: A low, creeping, hairy perennial. Leaves oval, short-stalked, serrated. Flowers lilac-blue, with darker veins, four joined petals and four sepals, in axillary spikes. Taste, bitter and astringent; odour slightly tea-like when dry.
Part Used: Herb.
Constituents: (i) Iridoid glycosides; aucubin, esters of catalpol such as veronicoside, minecoside and verproside [1244] (ii) Acetophenone gluco-sides; pungenin, isopungenin and its 6'-caffeate [1245] (iii) Flavonoids; apigenin, scutellarin, luteolin and their glycosides [1246].
Medicinal Use: Alterative, expectorant, diuretic.
Regulatory Status: GSL.

255

SPIKENARD, AMERICAN

Aralia racemosa L.
Fam. Araliaceae

Habitat: N. America.

Description: Rhizome up to 15 cm long, about 2.5 cm in diameter, with prominent concave scars. Roots about 2 cm thick at the base, pale brown, wrinkled. Fracture short and whitish. Taste and odour, aromatic.

Part Used: Rhizome and root.

Constituents: (i) Essential oil, contain the polyacetylenes falcarinone and falcarinolene [631] (ii) Araloside, a glycoside of undetermined structure [2].

Medicinal Use: Alterative, diaphoretic. Used also for rheumatic and cutaneous disorders, as an infusion.

Preparations: Liquid Extract, dose: 2–4 ml.

SQUAW VINE

Mitchella repens L.
Fam. Rubiaceae

Synonyms: Partridge Berry.

Habitat: North America.

Description: Stem slender with a deep furrow on one side; leaves opposite, dark green, coriaceous, round to ovate, about 2 cm long, shortly petiolate, with veins prominent on the upper surface. Flowers in pairs, pinkish, bearded inside. Taste, astringent; odourless.

Part Used: Herb.

Constituents: Largely unknown. Unspecified alkaloids, glycosides, tannins and mucilages have been reported. No recent or reliable research has been carried out.

Medicinal Use: Parturient, astringent. Used principally for amenorrhoea, dysmenorrhoea and in preparation for childbirth.

Preparations: Liquid Extract, dose: 2–4 ml.

Potter's Products: Motherhood Tea.

Regulatory Status: GSL.

SQUILL
INDIAN SQUILL

Drimia maritima (L.) Stearn
D. indica (Roxb.) Jessopp
Fam. Liliaceae

Synonyms: Scilla. Red and White Squill are derived from different varieties of *D. maritima* (= *U. maritima* (L.) Baker). Indian Squill was formerly *U. indica* (Roxb.) Kunth.

Habitat: *D. maritima* is native to the Mediterranean region; *D. indica* to India.

Description: The bulbs are pear-shaped, about 15–30 cm in diameter, but rarely seen whole in commerce as they tend to start growing; they are sliced transversely (longitudinally in the case of Indian squill) and dried.

White squill is cream coloured, red squill as the name suggests has a reddish tinge: Indian squill is usually darker in colour and several pieces may be joined together unlike the other types. Fracture short, tough, flexible. Taste, bitter and acrid.

Part Used: Bulb.

Constituents: (i) Cardiac glycosides, bufadienolides based mainly on the aglycone scillarenin (= scillaridin A). The most important glycosides are scillaren A, a rhamnoglucoside of scillarenin, and proscillaridin A, a glucoside of the same. The so-called scillaridin B is a mixture of glycosides [1, 5, 1247, 1248]. Both red and white squills contain similar compounds, however red squill contains scilliroside and scillirubroside in addition [1, 5, 1249]. Indian squill contains scilliglaucosidin in addition to the other glycosides [1249] (ii) Flavonoids and anthocyanidins; vitexin, isovitexin, dihydroquercetin and in red squill, a red pigment [1251].

Medicinal Use: Expectorant, emetic, diuretic, cardiac tonic. Squill is used mainly for its expectorant activity; it is a common ingredient of cough mixtures. In large doses it is emetic. Although it is cardioactive, the effect is not cumulative and the emetic properties prevent cardiotoxic problems with overdosage. Both squill and Indian squill have similar potencies and cardiotoxic activities in animals [1252]. Red squill was formerly used as a rat poison and has been used topically as a hair tonic for dandruff and seborrhoea; the active constituent is thought to be scilliroside. The diuretic effects, in common with other cardiac glycosides, are considerable, and squill had been used for dropsy. It is an ancient medicine; Pliny was conversant with it and knew the two varieties and Dioscorides described a method of making squill vinegar which is similar to that used today.

Preparations: Squill Liquid Extract BPC, dose: 0.06–2 ml; Squill Tincture BPC, dose: 0.3–2 ml; Squill Vinegar BPC, dose: 0.6–2 ml; Squill Oxymel BPC, dose: 2.5–5 ml.

Potter's Products: Balm of Gilead Cough Mixture.

Regulatory Status: GSL.

ST JOHN'S WORT

Hypericum perforatum L.
Fam. Hypericaceae

Habitat: A native European, including British, plant.

Description: Leaves opposite, sessile, oval to linear, with translucent oil glands on the surface and black dots on the lower surface in some cases. Flowers bright yellow, with numerous stamens, five petals, often black dotted along the margins. The stem has two raised lines along the stem. Taste, bitter and astringent; odour, aromatic, distinctive.

Part Used: Herb.

Constituents: (i) Essential oil, containing caryophyllene, methyl-2-octane, *n*-nonane, *n*-octanal, *n*-decanal, α- and β-pinene, and traces of limonene and myrcene [1252] (ii) Hypericins, prenylated phloroglucin derivatives; hypericin, pseudohypericin and hyperforin [1253, 1254] (ii) Miscellaneous; flavonoids, (+)- and (−)-epicatechin [1253, 1255].

Medicinal Use: Anxiolytic, sedative, antiinflammatory, astringent. St. John's Wort is used to treat menopausal problems, rheumatism, coughs and colds and can be used topically as a vulnerary. The hypericins have an anxiolytic effect by monoamineoxidase inibition [1256]. In a clinical trial of the standardized extract, significant improvement in symptoms of anxiety was noted in women after four to six weeks treatment [1257].
Preparations: Liquid Extract, dose: 2–4 ml.
Regulatory Status: GSL.

STAR ANISE

Illicium verum Hook, f.
Fam. Illiciaceae

Synonyms: Chinese Anise.
Habitat: Indigenous to S.E. Asia, cultivated extensively in China.
Description: Fruits about 2 cm in diameter, star-like, formed from eight boat-shaped carpels, open when ripe, each containing one smooth, polished brown seed. Pericarp brown and wrinkled below. Taste and odour, aniseed-like. It should not be confused with the smaller, deformed-looking Japanese star anise (*I. lanceolatum* A C Smith or *I. religiosum* Sieb. et Zucc.), which is poisonous.
Part Used: Fruit.
Constituents: Volatile oil, containing *trans*-anethole, 80–90%, with estragole, β-bisabolene, β-farnesene, caryophyllene, nerolidol and others [5].
Medicinal Use: Stimulant, carminative. Uses similar to those of aniseed (q.v.). It is an important spice in Chinese cookery.
Preparations: As for Aniseed.
Potter's Products: Lightning Cough Remover, Horehound and Aniseed Balsam.
Regulatory Status: GSL.

STAVESACRE

Delphinium staphisagria L.
Fam. Ranunculaceae

Habitat: Native to the Mediterranean region.
Description: Seeds greyish black, wrinkled and pitted, more or less triangular or four sided, convex at the back, about 2 cm long and rather less in width. Taste, bitter and tingling; odourless.
Part Used: Seeds.
Constituents: Diterpene alkaloids; delphidine, delphinine, delphirine, delphisine and neoline [800].
Medicinal Use: Parasiticide. Used for destroying lice etc. Care should be taken that the poisonous alkaloids are not ingested or absorbed.
Preparations: Stavesacre Lotion BPC 1949; Stavesacre Ointment BPC 1949.
Regulatory Status: P.

STOCKHOLM TAR

Pinus sylvestris L.
and other spp.
Fam. Pinaceae

Synonyms: Tar, Pine Tar, Pix Liquida.

Description: A viscous, dark brown or black liquid, obtained by the destructive distillation of the stems and roots of various species of *Pinus*. It has a characteristic odour and acid taste.

Constituents: A complex mixture of hydrocarbons and phenols [4].

Medicinal Use: Antiseptic, antipsoriatic, antipruritic, expectorant. It is an ingredient of some cough mixtures and ointments used for the treatment of eczema and psoriasis.

Preparations: Syrup of Tar BPC 1949, dose: 4–8 ml; ointment of Tar BPC 1949.

Regulatory Status: GSL Maximum dose, 20 mg.

STONE ROOT

Collinsonia canadensis L.
Fam. Labiatae

Habitat: Canada.

Description: Rhizome greyish-brown, very hard, up to 8 cm long, with knotty, short, irregular branches and numerous shallow stem scars. Bark very thin. Numerous brittle rootlets may be attached. Taste, bitter and unpleasant; odourless.

Part Used: Rhizome.

Constituents: Largely unknown. Essential oil, tannin, saponins and a possible alkaloid have been reported [2].

Medicinal Use: Stomachic, diuretic, tonic. Its main use is in kidney complaints such as stones and as a diuretic.

Preparations: Liquid Extract, dose: 1–4 ml; Collinsonia Tincture BPC 1934, dose: 2–8 ml.

Potter's Products: Compound Elixir of Collinsonia.

Regulatory Status: GSL.

STORAX

Liquidambar orientalis Mill.
Fam. Hamamelidaceae

Synonyms: Styrax, Sweet Gum, Levant Storax. American Storax is from *L. styraciflua* L.

Habitat: Native to Asia Minor.

Description: A viscid, treacly liquid, greyish brown, opaque, heavier than water. It is prepared by beating the tree, causing a flow of balsam which is then soaked up by the bark; this is boiled in water and pressed, and further purified by warming and straining or by dissolving in alcohol. American storax is collected from natural pockets in the trunk into which it exudes. Taste, sharply pungent and burning; odour, recalling that of the hyacinth.

Part Used: Balsam.

Constituents: Cinnamic acid, cinnamyl cinnamate (styracin), phenylpropyl cinnamate, triterpene acids such as oleanolic and their cinnamic esters, volatile oil. American storax is reported to have a similar composition with perhaps a greater proportion of volatile oil [1, 5, 1258].

Medicinal Use: Antiseptic, expectorant, stimulant. Its main use is as an ingredient for Friar's Balsam, a useful preparation which is used as an inhalation for coughs and colds and a soothing application for wounds and ulcers.

Preparations: Compound Benzoin Tincture BPC (Friar's Balsam).

Regulatory Status: GSL.

Biblical References: See Exodus 30 : 34. Could also be Balm of Gilead.

STRAMONIUM

Datura stramonium L.
Fam. Solanaceae

Synonyms: Thornapple, Jimson Weed, Jamestown Weed.

Habitat: Common in many parts of the world.

Description: Leaves petiolate, up to about 25 cm long, 15 cm broad, greyish-green when dried and usually found broken in commercial samples. Margins sinuous-dentate, with large irregular teeth, unequal at the base. Flowers white, tubular, with five teeth, funnel shaped when open, calyx tubular. Capsule, when present, spiny, containing black, flat, reticulated, kidney-shaped seeds. Taste, bitter and saline; odour, disagreeable when fresh, tea-like when dried. Other species of *Datura*, such as *D. metel* and *D. innoxia*, from India, are used as a source of the alkaloids. See [1].

Part Used: Leaves, flowering tops, seeds.

Constituents: Tropane alkaloids, about 0.2–0.45%; mainly hyoscyamine, hyoscine and to a lesser extent, atropine. The seeds contain about 0.2% alkaloids with 15–30% fixed oil [1, 4].

Medicinal Use: Spasmolytic, antiasthmatic, anticholinergic. Stramonium is used to control spasms of the bronchioles in asthma. Its anticholinergic effects are similar to those of atropine, as are the effects of overdosage (see Belladonna). It causes dryness of the mouth; this property can be used to control excessive salivation, for example in Parkinson's disease.

Preparations: Stramonium Liquid Extract BP 1968, dose: up to 0.6 ml daily; Stramonium Tincture BP, dose: up to 6 ml daily; Compound Lobelia Powder BPC 1949; Compound Stramonium Powder BPC 1934.

Regulatory Status: P.

STRAWBERRY

Fragaria vesca L.
and varieties
Fam. Rosaceae

Habitat: Widely cultivated in temperate countries.

Description: The strawberry plant is too well-known to require description.

Part Used: Leaves. The fruit is eaten.

Constituents: (i) Flavonoids; glycosides of kaempferol and quercetin [160] (ii) Ellagic acid tannins (iii) Essential oil [2].

Medicinal Use: Mild astringent and diuretic.

STROPHANTHUS

Strophanthus kombe Oliver
S. gratus.
Fam. Apocynaceae

Habitat: Tropical East Africa.

Description: A climbing plant producing greenish-brown seeds, about 1 cm long and 3 mm broad, elliptical, with appressed hairs and a long awn.

Part Used: Seeds.

Constituents: Cardiac glycosides, based on the aglycone strophanthidin, including K-strophanthoside, K-strophanthin-β- and cymarin and many minor glycosides; the mixture is known as Strophanthin-K. *S. gratus* contains ouabain (= strophanthin-G) [1, 4].

Medicinal Use: Cardiac tonic. The glycosides have a digitalis-like action (see Foxglove) but are poorly absorbed from the digestive tract and are not used orally. Ouabain has been used in the treatment of cardiac arrest since it acts very rapidly when given by injection. The seeds were formerly used in Africa as an arrow poison.

Regulatory Status: POM.

SUMACH, SMOOTH
SUMACH, SWEET

Rhus glabra L.
R. aromatica Ait.
Fam. Anacardiaceae

Synonyms: Sweet Sumach: Fragrant Sumach.

Habitat: Canada and the USA.

Description: The root-bark of both species occurs in quilled pieces, with scattered lenticels on the surface. The fracture shows transverse rows of minute, blackish oil glands. The surface of *R. glabra* is dull reddish-brown; that of *R. aromatica* is dull brown with exfoliating patches showing a reddish brown to whitish cortex. Taste, mucilaginous, with *R. glabra* more astringent; odourless.

Part Used: Root-bark. The berries of *R. glabra* are also used.

Constituents: Largely unknown. Both are reported to contain tannins. *R. aromatica* contains essential oil and resin [2]. The genus *Rhus* does not contain the poisonous urushiols present in the closely related genus *Toxicodendron* (formerly *Rhus*), for example Poison Oak and Poison Ivy, (q.v.) [1085].

Medicinal Use: Smooth Sumach: Astringent, tonic. The bark has been used for diarrhoea etc. as a decoction, and externally as a lotion. The berries are refrigerant and diuretic and are used for bowel complaints as an infusion. Sweet Sumach: Astringent, diuretic. It has a reputed antidiabetic activity. It is mainly used for urinary incontinence.

Preparations: Smooth Sumach: Liquid Extract (root bark), dose: 4–8 ml; Liquid Extract (berries) dose: 4–8 ml; Powdered Berries, dose: 0.6–2 g. Sweet Sumach: Liquid Extract, dose: 2–4 ml.

Regulatory Status: GSL.

SUMBUL

Ferula sumbul Hook
F. suaveolens
Fam. Umbelliferae

Synonyms: Musk Root.

Habitat: Far East, Eastern Europe.

Description: The root occurs in commerce cut into transverse slices about 2 cm thick and 2–5 cm in diameter, more rarely 12 cm. Pieces of the bristly crown and tapering lower part also occur. The external bark is thin, dark brown and papery, the transverse section brownish, resinous, marbled with white. Taste, bitter; odour, aromatic, musky.

Part Used: Root.

Constituents: F. sumbul: (i) Volatile oil, 0.2–0.4% (ii) Resin 5–15% (iii) Umbelliferone (iv) Sumbulic and angelic acids [2].

Medicinal Use: Antispasmodic, tonic. Formerly used for asthma, bronchitis, amenorrhoea etc.

Preparations: Liquid Extract, dose: 0.5–4 ml; Tincture, dose: 2–4 ml.

Regulatory Status: GSL.

SUNDEW

Drosera rotundifolia L.
Fam. Droseraceae

Habitat: Grows throughout Europe on wet heaths and moors and in sphagnum bogs.

Description: Sundew is an insectivorous plant. Leaves radical, six to ten in number, reddish, orbicular, fleshy, covered with stalked, sticky glands like tentacles. Flowering stem leafless, bearing small, white, five petalled flowers in a spike.

Part Used: Herb.

Constituents: (i) Naphthaquinones; plumbagin, its methyl ether, and methylnaphthazarin [218] (ii) Flavonoids [1259].

Medicinal Use: Antitussive, antiasthmatic, demulcent, antispasmodic. Used particularly for whooping cough and asthma and for gastric complaints. It is reported to be antispasmodic against bronchospasm induced by acetylcholine and barium chloride [33]. Plumbagin has a number of interesting actions; it is antimicrobial *in vitro* against some gram-positive and gram-negative bacteria, influenza virus, pathogenic fungi and parasitic protozoa [1260] and is active against some species of *Leishmania* [1261]. In large doses plumbagin is cytotoxic, but in small doses has immuno-stimulating activity *in vitro* [1262].

Preparations: Liquid Extract, dose: 0.5–1.5 ml.

Regulatory Status: GSL.

SUNFLOWER

Helianthus annuus L.
Fam. Compositae

Synonyms: Helianthus. *H. tuberosus* is the Jerusalem Artichoke, the tubers of which are a source of food.

Habitat: Widely grown throughout the world.

Description: The plant and its seeds are too well-known to require description.

Part Used: Seeds (fruits), oil expressed from them.

Constituents: (i) Fixed oil, high in polyunsaturated fatty acids, including α- and β-linoleic (ii) Protein. The tubers of *H. tuberosus* contain inulin.

Medicinal Use: The seeds have been used to prepare a decoction used as a demulcent in coughs and colds. They are used worldwide as a source of oil for cooking, salads and for the manufacture of modern, soft, "healthy", margarines. Jerusalem Artichokes have had a fashionable use as a slimming aid due to the inulin content. Unfortunately they can produce severe flatulence as a side effect.

SWAMP MILKWEED

Asclepias incarnata L.
Fam. Asclepiadaceae

Habitat: USA.

Description: Rhizome about 2–3 cm diameter, yellowish-brown, irregularly globular or elongated, hard, knotty, with a thin bark and tough, whitish wood. Rootlets about 10 cm long, light brown. Taste, sweetish, acrid and bitter; odourless.

Part Used: Root and Rhizome.

Constituents: Unidentified.

Medicinal Use: Emetic, cathartic.

T

TAMARAC

Larix laricina Koch.
Fam. Pinaceae

Synonyms: American Larch, L. americana Michx.
Habitat: USA.
Description: Dull purplish fragments, with irregular depressions on the
outer surface, smooth, finely striated on the inner. Fracture shortly
fibrous and laminate. Taste, mucilaginous, astringent; odour, slight.
Part Used: Bark.
Constituents: Tannins, 12–15% [2].
Medicinal Use: Formerly used as an alterative, diuretic and laxative, for
jaundice, rheumatism and cutaneous disorders.

TAMARIND

Tamarindus indicus L.
Fam. Leguminosae

Habitat: Native to tropical Asia and Africa, cultivated elsewhere, including
China, India, West Indies, Indonesia, Florida etc.
Description: The pods are about 6–15 cm long, with a thin brittle shell
containing a pulp, with up to twelve seeds. The pulp is a dark reddish-
brown, moist, stringy, sugary mass. The brittle shell may be removed and
the fruit preserved in syrup, or the whole fruit salted and pressed into
cakes. Taste, sweet, pleasant, acid; odour, aromatic, characteristic.
Part Used: Fruit, pulp.
Constituents: (i) Plant acids; nicotinic, d-tartaric, l-malic, with the presence
of citric acid disputed [4, 5, 1264] (ii) Volatile oil, containing geranial,
geraniol, limonene, α-terpineol, methyl salicylate, safrole, cinnamaldehyde, ethyl cinnamate, piperitone, alkylthiazoles and pyrazines [1264] (iii)
Sugars, pectin, fats, vitamins etc. [5].
Medicinal Use: Nutritive, laxative. Tamarind is reported to have mild
laxative effects which are destroyed on cooking. In China it is also used to
treat nausea in pregnancy [5]. Tamarinds are used in Indian and Far
Eastern cooking, and to make Worcestershire sauce and various pickles.
Preparations: Senna Confection BPC 1949, dose: 4–8 g.

TANSY

Tanacetum vulgare L.
Fam. Compositae

Habitat: A common European wild plant.
Description: Leaves dark green, pinnate, up to twelve pointed, toothed
segments on each side. Flowers yellow, rayless, button-like, in umbel-like
clusters. Taste, bitter; odour, strong, aromatic, characteristic.

Part Used: Herb.
Constituents: (i) Volatile oil, of variable composition depending on chemo-
type, containing possibly thujone, sabinene, camphor, 1,8-cineole, umbel-
lulone, α-pinene, bornyl acetate and germacrene D [1265, 1266] (ii)
Sesquiterpene lactones; parthenolide, artemorin, tatridin A and B, 11,13-
dehydrodesacetylmatricarin, *l-epi*ludovicin-C and others [1267, 1269]
(iii) Flavonoids; apigenin, diosmetin, quercetin, jaceidin, jaceosidin and
others [1267].
Medicinal Use: Anthelmintic, emmenagogue, bitter tonic. It has been used
for expelling worms in children, for amenorrhoea and nausea, and as a
lotion for scabies. It should be avoided during pregnancy.
Preparations: Liquid Extract, dose: 2–8 ml.
Regulatory Status: GSL.

TEA
Camellia sinensis (L.) Kuntze
Fam. Theaceae
Synonyms: C. *thea* Link, *Thea sinensis* L.
Habitat: Cultivated China, India, Sri Lanka, Kenya, Indonesia and
elsewhere.
Description: Tea is well-known. Green tea is the type produced in China and
Japan; it differs from black tea, produced in India, Sri Lanka and Kenya, in
that fermentation, which gives rise to the different flavour compounds, is
prevented by heating to inactivate the enzymes.
Part Used: Leaf buds and very young leaves.
Constituents: (i) Caffeine, with much smaller amounts of other xanthines
such as theophylline and theobromine [5] (ii) Tannins. The main tannin in
green tea is (−)-epigallocatechin [130]; those in black tea are oxidized and
more complex (ii) Flavonoids; quercetin, kaempferol and others [5, 33] (iii)
The flavour compounds are very complex, see [5] and references therein.
Medicinal Use: Stimulant, diuretic, astringent. The stimulant and diuretic
properties are due to the caffeine content, the astringency to the tannins.
Tea is useful in diarrhoea, and is used in China for many types of dysentery,
although in excess it can cause gastrointestinal upsets and nervous
irritability due to the caffeine. The tannins in green tea have recently been
shown to have antitumour-promoting ability [130]. Tea is drunk in nearly
every country in the world for its refreshing, stimulating and mildly
analgesic effects.

THUJA
Thuja occidentalis L.
Fam. Cupressaceae
Synonyms: Arbor Vitae, White Cedar.
Habitat: Native to northeastern N. America and cultivated elsewhere.
Description: Flattened, green twigs, bearing paired, decussate scale-like
leaves about 3 mm long, closely imbricated and appressed. Taste, bitter and
odour, juniper-like, camphoraceous, characteristic.

Part Used: Leaves and tops.

Constituents: (i) Volatile oil, containing thujone as the major component, with isothujone, borneol, bornyl acetate, *l*-fenchone, limonen, sabinene, camphor, *l*-α-thujene and others [5, 1269, 1270]. (ii) Flavonoids, mucilage, tannins [37].

Medicinal Use: Expectorant, stimulant, emmenagogue, anthelmintic. The main use of the infusion is as an expectorant in bronchial catarrh and for the treatment of cystitis and amenorrhoea. As it is a uterine stimulant it should be avoided during pregnancy. Thujone is toxic in large doses and should be taken internally only occasionally. Externally, as a tincture, thuja has antifungal and antiviral activity and is used as a treatment for warts. The antiviral activity has recently been demonstrated *in vitro*, however the active principles have not yet been identified [1271]. An extract has also been found to stimulate phagocytosis by erythrocytes of Kupfer cells in isolated rat liver [1272].

Preparations: Liquid Extract, dose: 2–4 ml.

THYME
WILD THYME

Thymus vulgaris L.
T. serpyllum L.
Fam. Labiatae

Synonyms: T. vulgaris: Common Thyme, Garden Thyme. *T. serpyllum:* Mother of Thyme, Serphyllum.

Habitat: Thyme is indigenous to the Mediterranean region, and cultivated widely; wild thyme is native to Britain and Europe.

Description: Both are small, bushy herbs; leaves opposite, elliptical, greenish-grey, shortly stalked, those of thyme are up to about 6 mm long and 0.5–2 mm broad; wild thyme being broader, about 2 mm, and a little longer. Margins entire, recurved in the case of thyme but not in wild thyme. Taste and odour characteristic; thyme being stronger.

Part Used: Herb.

Constituents: (i) Volatile oil, of highly variable composition; the major constituent is thymol, with lesser amounts of carvacrol, in both species although higher in *T. vulgaris*; with 1,8-cineole, borneol, geraniol, linalool, bornyl and linalyl acetate, thymol methyl ether and α-pinene. *T. serpyllum* contains more linalool and *p*-cymol [386, 1273, 1274, 1275] (ii) Flavonoids; apigenin, luteolin, thymonin, naringenin and others [648] (iii) Miscellaneous; labiatic acid, caffeic acid, tannins etc. [5]. No information on *T. serpyllum* appears be available on the flavonoids etc.

Medicinal Use: Carminative, antiseptic, antitussive, expectorant spasmolytic. Both species are used for coughs, bronchitis, whooping cough and similar complaints. Most of the activity is thought to be due to the thymol, which is expectorant and antiseptic. Thymol and carvacrol are spasmolytic; the flavonoid fraction has also been shown to have a potent effect on the smooth muscle of guineapig trachea and ileum [1276]. Thymol is a urinary tract antiseptic, anthelmintic; it is larvicidal, a counter irritant for use in topical antirheumatic preparations, and has many other useful actions. It is a popular ingredient of mouthwashes and toothpastes, however it is toxic in overdose and should be used with care. Thyme is a very useful culinary herb. Wild thyme has recently been shown to have an antithyrotropic effect in rats [225]; this may account for its reputed sedative activity, a property not ascribed to *T. vulgaris* [37].

Preparations: Thyme Liquid Extract BPC 1949, dose: 0.6–4 ml; Elixir of Thyme BPC 1949, dose: 4–8 ml; Thyme Oil BPC 1949, dose: 0.05–0.3 ml. (No preparations of this type for wild thyme).

Regulatory Status: GSL.

TOADFLAX, YELLOW
Linaria vulgaris Mill.
Fam. Scrophulariaceae

Habitat: A common European and British wild flower.

Description: Flowers pale yellow, two-lipped, the mouth closed, with an orange spot on the lower lip and a long straight spur. Leaves grass-like, bluish green.

Part Used: Herb.

Constituents: (i) Flavonoids; linarin and pectolinarin (ii) Peganine, an alkaloid (iii) Choline [2].

Medicinal Use: Astringent, hepatic.

TOBACCO
Nicotiana tabacum L
and other species
Fam. Solanaceae

Habitat: Cultivated worldwide.

Description: Needs no description.

Part Used: Leaf, cured.

Constituents: (i) Alkaloids; nicotine, cotinine, anabasine, nornicotine, corcotinine and others [112] (ii) Volatile oils, flavour ingredients etc.

Medicinal Use: None. Nicotine has interesting pharmacological actions, including stimulation, followed by paralysis, of autonomic ganglia and effects on skeletal muscle but these can hardly be referred to as medicinal. It is very toxic and often used as a horticultural insecticide; it is easily absorbed through the skin and this is the cause of most cases of poisoning. The addictive effects of tobacco are well known.

TOLU BALSAM
Myroxylon balsamum (L.) Harms
Fam. Leguminosae

Synonyms: Balsam Tolu, *M. toluiferum* H.B.K., *Toluiferum balsamum* L.

Habitat: South America, cultivated in the West Indies.

Description: The resin is collected from incisions in the bark and sap wood of the tree. It is a light brown, fragrant, balsamic resin, softening when warm and becoming brittle when cold. Taste, sweetish, acid; odour, aromatic, vanilla-like.

Part Used: Balsam.

Constituents: (i) Cinnamic acid, benzoic acid and their esters such as benzyl benzoate, cinnamyl cinnamate and esters with resin alcohols (ii) Miscellaneous; vanillin, ferulic acid, triterpenoids such as oleanolic acid, sumaresinolic acid, and others [1, 5, 1279].

Medicinal Use: Expectorant, stimulant, antiseptic. It is used as a mild expectorant and flavouring agent for cough mixture, as a lozenge base and as an ingredient in Friar's Balsam (see storax).

Preparations: Tolu Syrup BPC, dose: 2–8 ml; Tolu Tincture BPC 1959, dose: 2–4 ml.

Regulatory Status: GSL.

TONKA BEANS

Dipteryx odorata (Aubl.) Willd.
D. oppositifolia (Aubl.) Willd.
Fam. Leguminosae

Habitat: South America.

Description: The beans vary widely in appearance, they are usually 2–5 cm long, about 1 cm in diameter, greyish or black. Odour, like new-mown hay.

Part Used: Seeds.

Constituents: (i) Coumarin, about 1–3%, with 7-hydroxycoumarin (= umbelliferone) and coumarin glycosides [2, 1278] (ii) Fixed oil, sugars phytosterols etc. [2].

Medicinal Use: Formerly used as a tonic and aromatic. Rarely used medicinally now as coumarin has cardiotoxic effects but may be used for flavouring and perfumery.

TORMENTILLA

Potentilla erecta (L.) Raeuschel
Fam. Rosaceae

Habitat: Grows throughout Europe on moors and in grassy places.

Description: A creeping perennial; trefoil root-leaves, stem leaves with about five leaflets, serrate. Flowers bright yellow, with four petals and sepals and numerous stamens. Root hard, brown, cylindrical with a rough surface, pitted, showing stem and rootlet scars. Taste, astringent; odourless.

Part Used: Herb, rhizome.

Constituents: (i) Tannins, catechins and ellagitannins, including a dimeric ellagitannin [1279] (ii) Phlobaphene (= "tormentil red") [2].

Medicinal Use: Astringent, tonic. It has been used as an infusion for diarrhoea and as a lotion to sores and ulcers. The dimeric ellagitannin described above exhibited weak antiallergic, immunostimulating and interferon inducing activity *in vitro* [1279].

Preparations: Liquid Extract (root), dose: 2–4 ml.

Regulatory Status: GSL.

TRAGACANTH

Astragulus gummifer Labill.
and many other species
Fam. Leguminosae

Synonyms: Gum Tragacanth.

Habitat: Middle East, especially Turkey and Syria.

Description: It is the dried, gummy exhudation from the incised stem. In commerce it occurs as ribbon-like, translucent, horny, white or pale yellow flakes. Taste, mucilaginous; odourless.

Part Used: Gum.

Constituents: (i) Polysaccharides and proteinaceous polysaccharides. Tragacanthin is water-soluble, consisting of an arabinogalactan and tragacanthic acid; bassorin is an insoluble methylated fraction. Tragacanth yields on hydrolysis D-galactose, D-galacturonic acid, L-fucose, D-xylose, L-arabinose and others [4, 5]. Both contain residues of hydroxyproline, histidine, aspartic acid and arginine in variable amounts depending upon source [1290] (ii) Starch, cellulose, invert sugar, acetic acid [4, 5].

Medicinal Use: The main use of tragacanth is as a suspending or thickening agent for emulsions, mixtures, gels, low calorie syrups and various other pharmaceutical formulations. However, the polysaccharides have recently been shown to have immunostimulating activity such as stimulation of phagocytosis and an increase in plasma cell counts of T-lymphocytes [1281] and tragacanth has been shown to be active against a variety of tumours [1282]. Pretreatment in mice reduces the number of positive "takes" of translated Ehrlich ascites cells [1283].

Preparations: Compound Tragacanth Powder.

Regulatory Status: GSL.

TREE OF HEAVEN

Ailanthus altissima (Mill) Sw.
Fam. Simaroubaceae

Synonyms: Ailanto, Chinese Sumach, *A. glandulosa* Desf.

Habitat: Asia, Northern Australia, China.

Description: Bark brownish grey, with numerous warts, and on some pieces triangular scars. The inner surface is longitudinally striated. Fracture short, buff coloured; fibrous and porous in the inner part. Taste, bitter; odourless.

Part Used: Bark.

Constituents: (i) Quassinoids; ailanthone, ailanthinone, amarolide, acetylamarolide, shinjulactone B and others [306, 1284, 1285] (ii) Alkaloids; canthin-6-one, 1-methoxycanthin-6-one, methyl 6-methoxy β-carboline-1-carboxylate etc. [1286, 1287] (iii) Miscellaneous; flavonols, 2,6-dimethoxy-*p*-benzoquinone, tannins [2, 1286].

Medicinal Use: Febrifuge, astringent, antispasmodic, cardiac depressant. It has also been used for tapeworms, asthma and numerous other complaints, and for the treatment of dysentery. Many quassinoids are amoebicidal [1123], and recent work has shown that constituents of the bark and stem, particularly ailanthone, have antimalarial activity *in vitro* against *Plasmodium falciparum* and in mice against *P. berghei* [1124, 1125, 1284]. The alkaloids do not appear to have these properties [1125]. Some quassinoids are antineoplastic [1225]. *A. altissima* is currently the subject of a considerable amount of research which seems to be justifying the traditional use of the plant.

TURKEY CORN

Dicentra cucullaria (L.) Bernh
Fam. Papaveraceae

Synonyms: Turkey Pea, *Corydalis cucullaria*. Squirrel Corn is *D. canadensis* Walp.
Habitat: Canada and the USA.
Description: Tubers tawny yellow, about 0.5 cm diameter, subglobular, with a scar on both depressed sides. Taste, bitter; odourless.
Part Used: Root.
Constituents: Alkaloids; cularine, cularidine, cryptopine, bicuculline and others [2]. Squirrel corn contains protopine, corydaline, bulbocapnine, cancentrine, dehydrocancentrines A and B [2, 174].
Medicinal Use: Tonic, diuretic, alterative.
Preparations: Liquid Extract, dose: 2–4 ml.

TURMERIC

Curcuma longa L.
Fam. Zingiberaceae

Synonyms: *C. domestica* Val. or Loir.
Habitat: Southern Asia, cultivated in other tropical countries.
Description: The rhizomes are sold in both round and long pieces. The round pieces are pyriform, with transverse ridges or leaf scars, the longer pieces are the lateral rhizomes. Both are yellowish brown internally. In this country turmeric is imported ready prepared and ground into a bright, dark yellow powder. Taste and odour, characteristic.
Part Used: Rhizome.
Constituents: (i) Curcuminoids; the mixture known as curcumin consisting of at least four phenolic diarylheptanoids, including curcumin and monodesmethoxycurcumin [1288, 1289] (ii) Volatile oil, containing about 60% of turmerones which are sesquiterpene ketones, including arturmerone, α-atlantone, zingberene; with borneol, α-phellandrene and others [5, 1289] (iii) Miscellaneous; protein, sugars, fixed oil, vitamins etc [5].
Medicinal Use: Seldom used medicinally. However recent research has shown many useful properties of turmeric, particularly the antiinflammatory and antihepatotoxic effects. Curcumin inhibits carrageenin-induced inflammation in rats [1290], its antiinflammatory activity is

comparable in potency to that of phenylbutazone [1291] and has recently been shown to be due at least in part of cyclooxygenase inhibition [1292]. The curcuminoids are hepatoprotective, and although the mode of action is not fully understood it is known that they do not act by cleavage to caffeic acid, which is also hepatoprotective [1293]. In addition to these effects, turmeric has antifertility effects in rats [1294], and is antibiotic and antiprotozoal *in vitro* [1295, 1296]. Turmeric is important in the preparation of curry powders and is increasingly being used as a colouring agent because of the increased use of natural ingredients in foods.

TURPENTINE

Pinus palustris Mill.
and other species
Fam. Pinaceae

Part Used: Oil distilled or solvent extracted.

Constituents: Mainly monoterpene hydrocarbons, the main ones being α- and β-pinenes, with 3-carene, and to a much lesser extent camphene, dipentene, terpinolene, β-myrcene, β-phellandrene and others [5].

Medicinal Use: Rubifacient, counter-irritant. It is used externally in liniments and embrocations for rheumatism and muscle stiffness. Turpentine has been taken internally for a number of other complaints but is not recommended since it can cause toxic effects. It is used as a solvent and fragrance ingredient.

Preparations: Turpentine Oil BP; Turpentine Liniment BP, White Liniment BP.

Regulatory Status: GSL. For external use only.

TURPETH

Ipomoea turpeth R.Br.
Fam. Convolvulaceae

Habitat: India, Sri Lanka, Malaysia, Northern Australia.

Description: Variable. Wrinkled, dull grey-brown with a nauseous taste.

Part Used: Root.

Constituents: Resin, about 4–7%, containing turpethin about 50%, and the glycosides α- and β-turpethin [2].

Medicinal Use: Cathartic, purgative. Used like Jalap (q.v.)

Preparations: Powdered Root, dose: 0.3–1.2 g.

U

UNICORN ROOT, FALSE
Chamaelirium luteum A. Gray
Fam. Liliaceae

Synonyms: Starwort, Helonias Root, *Helonias dioica* Pursh.
Habitat: USA.
Description: The rhizome is about 2–3 cm long, 0.5–1 cm thick, nearly cylindrical, ringed transversely with a few stem scars on the upper surface and wiry rootlets on the lower. Fracture horny, greyish-white, showing numerous woody bundles in the centre. Taste, astringent at first, then bitter; odourless.
Part Used: Rhizome.
Constituents: Saponins; the glycosides chamaelirin and helonin, based on diosgenin [2].
Medicinal Use: Uterine tonic, diuretic, emetic, anthelmintic. Used particularly for dysmenorrhoea and amenorrhoea, for threatened miscarriage and also nausea of pregnancy; although modern thought is that all non-essential medication should be avoided during pregnancy. No pharmacological work has been carried out despite the useful indications for this plant.
Preparations: Liquid Extract, dose: 2–4 ml.
Potter's Products: Dysmenorrhoea Mixture No 88.
Regulatory Status: GSL.

UNICORN ROOT, TRUE
Aletris farinosa L.
Fam. Liliaceae

Synonyms: Stargrass, Colic Root, Ague Root.
Habitat: USA.
Description: Rhizome brownish-grey, flattened, up to 1 cm in diameter but usually less; tufted on the upper surface with leaf bases and marked with circular stem scars; numerous branched wiry rootlets on the lower. Fracture, mealy, white. Taste, sweet then bitter and soapy; odour, faint.
Part Used: Rhizome.
Constituents: Little information available. (i) Saponins, based on diosgenin [1297] (ii) Volatile oil, resin etc.
Medicinal Use: Tonic and stomachic. It has been used for anorexia and nervous dyspepsia and for debility. Aletris has been shown to be oestrogenic but the active constituents not identified [1298]. They are likely to be steroidal, based on diosgenin.
Preparations: Powdered root, dose: 0.3–0.6 g; Liquid Extract of Aletris BPC 1934, dose: 0.3–1 ml; Elixir of Aletris BPC 1934, dose: 2–4 ml.
Regulatory Status: GSL.

UVA-URSI

Arctostaphylos uva-ursi (L.) Spreng.
Fam. Ericaceae

Synonyms: Bearberry.

Habitat: Britain, Central and Northern Europe, N. America.

Description: A small, evergreen shrub. Leaves dark green on the upper surface, paler beneath, leathery, obovate, spatulate, about 2 cm long and 0.5–1 cm broad, margins entire, slightly revolute. Taste, astringent; odour, slight.

Part Used: Leaves.

Constituents: (i) Hydroquinones; mainly arbutin (= hydroquinone β-glucoside) and methylarbutin [386] (ii) Iridoids, monotropein [1299], and in the roots, unedoside [1300] (iii) Flavonoids, quercitrin, isoquercitrin, myricacitrin and others [386, 1301] (iv) Miscellaneous; tannins, volatile oil, ursolic, malic and gallic acids [2].

Medicinal Use: Urinary antiseptic, diuretic, astringent. It is used particularly for cystitis, urethritis and pyelitis. Uva-ursi extracts and arbutin have been shown to have antibacterial effects *in vitro* [1302]. Arbutin hydrolyses to hydroquinone which is an effective urinary antiseptic [1303], however large doses should be avoided.

Preparations: Liquid Extract, dose: 2–4 ml; Concentrated Infusion of Uva Ursi BPC 1934, dose: 2–4 ml.

Potter's Products: Antitis Tablets, Diuretab, Kasbah Remedy, Blood Pressure Medicinal Tea Bags, Liver and Bile Medicinal Tea Bags.

Regulatory Status: GSL.

V

VALERIAN

Valeriana officinalis L.
and other species
Fam. Valerianaceae

Habitat: Native to Europe and Asia, naturalized in N. America.

Description: The root consists of a short root-stock, about 2 cm long and 1 cm in diameter, with numerous short, lateral branches, and rootlets 2–10 cm long, the crown often showing scales from the stem base. The transverse section is horny with a narrow, woody ring and is pale grey-brown. Valerian is unmistakable due to its unpleasant, characteristic, nauseous odour. Tasting it is unnecessary.

Part Used: Root.

Constituents: Volatile oil, containing valerenic acid, valerenone, valerenal, hydroxyvalerenic acid, α-kessyl alcohol, isovaleric acid, citronellyl isovalerate, eugenyl and isoeugenyl isovalerate, bornyl acetate, bornyl isovalerate, faurinone and faurinols [1304, 1305, 1306, 1307, 1308, 1309] (ii) Iridoids known as valepotriates; mainly valtrate and didrovaltrate, with isovaltrate, deacetylisovaltrate, homovaltrate, acevaltrate, homodivaltrate, valechlorine, valeridine and possibly others [1310, 1311, 1312, 1313] (iii) Alkaloids; actinidine, valerine, valerianine and chatinine [1314, 1315] (iv) Miscellaneous; choline, flavonoids, sterols, tannins etc. [2,5].

Indian valerian contains valtrate and isovaltrate [1316]; V. thalictroides Graebn, V. edulis (H.B.K.) F G Mey and V. kilimandschatica Engl. also have high concentrations of valepotriates [1317]; however they do not contain valerenic acid [1306].

Medicinal Use: Sedative, hypnotic, nervine, hypotensive. Valerian is used widely, particularly in Europe, for insomnia, excitability and exhaustion. The sedative activity is thought to be due partly to the valepotriates and some of their degradation products [1318, 1319] and partly to valerenic acid, valerenone and other components of the volatile oil [1304, 1320], all of which have in vivo activity. It has also been suggested that there is an interaction between these constituents [1305], however they both have primary CNS depressant activity [1304]. Valerian, valerenic acid and the eugenyl and isoeugenyl esters are spasmolytic [1304]. The degradation products of the valepotriates had a higher therapeutic index in mice than didrovaltrate [1319], a significant finding since the valepotriates are notoriously unstable. Valerenic acid and derivatives have been shown to inhibit γ-amino-butyric acid (GABA) [1321].

The valepotriates have cytotoxic and antitumour activity in a number of in vitro systems [1316, 1322]; they inhibit the synthesis of DNA and proteins [1323] by covalent bonding [1322]. Tests in mice show that toxicity is low due to restricted distribution of the drug [1324], and no adverse reactions in humans have been noted [1322].

Clinical studies of valerian show that it improves the quality of sleep as measured by subjective assessment by the patients themselves; this is confirmed to some extent by EEG. It reduced the time taken to fall asleep, particularly in older people and in habitually poor sleepers, and did not cause somnolence in the morning or affect dream recall [1325, 1326]. Valerian extracts are sometimes used in skin creams for the treatment of eczema.

Preparations: Valerian Liquid Extract BPC 1963, dose: 0.3–1 ml; Simple Valerian Tincture BPC 1949, dose: 4–8 ml; Ammoniated Valerian Tincture BPC 1963, dose: 2–4 ml; Concentrated Valerian Infusion BPC 1963, dose: 2–4 ml.

Potter's Products: Nervine Medicinal Tea Bags, Nervous Debility and Uterine Disorder Mixture No. 98A, Headache and Nervous Exhaustion Mixture No. 101A, Neurelax Tablets, Valerian Tablets.

Regulatory Status: GSL.

VERNAL GRASS, SWEET

Anthoxanthum odoratum L.
Fam. Graminae

Habitat: Europe, including Britain, and temperate Asia.

Description: Flowers in dense spikes, tapering at both ends, about 3 cm long and 1 cm wide. It is distinguished from related species by having only two stamens in the flower and by its aromatic, hay-like odour.

Part Used: Flowers.

Constituents: Coumarin glycosides. These can be broken down to 4-hydroxycoumarin and further to dicoumarol if stored damp [2, 79].

Medicinal Use: Has been used for hay fever, internally as a tincture and as a nasal lotion. Dicoumarol is a potent anticoagulant.

VERVAIN

Verbena officinalis L.
Fam. Verbenaceae

Habitat: Grows throughout Europe, particularly in the south.

Description: Leaves pinnately lobed, rough, toothed, opposite, the upper unstalked. Flowers lilac two lipped, petals five lobed, in long, slender, leafless spikes. Taste, very bitter; odour, aromatic when rubbed.

Part Used: Herb.

Constituents: (i) Iridoids, verbenin, verbenalin and bastatoside (2, 1327] (ii) Miscellaneous; essential oil, mucilage and others [2].

Medicinal Use: Nervine, tonic, sudorific, emetic. The medicinal uses of verbena are varied, including antidepressant and anticonvulsant activity, and for jaundice, coughs and colds and as a digestive aid. Verbena is reputed to have weak parasympathomimetic activity and be of low toxicity. It may be taken as an infusion. Verbenalin is a mild purgative in animals [197].

Preparations: Liquid Extract, dose: 2–4 ml.

Regulatory Status: GSL.

VIOLET

Viola odorata L.
Fam. Violaceae

Synonyms: Sweet Violet.

Habitat: Widely found in Europe, including Britain, and Asia.

Description: A well-known plant. Leaves cordate or ovate, with long stalks. Flowers blue, with a hooked stigma and a short spur inflated at the end and channelled above. Taste, mucilaginous.

Part Used: Flowers, leaves.

Constituents: (i) Phenolic glycosides; gaultherin, violutoside (= salicylic acid methyl ester [2, 339] (ii) Saponins; myrosin and violin [339] (iii) Flavonoids; rutin and violarutin [1, 37] (iv) Miscellaneous; odoratine, an alkaloid [112], 2-nitroproprionic acid [339], mucilage [2].

Medicinal Use: Antiseptic, expectorant. It has been used in syrups for coughs and colds, bronchitis and catarrh. It has also been used for neoplasms [37], and a related species, *V. striata* has antitumour effects in murine tests [1328].

Regulatory Status: GSL.

W

WAFER ASH

Ptelea trifoliata L.
Fam. Rutaceae

Synonyms: Shrubby Trefoil, Swamp Dogwood.
Habitat: USA and Canada.
Description: The root-bark occurs in quilled or curved pieces, 3–20 mm thick, transversely wrinkled with a whitish-brown exfoliating surface of thin, papery layers. The inner surface is nearly smooth, with faintly projecting medullary rays. Transverse fracture short, yellowish white, the papery layer pale buff. Taste bitter; odourless.
Part Used: Root-bark.
Constituents: (i) Alkaloids, including kokusaginine (ii) Miscellaneous; bitters etc. [2].
Medicinal Use: Tonic, antiperiodic, stomachic. It has been used in the form of an infusion for fevers, as a tonic and to stimulate the appetite. The bitter substances are reported to have antibacterial activity [2].

WAHOO

Euonymus atropurpureus Jacq.
Fam. Celastraceae

Synonyms: Spindle Tree.
Habitat: Eastern and Central USA and Canada.
Description: Usually occurs in transverse curved pieces or occasionally quills, 2–4 mm thick, very light in weight. The outer surface is light brown, wrinkled, with patches of soft grey rhytidome and few lenticels. Root bark may have root scars and adhering rootlets; stem bark is smoother with lichens usually present. The inner surface is striated, porous, sometimes with adherent patches of yellow wood. Fracture short but friable, showing a narrow brown cork, a whitish cortex and a darker phloem. Taste, bitter and acrid; odour, faint.
Part Used: Stem and Root Bark.
Constituents: This often used remedy has not been well investigated. (i) Cardenolides based on digitoxigenin (ii) Alkaloids such as asparagine and atropurpurine (iii) Sterols; euonysterol, atropurpurol, homoeuonysterol (iv) Miscellaneous; ducitol, citrullol, fatty acids, tannins etc. [2, 37].
Medicinal Use: Cholagogue, laxative, diuretic, mild cardiac tonic and circulatory stimulant. It is reported to be a mild purgative and choleretic [4] and is used mainly in combination with other remedies for liver and gall bladder trouble and dyspepsia, and occasionally for skin problems where these conditions are thought to be a cause.
Preparations: Euonymus Tincture BPC 1949, dose: 0.6–2.6 ml; Elixir of Euonymus and Pulsatilla BPC 1934, dose: 4–16 ml.
Potter's Products: G B tablets (Gallstone Tablets), Indigestion Mixture.
Regulatory Status: GSL.

WALNUT
Juglans regia L.
Fam. Juglandaceae

Habitat: Native to the Middle East, cultivated widely for the walnuts, which ripen towards the end of September.

Description: Leaves composed of seven to nine leaflets of varying size, averaging 5–10 cm in length and 3–4 cm wide, greenish, parchment-like, turning brown with keeping. The bark is dull, blackish brown, with traces of a thin, whitish external layer, tough and fibrous and somewhat mealy. Taste, bitter and astringent; odour of leaves, characteristic and aromatic; bark, odourless.

Part Used: Leaves, bark.

Constituents: Leaves: (i) Naphthaquinones, mainly juglone (formerly known as nucin or regianin), often as the 4β-D-glucoside of α-hydrojuglone [218] (ii) Volatile oil, containing β-eudesmol, about 10%, eugenol, fatty acids including geranic acid, sesquiterpenes, diterpenes and others [1329] (iii) Miscellaneous; tannins, ellagic acid and gallic acids, flavonoids, inositol. No information on the constituents of the bark is readily available.

Medicinal Use: Alterative, laxative, antiseptic. An infusion has been used for herpes, eczema and other conditions, and externally to skin eruptions and ulcers etc. The volatile oil is antifungal *in vitro* [1329] and juglone has antimicrobial and antineoplastic activity [255]. The walnut has been used as food, and also medicinally, for many years: and because of its resemblance to the brain it was thought, according to the Doctrine of Signatures, to be good for headaches and epilepsy. A dye made from the shells has been used to darken the hair.

Preparations: Leaves: Liquid Extract: dose: 4–8 ml.

Biblical References: Song of Solomon 6 : 11; Genesis 43 : 11 (nuts)

WATER BETONY
Scrophularia aquatica L.
Fam. Scrophulariaceae

Synonyms: Water Figwort, *Betonica aquatica.*

Habitat: Common by streams or ponds and in wet places in Britain and parts of Europe.

Description: Stem four-angled, winged, bearing leaves in opposite pairs with winged petioles. The leaves are oval, with serrated margins, pointed at the apex, and sometimes with one or two small lobes at the base. The flowers are up to 1 cm across, brownish-purple with greenish undersides, with a tubular base opening into five small petal lobes, the upper two of which are joined. Taste, bitter; odourless.

Part Used: Herb.

Constituents: Undetermined.

Medicinal Use: Vulnerary. Used formerly as a poultice or ointment for ulcers, sores and wounds.

WATER DOCK
Rumex aquatica L.
Fam. Polygonaceae

Habitat: Northern Europe and Great Britain, mainly by rivers and ditches.

Description: The leaves are triangular, up to three times as long as wide, alternate, with a sheath round the stem at the base of the leaves. The root has a blackish or dark brown outer surface, the remains of a few branches, and transverse rings of rootlet scars. Taste, astringent and sweetish; odourless.

Part Used: Root.

Constituents: Anthraquinones, about 0.6%; tannins, about 20%, (unspecified) [2].

Medicinal Use: Alterative, deobstruent, detergent. An infusion has been used internally and the powdered root has been used as a dentifrice.

Preparations: Liquid Extract, dose: 4–8 ml.

WATER DROPWORT
Oenanthe crocata L.
Fam. Umbelliferae

Synonyms: Hemlock Water Dropwort, Dead Men's Fingers.

Habitat: Found in damp grassy places in Britain and France.

Description: A tall, hairless, perennial; flowers typical white umbels, leaves 3–4 pinnate, with broad, wedge-shaped toothed leaflets; stem, grooved. The root bears pale fleshy tubers, hence the synonym. Odour, parsely-like. Too poisonous to taste.

Part Used: Root.

Constituents: Oenanthetoxin, a polyunsaturated higher alcohol [79, 1330].

Medicinal Use: None. Formerly used for epilepsy but cannot be recommended. The plant has been responsible for numerous cases of poisoning, in mistake for parsley, celery etc. [79, 1330].

WATER FENNEL
Oenanthe aquatica (L.) Poir.
Fam. Umbelliferae

Synonyms: Fine-leaved Water Dropwort, *Oenanthe phellandrium* Lamk.

Habitat: In damp places throughout Europe.

Description: A much branched, hairless perennial. Leaves 3–4 pinnate, upper with pointed lobes, lower lobes linear to threadlike. Flowers white, umbels opposite to leaves as well as terminal. Fruits about 5 mm long and 2 mm in diameter, tapering towards the apex, and crowned with four teeth. Taste, acrid; odour, strong, aromatic, characteristic.

Part Used: Fruit.

Constituents: (i) Essential oil, about 1.5–2% [2] (ii) Flavonoids; tricetin, myricetin and rhamnetin [414] (iii) Fixed oil, about 20% [2]. The herb contains the poisonous oenanthetoxin (see Water Dropwort).

Medicinal Use: Expectorant, alterative, diuretic. Rarely used.

WATER GERMANDER
Teucrium scordium L.
Fam. Labiatae

Habitat: Europe, rarely in Britain.

Description: Leaves opposite and sessile, oval-oblong, about 2 cm long and 0.5 cm broad, narrowed at the base, coarsely serrate at the margin, softly hairy on both sides. Taste, bitter; odour, when the fresh leaves are rubbed, rather alliaceous.

Part Used: Herb.

Constituents: (i) Iridoids, including harpagide and acetyl harpagide [599] (ii) Diterpenes, of the clerodane type, teucrin F, teucrin G and 6α-hydroxyteuscordin [1331] (iii) Miscellaneous; tannins, essential oil etc. [2].

Medicinal Use: Antiseptic, diaphoretic, stimulant. It was recommended in ancient terms as a sudorific and antiseptic, and taken as an infusion. Gerard even declares that after battle the bodies found lying on these plants were much slower in decaying than those not.

Preparations: Liquid Extract, dose: 2–4 ml.

Regulatory Status: GSL.

WHITE POND LILY, AMERICAN
Nymphaea odorata Soland.
Fam. Nymphaceae

Synonyms: Water Nymph, Water Cabbage. *N. alba* and *N. tuberosa* are also used.

Habitat: USA.

Description: The rhizome occurs in irregular pieces up to about 5 cm in diameter. The outer surface is dark greyish brown to black, with the remains of leaf bases up to about 1 cm in diameter and root scars. Buds may also be present; these have a dense covering of fine grey hairs. Transverse surface yellowish brown with a ring of porous depressions immediately inside the cork. Fracture short. Taste, mucilaginous, slightly pungent; odour, faint.

Part Used: Rhizome.

Constituents: Unknown. *N. tuberosa* contains tannic acid and gallic acid; and alkaloids, sterols and flavonoids [1332] and *N. alba* the alkaloids nymphaeine and nupharine, glycosides and tannins [2].

Medicinal Use: Antiseptic, astringent, demulcent. It may be taken in the form of an infusion internally for chronic diarrhoea, as a douche for leucorrhoea and vaginitis, as a gargle for sore throat and as a poultice with Slippery Elm and Linseed for boils. *N. tuberosa* has some antitumour effects in hamsters. The tannic acid and gallic acid are antimicrobial [1332] and astringent. *N. alba* is hypotensive in animals and is reported to have low toxicity [1333].

Preparations: Liquid Extract, dose: 2–4 ml.

Regulatory Status: GSL.

WILD CARROT
Daucus carota L. subsp. *carota*
Fam. Umbelliferae

Synonyms: Queen Anne's Lace.

Habitat: Europe, Asia and N. Africa. This is the wild form of the garden carrot.

Description: Leaves oblong and obovate, bi- or tripinnate, hairy. The aerial parts resemble those of the garden carrot in appearance, taste and odour, but the root is small and white. Flowers white umbels, often with a central crimson or purplish flower. Fruit small, hairy, ridged.

Part Used: Herb, "seeds" (fruits).

Constituents: Herb: (i) Flavonoids; 3-O-methyl-kaempferol, apigenin, quercetin, myricetin and sakuranetin [414] (ii) Daucine, a volatile alkaloid (unconfirmed) [2] (iii) Volatile oil containing the terpenes carotol and geranyl acetate [313] (iv) Miscellaneous; petroselinic acid, tannins, [2]. Seeds: (i) Volatile oil consisting of asarone, cis-β-bergamotene, β-bisabolene, carotol, caryophyllene and its oxide, coumarin, daucol, β-elemene, geraniol, geranyl acetate, limonene, α-pinene, β-selinen, α-terpineol, terpinen-4-ol and others [5] (ii) Flavonoids; apigenin-4'-O-β-D-glucoside, kaempferol-3-O-β-D-glucoside and apigenin-7-O-B-D-galactomannoside [1334].

Medicinal Use: Herb: Diuretic, carminative, antilithic. It is used particularly for kidney stone, cystitis and gout. Seed: diuretic, emmanagogue, carminative, antiflatulent. Both may taken in the form of an infusion.

Preparations: Herb: Liquid Extract, dose: 2–4 ml.

Potter's Products: Sciargo Tablets, Sciargo Medicinal Tea Bags.

Regulatory Status: GSL.

WILD CHERRY BARK
Prunus serotina Ehrh.
Fam. Rosaceae

Synonyms: Virginian Prune Bark.

Habitat: Widely distributed throughout Canada and the USA.

Description: The bark occurs in flat, curved or channelled pieces, up to about 4 mm in thickness; larger pieces are considered to be of inferior quality. The external surface in the young bark is covered with a smooth, glossy, red-brown cork with white lenticels, often exfoliating to reveal the greenish brown cortex. The older bark is rougher and darker. The inner surface is brownish, longitudinally striated, often with adherent patches of yellowish wood. Taste, astringent and bitter; odour of benzaldehyde when damp.

Part Used: Bark.

Constituents: (i) Prunasin, a cyanogenetic glycoside which is hydrolysed by the enzyme prunase to hydrocyanic acid (ii) Benzaldehyde (iii) Miscellaneous; 3,4,5-trimethoxybenzoic acid (= eudesmic acid), *p*-coumaric acid, scopoletin, tannins, sugars etc [1, 4, 5].

Medicinal Use: Antitussive, sedative, astringent. Wild cherry bark has been used for centuries in cough syrups, particularly for irritable and persistent coughs such as those due to bronchitis and whooping cough. It is also used for nervous dyspepsia and as an astringent in diarrhoea.

Preparations: Wild Cherry Syrup BP, dose: 2.5–10 ml; Tincture of Wild Cherry BPC 1949, dose: 2–4 ml.

Potter's Products: Horehound and Aniseed Balsam.

Regulatory Status: GSL.

WILD INDIGO

Baptisia tinctoria R.Br.
Fam. Leguminosae

Synonyms: Indigoweed..

Habitat: Indigenous to Canada and the USA.

Description: Crown of root with knotty branches; the roots vary in diameter from 0.2–1.5 cm, external surface brownish, longitudinally wrinkled and grooved, somewhat warty due to detached rootlets. Fracture tough and fibrous, showing a thick bark and whitish wood with concentric rings. Taste, bitter, acrid, disagreeable; odour, faint.

Part Used: Root, leaves.

Constituents: (i) Isoflavones; genistein, biochanin A etc. (ii) Flavonoids (iii) Alkaloids such as cytisine (v) Coumarins [2, 37, 1335] (iv) Polysaccharides [1336].

Medicinal Use: Antimicrobial, antiseptic, antipyretic, laxative. Wild indigo is used as an infusion for tonsillitis, pharyngitis and other infections; boils, internally and as a mouthwash for aphthous ulcers and sore gums; in the form of an ointment for sore nipples, indolent ulcers etc, and as a douche in vaginitis. The isoflavones are oestrogenic. The polysaccharide fraction has been shown to enhance antibody production in sheep red blood cells [1335] and stimulate phagocytosis of erythrocytes in isolated perfused rat liver [1272].

Preparations: Tincture of Baptisia BPC 1934, dose: 2–5 ml.

Potter's Products: Compound Elixir of Echinacea.

Regulatory Status: GSL.

WILD MINT

Mentha aquatica L.
Fam. Labiatae

Synonyms: Water Mint, Marsh Mint, Hairy Mint, *M. sativa* L.

Habitat: Europe and the British Isles.

Description: Similar to Peppermint (q.v.), which is a hybrid of this species. The leaves are wider, less sharply toothed and the flowers more hairy. Odour and taste, characteristic.

Part Used: Herb.

Constituents: Essential oil, about 0.3–0.85%, composed of 40–50% methofuran, with menthol, menthyl acetate, pulegone etc. [2].

Medicinal Use: Stimulant, emetic, astringent; it has been used for difficult menstruation and diarrhoea.

WILD YAM

Dioscorea villosa L.
Fam. Dioscoriaceae

Synonyms: Colic Root, Rheumatism Root.

Habitat: Common in Eastern and Central USA and in some tropical countries.

Description: Tubers cylindrical, pale brown, compressed, about 10–15 cm long and 1–2 cm thick, curved, branched at intervals, showing stem scars on the upper surface and rootlets on the other. Occurs in commerce as hard, pale yellowish-brown chips of rhizome and narrow, fibrous roots. Fracture short, hard. Taste, insipid at first, then acrid; odourless.

Part Used: Root and rhizome.

Constituents: Steroidal saponins, based on diosgenin: dioscin, dioscorin, and others [2]. Many other species of *Dioscorea* are used as sources of saponins for the preparation of steroids for the pharmaceutical industry.

Medicinal Use: Antiinflammatory, cholagogue, spasmolytic, mild diaphoretic. The main use is in various types of rheumatism and for bilious and intestinal colic. It is also used for dysmenorrhoea and cramps.

Preparations: Liquid Extract, dose: 2–4 ml.

WILLOW

Salix alba L.
S. fragilis L.
S. cinerea L.
and other species
Fam. Salicaceae

Synonyms: White Willow, European Willow.

Habitat: Indigenous to Britain, Central and Southern Europe.

Description: The bark occurs in thin channelled pieces up to about 2 cm wide and 2 mm thick. Outer surface glossy in young bark, wrinkled and duller in older bark, greenish or greyish brown; inner surface striated, fibrous, yellowish or reddish brown. Taste, astringent and bitter; odour, faint.

Part Used: Bark.

Constituents: (i) Phenolic glycosides; salicin, picein and triandrin, with esters of salicylic acid and salicyl alcohol, acetylated salicin, salicortin and salireposide; concentrations etc. depending on species [2, 4, 386] (ii) Miscellaneous; tannins, catechin, *p*-coumaric acid and flavonoids [2, 386].

Medicinal Use: Analgesic, antiinflammatory, febrifuge, tonic. Willow is an ancient remedy which has been used in various forms for rheumatism and gout, fevers and aches and pains of all kinds. It is usually considered to be the natural form and origin of the modern aspirin.

Potter's Products: Rheumatism Mixture No. 92A, Sciatica Mixture No. 124A, Herbprin Tablets.

Regulatory Status: GSL.

Biblical References: Leviticus 23 : 40; Job 40 : 22; Psalm 137 : 2; Isaiah 15 : 7 and 44 : 4; Ezekiel 17 : 5.

WINTER'S BARK

Drimys winteri Forst.
Fam. Winteraceae

Synonyms: True Winter's Bark, Pepper Bark. *D. granadensis* is often substituted. False Winter's Bark is *Cinnamodendron corticosum*.

Habitat: Central and South America.

Description: Rare in commerce. In short pieces, 5–8 mm thick, dark brown throughout. Fracture short and granular, showing pale medullary rays which project on the inner surface, giving it a striated appearance. Taste, pungent; odour, faint.

Part Used: Bark.

Constituents: Acrid resin, volatile oil, tannins. The leaf contains eudesmane sesquiterpenes [183].

Medicinal Use: Rarely used except locally, for indigestion, flatulence and colic; usually as an infusion. False Winter's Bark is used for similar purposes.

WINTER CHERRY

Physalis alkekengi L.
Fam. Solanaceae

Habitat: Indigenous to Asia and parts of Europe, cultivated in gardens in Britain and America.

Description: The dried berries are dull red, about 0.5 cm in diameter, globular, bilocular, containing numerous whitish, ovoid flattened seeds. Taste, sweet and bitterish; odourless. The plant sold in pots as Winter Cherry is *Solanum pseudocapsicum*.

Part Used: Berries.

Constituents: (i) Flavonoids, including luteolin-7-glucoside [1337] (ii) Sterols; the physalins A, B and C [1338] (iii) In the roots at least, tropane alkaloids; cuscohygrine, tropine and tigloidine [1339].

Medicinal Use: Diuretic, febrifuge. Has been employed in intermittent fevers, in urinary disorders and gout.

WINTERGREEN

Gaultheria procumbens L.
Fam. Ericaceae

Synonyms: Teaberry, Checkerberry.

Habitat: Native to N. America and Canada.

Description: Leaves obovate or broadly elliptical, short-stalked, faintly serrate at the margin, leathery, glossy green above, paler beneath. Taste astringent and aromatic; odour, characteristic.

Part Used: Leaves.

Constituents: (i) Phenolic compounds; gaultherin, salicylic acid, *o*-pyrocatechuic, gentisic, vanillic, caffeic and other acids [1340] (ii) Volatile oil, 0.5–1%, containing methyl salicylate, about 98%, which is produced by enzymatic hydrolysis of gaultherin during maceration and steam distillation [5].

Medicinal Use: Antiinflammatory, antirheumatic, diuretic. An infusion of the leaves is occasionally taken internally but oil of wintergreen is used mainly in the form of an ointment or liniment for rheumatism, sprains, sciatica, neuralgia and all kinds of muscular pain.

Preparations: Methyl Salicylate Liniment BPC; Compound Methyl Salicylate Ointment BPC; Methyl Salicylate Ointment BPC.

Potter's Products: Nine Rubbing Oils.

Regulatory Status: GSL.

WITCH HAZEL

Hamamelis virginiana L.
Fam. Hamamelidaceae

Habitat: Indigenous to N. America and Canada.

Description: Leaves broadly oval, up to 15 cm long, 7 cm broad, the margin dentate or crenate, the apex acute and the base asymmetrically cordate. When dried the lamina is papery, dark greenish brown. Venation pinnate, very conspicuous on the lower surface. Bark quilled or channelled, usually in pieces up to 10 cm long and 2 cm broad, 1–2 mm thick, with a silvery grey external surface with numerous lenticels and a pinkish-brown striated inner surface. Fracture fibrous and laminated. Taste of both leaves and bark, very astringent; odour, slight.

Part Used: Leaves, twigs, bark.

Constituents: Leaves: (i) Tannins; 8–10%, composed mainly of gallotannins with some condensed catechins and proanthocyanins. The presence of hamamelitannin is disputed [1, 5, 1341] (ii) Miscellaneous; flavonoids; quercetin, kaempferol, astragalin, myricitrin and others, volatile oil, containing hexenol, *n*-hexen-2-al, α- and β-ionones and others [5, 1342, 1343, 1344]. Bark: (i) Tannins; 1–7%, mainly the α-, β- and γ-hamamelitannins, with some condensed tannins such as *d*-gallocatechin, *l*-epigallocatechin and *l*-epicatechin [1, 5, 1341] (ii) Miscellaneous; saponins, volatile oil, resin etc. [5].

Medicinal Use: Astringent, haemostatic. Witch hazel extract is very highly regarded for the treatment of haemorrhage, piles and varicose veins. The distilled extract, known as witch hazel water, is widely used as a treatment for sprains and bruises, spots and blemishes, in eye drops, aftershave lotions and in cosmetic preparations; for example mixed with equal parts of rose water (see Rose) as a skin tonic. Distilled witch hazel water is reputed not to contain tannins; however its astringency is not otherwise explained [5].

Preparations: Leaves: Hamamelis Dry Extract BPC; Hamemelis Liquid Extract BPC; Hamemelis Ointment BPC. Bark: Hamamelis Tincture BPC 1949; dose: 2–4 ml. Twigs: Distilled Extract of Witch Hazel BPC 1949.

Potter's Products: Varicose Ointment.

Regulatory Status: GSL.

WOOD BETONY
Stachy officinalis (L.) Trev.
Fam. Labiatae

Synonyms: Bishopswort, *Betonica officinalis* L.

Habitat: Europe, including Britain, in open woods, hedgebanks, grasslands and heaths.

Description: Basal leaves up to 7 cm long, ovate or oblong, obtuse, cordate at base, coarsely crenate. Stems upright and hairy, bearing smaller leaves, 2–3 pairs. Flowers bright reddish-purple, in tight oblong spikes, the tube longer than the calyx. Taste slightly bitter; odour, faint.

Part Used: Herb.

Constituents: (i) Alkaloids; stachydrine and betonicine (ii) Miscellaneous; betaine, choline, tannins etc. [2].

Medicinal Use: Sedative, bitter, aromatic, astringent. Used, often in combination with other remedies, for nervous headache, neuralgia and anxiety. Parkinson states ". . . it is said also to hinder drunkenness being taken beforehand and quickly to expell it afterwards". This use has not been tested in modern times and cannot be relied upon.

Preparations: Liquid extract, dose: 2–4 ml.

Regulatory Status: GSL.

WOODRUFF
Galium odoratum (L.) Scop.
Fam. Rubiaceae

Synonyms: *Asperula odorata* L.

Habitat: Grows in woods in Britain and Europe.

Description: A short perennial, unbranched, with slender, quadrangular, brittle stems and whorls of 6–9 elliptical, pointed leaves edged with tiny, forward-pointing bristles. Flowers small, with four petal lobes, white, in loose clusters. Odour, when dry, of new-mown hay.

Part Used: Herb.

Constituents: (i) Iridoids; asperuloside (about 0.05%) and monotropein [5, 1345] (ii) Miscellaneous; tannins, anthraquinones, flavonoids, nicotinic acid. The presence of coumarin has been disputed [5, 356].

Medicinal Use: Diuretic, tonic, antispasmodic, sedative, hepatic. Asperuloside and monotropein are mildly purgative in animals [197] and asperuloside has been suggested as a useful starting material for the production of prostaglandins [360]. Woodruff has recently been shown to have antiinflammatory activity in animals [403]. It is sometimes used as a fragrance ingredient.

WOOD SAGE
Teucrium scorodonia L.
Fam. Labiatae

Synonyms: Garlic Sage.

Habitat: Grows in open woods and on heaths and scrubs throughout Western Europe.

Description: A short, downy perennial. Leaves cordate, bluntly toothed, wrinkled, sage-like. Flowers greenish-yellow, two-lipped, with prominent maroon stamens. Taste bitter; odour, slightly aromatic.

Part Used: Herb.

Constituents: (i) Iridoids; harpagide and acetyl harpagide [599] (ii) Diterpenes of the clerodane type; teupolin, teuscorolide, teuscorodol, teuscorodin, teuflin [1346,1347] (iii) Flavonoids; luteolin [1346].

Medicinal Use: Antirheumatic, astringent, carminative, antimicrobial, diaphoretic, vulnerary. It is used for feverish colds, rheumatic conditions and flatulent dyspepsia, normally as an infusion. As a poultice it is applied to boils and abscesses.

Preparations: Liquid Extract, dose: 2–4 ml.

Regulatory Status: GSL.

WOOD SORREL

Oxalis acetosella L.
Fam. Oxalidaceae

Habitat: Common in woods throughout Europe.

Description: Leaves, bright green, trifoliate, stalked, the leaflets broadly obcordate. Flowers white, bell-shaped, with purplish veins. Taste acid; odourless.

Part Used: Herb.

Constituents: Flavonoid glycosides; orientin, vitexin and isovitexin [1348].

Medicinal Use: Diuretic, refrigerant. Has been used for fevers and urinary disorders, in the form of an infusion and boiled in milk.

WORMSEED

Chenopodium ambrosioides L.
C. ambrosioides L. var *anthelminticum* (L.) A Gray
Fam. Chenopodiaceae

Synonyms: American Wormseed.

Habitat: Tropical America; also cultivated in India and China.

Description: Fruit subglobular, about 2 mm in diameter, greenish or brown. The single seed is glossy, black, lenticular, with an obtuse edge. Taste, acrid, astringent; odour, camphoraceous and terebinthinate.

Part Used: Seeds.

Constituents: (i) Oil, containing ascaridol, an unsaturated terpene peroxide, in highly variable amounts up to 90%, with geraniol, cymene, terpinene, methyl salicylate, and butyric acid (ii) Triterpenes; "chenopodium sapogenin", triacontyl alcohol, α-spinasterol [5, 3, 185, 1349].

Medicinal Use: Anthelmintic. The active constituent is ascaridol; it is highly active against roundworms, hookworms and small, but not large, tapeworms. It is used in conjunction with a purgative. It must be used with care as it is highly toxic and can cause unpleasant side effects such as headache, dizziness, vomiting, convulsions and even death in overdose.

Preparations: Powdered seed, dose: 1–4 g; Liquid Extract, dose: 2–4 ml.

Regulatory Status: P.

WORMSEED, LEVANT

Artemisia cina Berg.
Fam. Compositae

Synonyms: Santonica.

Habitat: Native to Eastern Europe and Russia, cultivated elsewhere.

Description: Dried, unexpanded flowerheads containing three to five minute, tubular flowers without pappus. The flowerheads are about 3 mm long and 1.5 mm in diameter, greenish-yellow when fresh, brown when kept for some time; each has numerous oblong-obtuse scales closely overlapping each other. Taste, bitter; odour; aromatic, characteristic.

Part Used: Unexpanded flowerheads.

Constituents: (i) Volatile oil, containing 1,8-cineole as the major component, up to about 80%, with α-terpineol and carvacrol [386] (ii) Sesquiterpene lactones; about 2–6% L-α-santonin and α-hydroxysantonin (= artemisin) [4, 386].

Medicinal Use: Vermifuge. Santonin is particularly active against roundworms, and to some extent against threadworms, but is ineffective against tapeworm. Wormseed has been taken combined with honey or treacle or as a decoction or infusion, it must be used with care as high doses are toxic.

Preparations: Santonin BP 1963.

Regulatory Status: P.

WORMWOOD

Artemisia absinthium L.
Fam. Compositae

Synonyms: Absinthium.

Habitat: Native to Europe, N. Africa and Western Asia, cultivated in the USA and elsewhere.

Description: A shrubby perennial reaching about 1 m; leaves pinnately divided, up to 12 cm long, the lobes obovate or lanceolate, entire or toothed. Both surfaces are covered with fine, whitish, silky hairs. The flowers are small, nearly globular, with no pappus, greenish-yellow, arranged in an erect leafy panicle. Taste, very bitter; odour, characteristic, aromatic.

Part Used: Herb.

Constituents: (i) Volatile oil, of variable composition, usually containing α- and β-thujone as the major component, up to about 35%; with thujyl alcohol, azulenes including chamazulene, 3,6- and 5,6-dihydrochamazulene; bisabolene, cadinene, camphene, sabinene, *trans*-sabinylacetate, pinene, phellandrene and others [5, 1360, 1351] (ii) Sesquiterpene lactones; artabsin, absinthin, anabsinthin, artemetin, arabsin, artabin, artabsinolides A, B, C and D, matricin, isoabsinthin, artemolin and others [5, 1352, 1353, 1354, 1355, 1356, 1357] (iii) Acetylenes, in the root; *trans*-dehydromatricaria ester, C_{13} and C_{14}-*trans*-spiroketalenol ethers and others [1358] (iv) Flavonoids; quercetin 3-glucoside and 3-rhamnoglucoside, spinacetin 3-glucoside and 3-rhamnoglucoside and others [1359] (v) Phenolic acids; *p*-hydroxyphenylacetic, chlorogenic, *p*-coumaric, protocatechuic, syringic, vanillic and other acids [1360] (vi) Lignans; diayangambin and epi-yangambin [1361].

Medicinal Use: Choleretic, anthelmintic, stomachic, antiinflammatory. Wormwood has been used for hundreds of years for many types of disorders; for colds, rheumatism, as a cardiac stimulant, carminative, antispasmodic, emmenagogue, pain reliever during childbirth, tonic and antiseptic. The azulenes are antiinflammatory (see Chamomile), and the choleretic effects have been demonstrated in man [1362]. Thujone however is toxic, it has hallucinogenic and addictive properties which have led to the suggestion that it interacts with a common receptor in the central nervous system to that of tetrahydrocannabinol, the active constituent in Indian Hemp (q.v.) [1363]. Wormwood was the basis for the alcoholic drink "absinthe", which was popular in the 19th century but subsequently banned because of its dangerous properties. In large doses it causes insomnia, nightmares, vomiting, and convulsions [1364]. However it is possible to make a thujone-free extract of the herb [1365]. The anthelmintic properties are probably due to the sesquiterpene lactones present. Wormwood is widely used as a flavouring agent in liqueurs.

Preparations: Dried herb, dose: 1–2 g; Tincture Absinthium BPC 1934, dose: 4–16 ml; Liquid Extract, dose: 1–2 ml.

Regulatory Status: GSL.

Biblical References: Deuteronomy 29 : 18; Proverbs 5 : 4; Jeremiah 9 : 15 and 23 : 15; Lamentations 3 : 15, 19; Amos 5 : 7; Revelations 8 : 11 and similar species.

WOUNDWORT

Stachys palustris L.
Fam. Labiatae

Synonyms: Marsh Woundwort. Hedge Woundwort is *S. sylvatica* L.

Habitat: Grows in damp places throughout Europe, including Britain.

Description: Leaves narrowly lanceolate, nearly sessile, hairy. Flowers purple. *S. sylvatica* has ovate and cordate leaves, long stalked, hairy; and reddish-purple flowers. Both taste astringent; odour unpleasant.

Part Used: Herb.

Constituents: *S. palustris:* (i) Iridoids, harpagide and acetyl harpagide [62] (ii) Flavonoids; based on isoscutellarein and oroxylin A [648]. *S. sylvatica:* (i) Alkaloids; betonicine, stachydrine and trigonelline (ii) Allantoin (iii) Betaine and choline [2].

Medicinal Use: Antiseptic, antispasmodic, vulnerary. Both are used for gout, cramp, vertigo, and haemorrhage, and as a poultice applied to wounds. Betonicine (= achilleine) has been shown to be haemostatic [1366].

Y

YARROW

Achillea millefolium L.
Fam. Compositae

Synonyms: Milfoil, Nosebleed.

Habitat: Native to Eurasia and naturalized in N. America, found in most temperate zones of the world.

Description: A widely varied aggregate species. Stem angular, tough. Leaves opposite, dark green, bipinnatifid, about 6–10 cm long, clasping the stem at the base, the segments very narrow, downy, and feathery in appearance. Flowers in terminal, flattened, corymbose cymes, ray florets usually white or pinkish, disc florets cream. Taste, insipid; odour, faintly aromatic.

Part Used: Herb.

Constituents: (i) Volatile oil, containing α- and β-pinenes, borneol, bornyl acetate, camphor, caryophyllene, eugenol, farnesene, myrcene, sabinene, salicylic acid, terpineol, thujone and many others, and including the sesquiterpene lactones. Many samples contain high concentrations of azulenes, up to about 50%, including chamazulene (= "achillea azulene") and guajazulene, and although these are now thought to be absent from true *A. millefolium*, they are present in closely related species which are supplied for this. [1367, 1368, 1369 (review)] (ii) Sesquiterpene lactones; achillin, achillicin, hydroxyachillin, balchanolide, leucodin, millifin, millifolide and many others [1369, 1370, 1371] (iii) Flavonoids; apigenin, luteolin, quercetin and their glycosides, artemetin, casticin, rutin and others [1369, 1372] (iv) Alkaloids and bases; betonicine (= achilleine), stachydrine, achiceine, moschatine, trigonelline and others [1369] (v) Miscellaneous; acetylenes, aldehydes, cyclitols, plant acids etc [1369]. For full review see [1369].

Medicinal Use: Antipyretic, antiinflammatory, haemostatic, spasmolytic, diuretic, diaphoretic, hypotensive. Yarrow is used for very many complaints, throughout the world, with justification; and particularly for rheumatism, colds, catarrh, fevers, amenorrhoea, and hypertension. Apigenin is antiinflammatory, antiplatelet and spasmolytic [436, 437]; the azulenes where present are antiinflammatory, as is salicylic acid. Eugenol has local anaesthetic activity. The alkaloid betonicine (achilleine) has been shown to be haemostatic [1366]. It has also been used as an eyewash, for diarrhoea, dyspepsia, ulcers and rashes. Yarrow is generally regarded as non-toxic. For full review see [1369].

Preparations: Liquid Extract, dose: 2–4 ml.

Potter's Products: Tabritis Remedy for Arthritis, Catarrh Herbs, Herbprin.

Regulatory Status: GSL.

YELLOW DOCK
Rumex crispus L.
Fam. Polygonaceae

Synonyms: Curled Dock.

Habitat: A common European weed.

Description: Leaves large, typically dock-like, lanceolate, with strongly wavy margins. The root is found in commerce cut and split; with a thick grey-brown cork, yellowish cortex and pale wood, showing concentric rings and a radiate structure. Taste, mucilaginous, bitter; odourless.

Part Used: Root.

Constituents: (i) Anthraquinone glycosides, about 3–4%, including nepodin, and others based on chrysophanol, physcion and emodin [1373, 1374] (ii) Miscellaneous; tannins, rumicin and oxalates [183].

Medicinal Use: Laxative, cholagogue, alterative, tonic. It is used for chronic skin disease, jaundice and constipation. Large doses should be avoided due to the oxalate content.

Preparations: Liquid Extract, dose: 2–4 ml.

Regulatory Status: GSL.

YELLOW FLAG
Iris pseudoacorus L.
Fam. Iridaceae

Synonyms: Yellow Iris, *I. lutea*, Fleur-de-Lys.

Habitat: Native to Europe and Africa and a world-wide garden plant.

Description: The flowers and leaves are well known. Rhizome brownish externally, cylindrical, compressed, with transverse leaf scars above and root scars beneath. Taste, very acrid; odourless.

Part Used: Rhizome.

Constituents: Not well investigated. A glycoside, irisin, iridin or irisine, is reportedly present, with myristic acid [2, 79].

Medicinal Use: Astringent. Has been used in dysmenorrhoea and leucorrhoea as a lotion.

YERBA SANTA
Eriodictyon californicum (Hook. et Arn.) Torr.
Fam. Hydrophyllaceae

Synonyms: Eriodictyon, Mountain Balm, Bearsweed, *E. glutinosum* Benth.

Habitat: California, Oregon and parts of Mexico.

Description: A low, evergreen shrub, with woody rhizomes from which arise lanceolate leaves, up to 15 cm long and about 2 cm broad, irregularly dentate at the margins. The upper surface is green and appears to be varnished with resin, the lower surface is reticulated and white with hairs. Taste, balsamic; odour, pleasant and aromatic.

Part Used: Leaves.

Constituents: (i) Flavonoids; homoeriodictyol (= eriodictyone), eriodictyol, chrysoeriodictyol, xanthoeriodictyol [5, 386] (ii) Resin, containing triacontane, pentatriacontane, cerotic acid, eriodonol [5].

Medicinal Use: Aromatic, tonic, expectorant. It is used for bronchitis and asthma; and to mask the taste of quinine in syrups.

Preparations: Liquid Extract, dose: 2–4 ml.

YEW
Taxus baccata L.
Fam. Taxaceae

Habitat: Grown as an ornamental in Britain, America and other parts of the world.

Description: A large evergreen tree, with male and female flowers on separate plants. The leaves are 1–2 cm long, lanceolate, dark green; the flowers small and green, followed by pink, waxy, cup-like berries. All parts of the plant, excepting the pulp of the fruit, are poisonous.

Part Used: Leaves.

Constituents: (i) Alkaloids; the mixture is known as taxine and contains taxine A, taxagifine and others [749] (ii) Diterpenes; taxol [749] (iii) Lignans; isotaxiresinol and others [1375].

Medicinal Use: None. Yew is very poisonous, it is a CNS depressant and reduces motor activity, with being either analgesic or anticonvulsant [1376]. Taxol is an antimitotic with a unique mode of action and has completed phase III of anti-cancer clinical trials; like most drugs of this class it has unpleasant side effects including leucopenia, nausea etc. [749].

YOHIMBE BARK
Pausinystalia yohimbe (K. Schum) Pierre
Fam. Rubiaceae

Habitat: Cameroon.

Description: The bark occurs in flat or slightly quilled pieces up to 75 cm long and 2 cm thick; the outer surface is grey-brown, cracked and fissured, often covered with lichen; the inner surface is reddish-brown and striated. Taste, bitter; odourless.

Part Used: Bark.

Constituents: Indole alkaloids; the major one is yohimbine, minor ones include α- and β-yohimbane, pseudoyohimbine and coryantheine [386].

Medicinal Use: Aphrodisiac. Yohimbine is an α-adrenergic blocker and has a long-standing reputation as a sexual stimulant. A recent study in rats has shown this to be justifiable [1377] despite earlier clinical studies which gave equivocal results [1378]; the dose of yohimbine is very important as too high a dose leads to general depression.

Preparations: Liquid Extract, dose: 2–4 ml.

Regulatory Status: POM.

Z

ZEDOARY

Curcuma zedoaria Rosc.
Fam. Zingiberaceae

Habitat: India, cultivated elsewhere in the Far East.

Description: The rhizome usually occurs in transverse slices, about 2–4 cm in diameter and 0.5–1 cm thick; outer surface greyish, with a few circular striae and small, spiny points of root bases. The transverse section is greyish-white, hard and horny. Taste, bitter; odour, camphoraceous, and recalling that of cardamoms and ginger.

Part Used: Rhizome.

Constituents: Sesquiterpenes; curcumenone, curcumanolide A and B, (+)-germacrone-4,5-epoxide, isofuranogermacrene and others [1379, 1380].

Medicinal Use: Aromatic, stimulant. Used in a similar manner to ginger (q.v.). The rhizome is used to treat certain types of tumour in China and has shown cytotoxicity in some systems [1381].

Glossary of Medical Terms

This glossary has been only slightly changed from the original. It is included to explain some of the terms used in herbal medicine as these are often of a more vague or general nature than those used in conventional medicine and are in accordance with the more holistic methods of treatment used. They are not intended as a recommendation to particular remedies where used in the text but are an indication of the current and historical usage of the plant, whether or not the claims can be validated.

Abortifacient Causing abortion
Adaptogen Aiding adaptation of the body, particularly to stress
Alterative A vague term to indicate a substance which hastens the renewal of the tissues so that they can better carry out their function
Analgesic Pain-relieving
Anodyne Pain-easing
Anthelmintic Causing death or removal of worms in the body
Antibilious Against biliousness or excess bile
Antilithic Against stones, e.g. kidney or bladder
Antiperiodic Preventing the return of recurrent fevers, e.g. malaria
Antiscorbutic Preventing scurvy, i.e. a source of vitamin C
Antiphlogistic Relieving pain and inflammation
Antiscrophulous Preventing or curing scrophula, an old fashioned term for diseases causing swelling of the lymph glands, especially in the neck, also known as king's evil
Antiseptic Preventing putrefaction or infection
Antispasmodic Preventing spasm
Aperient Promoting a mild or natural movement of the bowels
Aphrodisiac Exciting the sexual organs
Aromatic Having an aroma
Astringent Causing contraction of the tissues, binding
Bitter Applied to bitter tasting substances used to stimulate the appetite
Cardiac Having an effect on the heart
Carminative Easing griping pains and expelling flatulence
Cathartic Producing evacuation of the bowels
Cholagogue Producing a flow of bile
Choleretic Preventing excessive bile
Corrective Restoring to a healthy state
Demulcent Applied to drugs which soothe and protect the alimentary canal
Deobstruent Clearing away obstructions by opening the natural passages of the body
Depurative A purifying agent
Dermatic Applied to drugs with an action upon the skin
Detergent Cleansing
Diaphoretic Promoting perspiration

Diuretic Increasing the flow of urine
Digestive Aiding digestion
Emetic Causing vomiting
Emmenagogue Promoting menstrual flow
Emollient Softening and soothing, usually the skin
Expectorant Aiding expectoration, loosening phlegm
Febrifuge Reducing fever
Flatulence Having gases in the intestine, distension; windiness
Galactagogue Milk-inducing
Haemostatic Controlling or stopping bleeding
Hallucinogen Producing visions or hallucinations
Hepatic Affecting the liver
Hypnotic Producing sleep
Insecticide A substance which kills insects
Irritant Causing irritation **Counter Irritant**, against irritation, often by
　　having a warming or rubifacient effect (q.v.)
Laxative Bowel stimulant
Mydriatic Causing dilation of the pupil of the eye
Myotic Causing contraction of the pupil of the eye
Narcotic Applied to drugs producing stupor or insensibility
Nervine Restoring the nerves, mildly tranquillizing
Nutritive Nourishing
Orexigenic Stimulating the appetite
Oxytocic Stimulating contractions of the womb
Parasiticide A substance which kills parasites
Parturient Applied to substances used to facilitate childbirth
Pectoral having an effect upon the lungs
Protozoicidal A substance which kills protozoa, e.g. amoebae
Purgative A substance which evacuates the bowels, more drastic than an
　　aperient or laxative
Refrigerant Relieving thirst and giving a feeling of coolness
Rubefacient Causing reddening of the skin, applied to substances producing
　　inflammation and sometimes used as a rub for muscular pain
Sedative Causing sedation, reducing nervous excitement
Sternutatory Producing sneezing by irritation of the mucous membranes
Stimulant Energy producing
Stomachic Applied to drugs which ease stomach pain
Styptic A substance which stops bleeding by clotting the blood, applied
　　externally to cuts or wounds
Sudorific Producing copious perspiration
Taenicide A substance which expels tape-worms
Tonic A substance which gives a feeling of well-being to the body
Vermifuge A substance which expels worms from the body
Vulnerary Used in healing wounds

Forms of Medicinal Preparations

Infusions

Infusions are aqueous preparations made by pouring boiling water over finely chopped botanical drugs, herbs, roots, barks, flowers, or seeds. The usual quantities used for infusion are 500 ml (1 pint) of water to 30 g (1 oz) of drug. The infusion is then allowed to stand for up to 30 minutes with occasional stirring. The clear liquid is then decanted or strained. Being extemporaneous preparations, infusions should be taken in divided doses during the day of preparation. The amount of infusion to be taken would be proportionate to the amount of the drug dosage required. A few medicinal drugs such as Calumba and Quassia having only water soluble constituents, may be infused with cold water. Infusions are mainly used when the drug to be extracted is of light structure as with leafy herbs.

Decoctions

These are made by pouring cold water on to the finely divided botanical drug and then allowing the mixture to simmer. This method is used for hard materials such as roots and barks. Decoctions are generally made in a strength of 30 g (1 oz) to 500 ml (1 pint) but, as the water boils away, it is best to use 800 ml (1½ pints) and allow to simmer down to 500 ml (1 pint). When cool the decoction is strained and taken in divided doses proportionate to the required dosage of the drug. As with infusions, decoctions are not permanent preparations and should be prepared fresh daily.

Liquid Extracts

Liquid extracts provide a more permanent and convenient form of preserving the constituents of vegetable drugs in a concentrated form. They are prepared by percolating or macerating the comminuted drug with sufficient of the solvent best suited for the extraction of the drug constituents. This may be water or a mixture of water and alcohol. When extraction is complete this is then evaporated under vacuum down to a point where the liquid extract will, in 30 ml (1 fl.oz.), represent the medicinal value of 30 g (1 oz) of the drug (1 in 1).

Solid Extracts (Soft Extracts)

Are prepared by evaporating down (to the consistency of a paste) the fresh expressed juices, or the liquors used as extractives of a vegetable drug. If alcohol/water mixtures are used as solvents the alcohol is distilled off and recovered before evaporating the residual extract to the required consistency.

Dry Extracts

Are prepared by removing the remaining water in the solid (soft) extract by drying under vacuum.

Solid extracts and dry extracts represent a much larger quantity of the drug from which they are prepared than do liquid extracts, tinctures, or infusions.

Tinctures

Are spirituous preparations, which use differing strengths of alcohol as their solvent for extracting the botanical drugs to be converted into tinctures. Tinctures, like liquid extracts, are permanent preparations. They are particularly suitable for extracting drugs containing resinous and volatile principles. Tinctures are prepared at room temperature when the solvent acts selectively. Alcohol precipitates unwanted gums and albuminous matter so that tinctures may be filtered to yield clear, elegant, preparations which are well preserved from deterioration.

Tinctures are usually made in strengths of 1 in 5 to 1 in 10, 100 g (3½ oz) in 500 ml (1 pint) or 50 g (1¾ oz) or 500 ml (1 pint).

Pills

Pills have been widely used as a convenient and tasteless method of taking unpleasant substances. They are small spherical bodies usually containing concentrated herbal extracts, often combined powdered crude herbs, and an excipient to form a firm plastic mass, soluble in the stomach. Pills may be sugar-coated or, more usually, pearl-coated.

Tablets

Are made by compressing vegetable drug extracts and powders using the necessary excipients for combination and disintegration. Tablets have now largely superseded pills because they are more readily absorbed and quicker in their action.

Capsules

Are hard or soft gelatin enclosures provided in convenient sizes for swallowing. They are used for taking nauseous substances, such as Cod Liver Oil, Garlic Oil or other drugs difficult to administer in their naturally occurring form.

Suppositories

Are small cone shaped, or torpedo shaped moulds, usually of a cocoa butter, or glyco-gelatin base carrying the medicament to be introduced into the rectum. The base is easily soluble at body temperature. They provide a valuable treatment for haemorrhoids and other disorders of the rectum.

Pessaries

Use a similar base to that used for suppositories and are used to introduce medicaments into the vagina when it is necessary to apply remedies to the walls of these internal passages.

Conversion Table for Metric and Imperial Weights and Measures with Approximate Domestic Equivalents and Abbreviations

IMPERIAL:	*METRIC:*	*APPROXIMATE DOMESTIC EQUIVALENT*
1 drachm (60 grains)	3.888 grammes	4 g
1 ounce (oz)	28.3495 grammes (g)	30 g
1 pound (lb)	453.59 g	500 g (0.5 kg)
1 fluid drachm (60 minims)	3.552 ml	4 ml
1 fluid ounce (fl.oz;	28.4123 millilitres (ml)	30 ml
1 pint (pt) (20 oz)	0.5682 litres (l)	500 ml (0.5 l)
1 gallon (gal) (8 pt)	4.5459 l	4 l
1 inch (in)	2.54 centimetres (cm)	2.5 cm, 25 millimetres (mm)
1 foot (ft)	30.48 cm	30 cm
1 yard (yd)	0.9144 metres (m)	1 m
	5 ml	1 teaspoonful (tsp)
	10 ml	1 dessertspoonful (dsp)
½ fl.oz.	15 ml	1 tablespoon (tblsp)
1½–2 fl.oz (3–4 tblsp)		1 wineglassful
4–5 fl.oz. (5–10 tblsp)		1 teacupful

N.B.
10 millimetres	= 1 centimetre
100 centimetres	= 1 metre
1000 millilitres	= 1 litre

Glossary of Botanical Terms

Achene A one-seeded fruit, or part of a compound fruit, dry, not opening when ripe, distinguished from a seed by the remains of a stigma or style

Acrid Leaving a burning sensation in the mouth

Acuminate Tapering to a fine point

Acute Pointed

Alliaceous Garlic or onion-like

Alternate Arranged in two rows, not opposite, often including a spiral arrangement

Amplexicaul Clasping the stem

Anastomosing Joining up to form loops

Annular, Annulated Ring-like, ringed

Anther Part of the stamen containing the pollen grains

Apetalous Without petals. When only one layer of floral leaves is present, even if coloured, this is considered to be the calyx.

Apiculate With a small, broad point at the apex

Apocarpous Having the carpels free from one another

Appressed Pressed close to but not united with another organ, e.g. hairs against the stem

Arillus A fleshy growth from the point of attachment of a seed, e.g. mace around a nutmeg

Ascending Sloping or curving upwards

Awn A stiff, bristle-like projection e.g. terminating the flower scales in grasses

Axillary Arising from the axil or angle of a leaf or bract

Balsamic Balsam-like, e.g. odour, sweet, like benzoin

Barbed Furnished with sharp points, curved backwards

Berry A fleshy fruit, usually containing many seeds, without a stony layer surrounding them

Biennial Completing the life cycle within two years, without flowering in the first year

Bifid Deeply split into two division

Bipinnatifid Twice divided, in a pinnate or feather-like way, in a leaf about halfway to the stalk or midrib

Bract A leaf-like structure under a flower

Bracteole The bracts under the flower, when there are other bracts present under the inflorescence

Bristles Stiff or rigid hairs

Bulb An underground organ composed of fleshy modified leaves, often with thin or membranous outer scales, containing the next year's plant

Bulbil A small bulb rising in an axil in the aerial parts

Calyx The sepals or outer layer of floral leaves

Campanulate Bell-shaped

Capsule A dry fruit, opening when ripe, composed of more than one carpel

Carpel A unit of the ovary which may be separate and distinct, or joined or fused

Catkin A spike of male or female flowers, usually from a tree and without petals or calyx

Cauline Of leaves, borne on the aerial part of the stem, not subtending a flower or inflorescence

Chlorophyll The green pigment of plants

Clavate Club-shaped

Compound Of an inflorescence, with the axis branched: of flowerheads, made up of many small florets; of leaves, composed of several distinct leaflets

Conchoidal Shell-like, e.g. of a fracture, concave with curved lines

Cordate Heart-shaped

Coriaceous Having a leathery texture

Corm A short, swollen, underground stem, often with membranous scales, from which the next year's plant arises, e.g. crocus

Corolla The petals, or inner row of floral leaves, either distinct or united, e.g. into a tube

Cortex The outer, separable portion of the stem or fruit

Corymb A raceme of flowers where the pedicels are of different lengths, so that all the flowers are at the same level at the top, the outer flowers opening first *adj.* corymbose

Cotyledons The first leaves of a plant, present in the seed, containing nourishment for the seedling and usually different from subsequent leaves

Crenate Having rounded teeth

Crenulate Diminutive form of crenate

Cruciform Cross-shaped, e.g. wall-flower

Cuneate Wedge-shaped

Cuneiform Wedge-shaped with the thin end at the base

Cuticle The waxy layer outside the epidermis, e.g. in leaves

Cyme An inflorescence where the growing points terminate in a flower, hence the central flower opens first and the oldest branches or flowers are normally at the apex *adj.* cymose

Deciduous Dropping off, losing the leaves in autumn

Decumbent Lying on the ground, usually rising at the end

Decurrent Having the base prolonged down the axis, e.g. in leaves where the base continues down the petiole to form a winged stem

Decussate Of leaves, opposite but with pairs oriented at right angles to each other

Dehiscence Opening to shed seeds or spores

Dentate Sharply toothed

Denticulate Diminutive of dentate

Digitate Finger-like, having five or more narrow segments, e.g. like the leaves of the lupin

Dioecious Having the sexes on different plants

Disc, disk The fleshy part of the receptacle, e.g. in the Compositae

Divaricate Diverging at a wide angle

Drupe A more or less fleshy fruit, with one or more seeds, each surrounded with a stony layer, e.g. sloe

Elliptic Shaped like an ellipse

Emarginate Notched or indentated at the apex

Embryo The young plant in the seed

Endocarp The inner layer of the fruit, corresponding to the inner layer of the carpel, e.g. in the plum, the endocarp is the stone, the mesocarp forms the flesh and the epicarp the skin

Endosperm The nutritive tissue in the seed

Entire Not toothed or cut at the margin

Epicalyx A calyx-like structure outside the true calyx

Epicarp See endocarp

Epidermis The outer skin, e.g. of the leaf

Epigeal Above ground, e.g. germination where the cotyledons are raised above ground

Epigynous Where the stamens etc. are inserted on a level with or above the top of the ovary, e.g. into the pistil

Epipetalous Inserted upon the corolla

Exfoliating Splitting off in layers, e.g. some barks

Falcate Scythe-shaped

Filament The stalk of the anther

Filiform Thread-like

Fimbriate Fringed

Florets The small individual flowers in the flowerheads of the Compositae; the central ones being the tubular or disc florets, the outer, long ones being the ray or ligulate florets

Fracture The way in which an organ breaks, e.g. tough, layered, fibrous, short (= brittle or not fibrous) and its appearance

Fusiform Spindle-shaped

Gamopetalous Having the petals joined, into a tube or at the base

Gamosepalous Having the sepals joined

Gibbous Having a rounded, solid projection

Glabrous Without hairs

Gland A small, globular or oblong vesicle containing oil, resin etc.

Glandular Furnished with glands

Glaucous Bluish

Gynoecium The female part of the plant, made up of the ovary or ovaries, stigma and style

Hastate Shaped like a halberd or arrow-tip

Heartwood The central portion of a tree trunk, sometimes filled with resin or colouring matter

Hermaphrodite Having both stamens and ovary

Hilum The scar on a seed where it has been attached by a stalk to the ovary; also applied to the more or less central spot or marking on a starch grain

Hirsute Clothed with long, not stiff, hairs

Hispid Clothed with coarse, stiff hairs

Hybrid A plant originating by fertilization of one species or subspecies by another

Hypogeal Below ground, e.g. in germination where the cotyledons remain below ground

Hypogynous Calyx or corolla situated below the ovary

Imbricate Having the edges overlapping, like roof tiles

Imparipinnate A pinnate leaf having an odd leaf at the apex

Indehiscent Not opening to release seeds or spores

Inferior When the ovary is inserted into or fused with the receptacle

Inflorescence Flowering branch, above the last stem leaves, including bracts and flowers

Internodes The interval between branches or leaves on a root or stem

Involucre A ring of bracts forming a calyx-like structure around or below an inflorescence or flowerhead, e.g. in the Compositae

Involute With the margins rolled upwards

Keeled Having a projecting line resembling the keel of a boat

Lamina Layer, the flat part or blade of a leaf etc.

Lanceolate Oval and pointed at both ends

Latex Milky juice, e.g. of poppies

Leaflet Each individual part of a compound leaf

Legume A fruit consisting of one carpel, opening on one side, e.g. pea

Lenticel Breathing pores in the bark

Lenticular Lens-shaped, e.g. lentil

Lichen Cryptogamic plants, usually greyish or yellowish, growing on rocks and tree trunks.

Ligulate Strap-shaped

Linear Of leaves, narrow and short with parallel margins

Lobed Of leaves, divided, but not into separate leaflets

Membranous Thin, dry and flexible, not green

Medullary Ray Slender lines of parenchyma tissue connecting the pith with the bark, seen as radiating lines in the wood

Mericarp A one-seeded portion split off from a syncarpous ovary at maturity, e.g. caraway, fennel

Micropyle The pore of a seed through which the embryo emerges

Monoecious Having unisexual flowers, but both sexes on the same plant

Mucronate Having a short, narrow point

Mycelium The thread-like mass of fungi from which the fruiting body emerges; in mushrooms it is cottony and known as mushroom spawn, in ergot it is compacted into a hard mass and known as a sclerotium

Node The point on a stem from which leaves arise

Nodule A small, more or less globular, swelling

Nut A fruit composed of three fused carpels, containing one seed

Ob- *prefix:* Inverted, e.g. an ovate leaf is broader above the middle, an obovate leaf below the middle

Obtuse Blunt

Ochrea A sheath, formed from fused stipules, e.g. Polygonaceae

Opposite Applied to leaves where two arise from opposite sides of the same stem node

Ovary The part of the gynoecium containing the ovules and young seeds, composed of one or more carpels

Ovate Egg-shaped

Ovoid Nearly egg-shaped

Paleae Delicate, membranous bracts; in the Compositae forming the bracts of the disc florets and in grass flowers enclosing the pistils and stamens

Palmate Consisting of more than three leaflets arising from the same point

Panicle A branched, racemose inflorescence

Papillae Small raised points or elongated projections

Pappus The calyx in a composite flower developed in the form of simple or feathery hairs, membranous scales, teeth or bristles. May or may not be present.

Pedicel The stalk of a single flower

Peduncle The stalk of an inflorescence

Peltate Of a leaf, when the stalk is inserted on the under surface, not at the edge

Perennial Living for more than two years, normally flowering every year

Perianth The floral leaves as a whole, including petals and sepals

Perianth segment The separate leaves of the perianth, especially when petals and sepal cannot be distinguished

Perigynous Arising from a ring between the ovary and the floral parts

Petals The corolla or inner, usually coloured, layer of floral leaves

Petiole The stalk of a leaf

Pilose Hairy, with long, soft hairs

Pinnate A leaf composed of more than three leaflets arranged in two rows along a common stalk or rhachis. The primary divisions may also be divided in a pinnate manner, e.g. bipinnate or 2-pinnate, 3-pinnate etc.

Pinnatifid Pinnately cut but not completely, the lobes still being joined at the lamina

Pinnatisect As pinnatifid but cut more deeply, some leaflets may be free

Placenta The part of the ovary to which the ovules are attached

Pollen The male gamete, produced by the anthers

Polypetalous Having many petals

Polysepalous Having many sepals

Procumbent Lying loosely along the ground, rising at the ends

Prostrate Lying flat on the groud

Pubescent Shortly and softly hairy

Punctate Dotted or shallowly pitted, usually with glands

Pungent Biting or piercing

Pyriform Pear-shaped

Quill Applied to a bark which is inrolled into a tube, e.g. cinnamon

Raceme An inflorescence, usually conical in outline, in which the pedicels are of approximately equal length, and the lowest flowers open first *adj.* racemose

Rachis or rhachis The central rib or axis of a pinnate leaf

Radical Of leaves, arising from the base of the stem or rhizome

Receptacle The upper part of the stem from which the floral parts arise

Recurved Bent backwards in a curve

Reniform Kidney-shaped

Reticulate Marked with a network, usually of lines or veins

Revolute Rolled back at the edges

Rhizome An underground stem lasting more than one growing season

Rhomboid More or less diamond-shaped

Rosette Of leaves, closely and spirally arranged

Rotate Of a corolla, wheel-like

Rugose Wrinkled

Ruminate Usually of seeds, looking as though chewed, infolded

Scarious Thin, rather stiff and dry, not green

Schizocarp A dry fruit which splits into separate one-seeded parts when mature, e.g. caraway, dill

Scyphi The wineglass-shaped reproductive organ bearing fruit in some lichens

Sepals The leaves of the calyx

Serrate Having oblique teeth like a saw

Sessile Without a stalk

Sinuate Having a wavy outline

Spathulate or spatulate Paddle-shaped

Spike An inflorescence in which sessile flowers are arranged in a raceme

Spine The hardened, projecting vein of a leaf, e.g. holly or thistle

Spore A small, asexual reproductive body

Spur A tubular projection at the base of the corolla, e.g. toadflax

Stamen The male reproductive organ, consisting of the two anthers containing pollen, and the filament

Staminode An infertile, often reduced stamen, e.g. Scrophulariaceae

Stellate Star-shaped

Stigma The sticky apex of the style to which the pollen grains adhere

Stipule A small, leaf-like structure usually at the base of the petiole

Stipulet or Stipel A stipule-like structure at the base of a leaflet in a compound leaf

Stolon A creeping stem of short duration produced from a central rosette or erect stem, usually above ground

Stoma, Stomata Pore(s) in the leaf through which exchange of gases takes place.

Striations More or less parallel line markings

Style The thread connecting the stigma and ovary

Sucker Underground shoots which arise some distance away from the plant

Superior Of ovary, with the perianth inserted below the base

Syncarpous Of ovary, having the carpels united to one another

Tendril A climbing organ derived from the stem, leaf or petiole, e.g. pea

Terebinthinate Turpentine-like

Terminal At the end of a shoot or branch

Ternate Divided into three distinct segments

Thallus A flat, branching, undifferentiated plant body, e.g. seaweed

Tomentose Covered with dense, short, cottony hairs

Tortuous Twisted and undulating

Trifid Split into three

Trifoliate Having three distinct leaflets, e.g. clover

Truncate Appearing as if cut off at the end

Tuber A swollen part of an underground stem, of one year's duration, bearing leaf buds and capable of new growth, e.g. potato

Tubercle A more or less spherical or ovoid swelling

Umbel An inflorescence where the petioles all arise from the top of the stem, umbrella-like

Unisexual Flowers having either stamens or pistils, but not both

Vascular Consisting of the conductive tissue, vessels or tubes

Villous Shaggy

Viscid Sticky

Vitta The oil gland of an umbelliferous fruit, seen as a dark line between the ridges

Whorl A circle of leaves around a node

References

1 "Pharmacognosy", 12th Ed. Trease, G. E. and Evans, W. C. Pub. Bailliere Tindall (1983) UK
2 "Drogenkunde", 8th Ed. Heinz, A., Hoppe. Pub. W. de Gruyter (1975) Berlin
3 "Botanicum Officinale, or a Compendious Herbal", J. Miller (1722)
4 "Martindale. The Extra Pharmacopoeia", 27th Ed. Pub. The Pharmaceutical Press (1977) UK
5 "Encyclopedia of Common Natural Ingredients used in Food Drugs and Cosmetics", Albert Y. Leung. Pub. John Wiley & Sons Inc. (1980) NY
6 Rao, M. R. (1966) *Acta Pharm. Sinica* **3**, 195
7 "Pharmacology and Applications of Chinese Materia Medica Vol 1", Ed. H. Chan and P. But, Pub. World Scientific (1986) Singapore
8 "An Atlas of Common Chinese Drugs", Farnsworth, N. R. Pub. University of Illinois Medical Center, Chicago Ill. (1975) USA
9 Cavallito, *et al.* (1946) *J. Am. Chem. Soc.* **66**, 2332
10 Pinder, A. R. (1976) *Tetrahedron* **23**, 2172
11 Valisolado, J. *et al.* (1980) *Bull. Soc. Chem. Fr.* 473
12 Yamazaki, M. and Shirota, H. (1981) *Shoyakugaku Zasshi* **35**, 96
13 Drozd, G. A. *et al.* (1983) *Khim. Prir. Soed.* **1**, 106
14 Patrascu, V. *et al.* (1984) *Ser. Dermato-Venerol.* **29** (2), 153–157
15 Peter-Horvath, M. *et al.* (1964) *Rev. Med.* **10** (2), 190–3
16 Chon, S. C. *et al.* (1987) *Med. Pharmacol. Exp.* **16** (5), 407–413
17 Freudenberg, K. and Weinges, K. (1967) *Tet. Lett.* **17**, 19
18 Papageorgiou, V. P. (1980) *Planta Med.* **38** (3), 193
19 Wiedenfield, H., Kirfield, A. *et al.* (1985) *Arch. Pharm.* **318** (4), 294
20 Majlathova, L. (1971) *Nahrung* **15**, 505
21 Hogg, J. W. *et al.* (1971) *Am. Perf. Cosmet.* **86**, 33
22 Oishi, K. *et al.* (1974) *Nippon Suisan Gakaishi* **40**, 1241 (via [5])
23 Saito, Y. *et al.* (1976) *Eiyo To Shokuryo* **29**, 505 (via [5])
24 Kato, Y. (1975) *Koryo* **113**, 17 and 24 (via [5])
25 "The Merck Index", 9th Ed. (1976) Pub. Merck Inc. Rahway, NJ, USA
26 Opdyke, D. L. J. (1976) *Food Cosmet. Toxicol.* **14**
27 Kupchan, S. M. and Karim, A. (1976) *Lloydia* **39** 223
28 Shida, T. *et al.* (1985) *Planta Med.* **51** (3), 273
29 "Alkaloids". Vol. 1. Ed. S. W. Pelletier. Pub. John Wiley (1983)
30 Atta-ur-Rahman, A. M. *et al.* (1985) *Phytochem.* **24**, 24(II), 2771
31 Kucera, M. V. *et al.* (1973) *Afric. J. Pharm. Pharm. Sci.* 3228
32 "Chopra's Indigeneous Drugs of India" Vol 1. R. N. Chopra *et al.* Pub. Dhur and Sons (1938) Calcutta
33 "Medicinal Plants of Tropical West Africa" B. Oliver-Bever. Pub. Cambridge University Press (1986) UK

34 Goyal, H. *et al.* (1981) *J. Res. Ayur. Siddha.* **2** (3), 286
35 Sharp, T. M. (1934) *J. Chem. Soc.* 287
36 Khan, I. and Qureshi, Z. (1967) *J. Pharm. Pharmacol.* **19**, 815
37 "British Herbal Pharmacopoeia". Pub British Herbal Medicine Association (1983) UK
38 Ashraf, M. *et al.* (1977) *Pak. J. Ind. Res.* **20** (4–5), 298
39 Escher, S., Keller U. *et al.* (1979) *Helv. Chim. Acta* **62** (7), 2061
40 'Taskinen, J. (1975) *Acta. Chem. Scand.* **29** (5), 637
41 Ashraf, M. *et al.* (1980) *Pak. J. Sci. Ind. Res.* **23** (1–2), 73
42 Lemmich, J. *et al.* (1983) *Phytochem.* **23** (2), 553
43 Tastrup, O. *et al.* (1983) *Phytochem.* **22** (9), 2035
44 Zotikov, Y. M. *et al.* (1978) *Rastit. Resur.* **14** (4), 579
45 Opdyke, D. L. J. (1975) *Food Cosmet. Toxicol.* **13**, Suppl. 713
46 Sethi, O. P. and Shah, A. K. (1979) *Ind. J. Pharm. Sci.* **42** (6), C11
47 Musago, L. and Rodeghiero, G. in "Photophysiology" Vol. II. p 115. Ed. A. C. Giese. Pub. Academic Press (1972)
48 "Advances in Chinese Medicinal Materials Research", Eds H. M. Chang *et al.* Pub. World Scientific Pub. Co. (1985) Singapore
49 Brieskorn, C. H. and Beck, V. (1971) *Phytochem.* **10**, 3205
50 "Fenaroli's Handbook of Flavor Ingredients", Vol. 1. 2nd Ed. Pub. CRC Press (1975)
51 Albert Puleo, M. (1980) *J. Ethnopharmacol.* **2** (4), 337
52 Nofal, M. A. (1981) *Ain. Shams Univ. Fac. Agric. Res. Bull.* **0** (1602), 1–10
53 Kartnig, T. *et al.* (1975) *Planta Med.* **27**, 1
54 Kunzemann, J. and Herrmann, K. (1977) *Z. Leb.-Unters. Forsch.* **164**, 194
55 Kubeczka, K. H. *et al.* (1976) *Z. Naturforsch.* **31b**, 283
56 Mueller-Limmroth, W. and Froenlich, H. H. (1980) *Fortschr. Med.* **98** (3), 95
57 Gershbein, L. L. (1977) *Food Cosmet. Toxicol.* **15** (3), 173
58 Adrian, J. and Jacquot, R. in "Valeur Alimentaire de l'Arachide et ses Derives", Pub. Maisonneuve et Larose, Paris. (1968). via [33]
59 Boudreaux, H. B. and Frampton, V. L. (1960) *Nature* **185**, 469
60 Bezanger-Beauquesne, L. *et al.* in "Les Plantes Dans La Therapeutique Moderne" Pub. Malone (1975) Paris
61 Schaunberg, P. and Paris, F. in "Guide to Medical Plants", Pub. Lutterworth (1977) UK
62 Kooiman, P. (1972) *Acta. Bot. Neerl.* **21** (4) 417
63 Juptner, H. (1968) *Z. Tropenmed. Parasit.* **19**, 254 via [4]
64 Halub, M. *et al.* (1975) *Phytochem.* **14**, 1659
65 Willuhn, G. *et al.* (1984) *Planta Med.* **50** (1), 35
66 Merfort, I. (1985) *Planta Med.* **51** (2), 136
67 Merfort, I. (1984) *Planta Med.* **50** (1), 107
68 Wagner, H. in "Advances in Chinese Medicinal Materials Research", Eds H. M. Chang *et al.* Pub. World Scientific (1986) Singapore
69 Brandt, L. (1967) *Scand. J. Haematol. Suppl.* **2**

70 Hall, I. H. *et al.* (1979) *J. Pharm. Sci.* **68**, 537
71 Kaziro, G. S. N. *et al.* (1984) *Br. J. Oral Maxillofacial Surg.* **22**, 42
72 Rajanikanth, B. *et al.* (1984) *Phytochem.* **23** (4), 899
73 Buddrus, J. *et al.* (1985) *Phytochem.* **24** (4), 869
74 Naimie, H. *et al.* (1972) *Collect. Czec. Chem. Commun.* **37**, 1166
75 Mansurov, M. M. (1967) *Med. Zh. Uzb.* **6**, 46 via [5]
76 Gracza, L. (1987) *Pharmazie* **42** (2), 141
77 Mose, J. R. and Lukas, G. (1961) *Arzneim.-Forsch.* **11**, 33
78 Rosch, A. (1984) *Z. Phytother.* **5** (6), 964
79 "Poisonous Plants in Britain and their effects on Animals and Man", Ministry of Agriculture Fisheries and Food. Pub; HMSO (1984) UK
80 Delaveau, P. *et al.* (1980) *Planta Med.* **40**, 49
81 Goryanu, G. M. *et al.* (1976) *Khim. Prir. Soed.* **3**, 400, and **6**, 762
82 Kawano, K. *et al.* (1975) *Agric. Biol. Chem.* **39**, 1999
83 Tagasuki, M. *et al.* (1975) *Chem. Lett.* **1**, 43 via [5]
84 Woeldecke, M. and Hermann, K. (1974) *Z. Lebensm.-Forsch.* **25**, 459
85 Shiomi, N. *et al.* (1976) *Agric. Biol. Chem.* **40**, 567
86 Pšenák, M. *et al.* (1970) *Planta Med.* **19** (2) 154
87 Ekong, D. E. U. (1967) *Chem. Comm.* 808
88 Ekong, D. E. U. and Ibiyemi, S. A. (1971) *Chem. Comm.* 1177
89 El Said *et al.* (1968) "Study of certain Nigerian plants used in Fever". Communication at the Inter-African Symposium. Dakar. (via [33])
90 Okpanyi, S. N. and Ezenkwu, G. .C. (1981) *Planta Med.* **41**, 34
91 Bray, D. H. *et al.* (1985) *Trans. Royal Soc. Trop. Med. Hyg.* **79**, 426
92 Lavie, D. and Levy, E. C. (1969) *Tet. Lett.* 3525
93 Kraus, W. and Bokel, M. (1981) *Chemische Berichte* **114**, 267
94 Andrei, G. M. *et al.* (1986) *Experientia* **42** (7), 843
95 Pat. Appl. 83/234, 294 Japan (1983)
96 Sharma, B. R. and Sharma, P. (1981) *Planta Med.* **43**, 102
97 Enjalbert, F. *et al.* (1983) *Fitoterapia* **2**, 59
98 Thieme, H. and Kitze, C. (1973) *Pharmazie* **28** (1), 69
99 Kucera, L. S. and Hermann, E. C., Jnr. (1967) *Proc. Soc. Exp. Biol. Med.* **124**, 865 and 874
100 Brieskorn, C. H. and Krause, W. (1974) *Arch. Pharm.* **307** (8), 603
101 Wolbling, R. H. and Milbradt, R. (1984) *Therapiewoche* **34** (9), 1193
102 Ozarowski, A. (1982) *Wiad. Ziel.* **4**, 7
103 Chlabicz, J. *et al.* (1984) *Pharmazie* **39** (11), 770
104 Buechner, K. H. *et al.* (1974) *Med. Klin.* **69** (23), 1032
105 De Jong, C. A. G. (1978) *Ned. Tijdschr. Geneeskd.* **112** (3), 82
106 Auf'mkolk, M. *et al.* (1984) *Endocrinology* **115** (2), 527
107 Auf'mkolk, M. *et al.* (1984) *Horm. Metab. Res.* **16** (4), 183
108 Auf'mkolk, M. *Endocrinology* **116** (5), 1687
109 Forster, H. B. *et al.* (1980) *Planta Med.* **40** (4), 309
110 Thieme, H. and Benecke, R. (1969) *Pharmazie* **24**, 567
111 Ikram, M. (1975) *Planta Med.* **28**, 253
112 Willaman, J. J. and Hui-Li, L. (1970) *Lloydia* **33** (3A), 1
113 Andronescu, E. *et al.* (1973) *Clujul. Med.* **46**, 627 (via [5])

114 Naidovich, L. P. *et al.* (1976) *Farmatsiya* **24**, 33 (via [5])
115 Subbaiah, T. V. and Amin, A. H. (1967) *Nature* **215**, 527
116 Ubebaba, K. *et al.* (1984) *Jpn. J. Pharmacol.* **36** (Suppl.), 352
117 Preininger, V., in "The Alkaloids Vol. 15" Ed. R. H. F. Manske. Pub. Academic Press (1975) UK
118 Lahiri, S. C. *et al.* (1958) *Ann. Biochem. and Exp. Med. India* **18**, 95
119 Liu, C. X. *et al.* (1979) *Chinese Traditional and Herbal Drugs Communications* **9**, 36 (via [7])
120 Chen, M. Q. *et al.* (1965) *Acta Pharm. Sinica* **12** (3), 185
121 Cordell, G. A. and Farnsworth, N. R. (1977) *Lloydia* **40**, 1
122 Dhar, M. L. *et al.* (1968) *Indian J. Exp. Biol.* **6**, 232
123 Labbe, M. (1936) *J. Canad. Med. Assoc.* **34**, 141
124 "Herbs. An Indexed Bibliography 1971–80" Eds. J. E. Simon, A. F. Chadwick and L. E. Craker. Pub. Archon Books (1984) USA
125 Jain, M. L. and Jain, S. R. (1972) *Planta Med.* **22**, 66
126 Balambal, R. *et al.* (1985) *J. Assoc. Phys. (India)* **33** (8), 507
127 Opdyke, D. L. J. (1973) *Food Cosmet. Toxicol.* **11**, 867
128 Miller, E. C. *et al.* (1983) *Cancer Res.* **43**, 1124
129 Paul, B. D. *et al.* (1974) *J. Pharm. Sci.* **63**, 958
130 Yoshizawa, S. *et al.* (1987) *Phytother. Res.* **1** (1), 44
131 Phillipson, J. D. *et al.* (1975) *Phytochem.* **14**, 999
132 Das, P. C. and Sarkar, A. K. (1979) *Acta Physiol. Pol.* **30** (3), 389
133 Fukuda, N. *et al.* (1981) *Chem. Pharm. Bull.* **29** (2), 325
134 Nakano, K. *et al.* (1982) *Yakugaku Zasshi* **102** (11), 1031
135 Nakano, K. *et al.* (1983) *Phytochem.* **22** (5), 1249
136 Nakano, K. *et al.* (1982) *J. Chem. Soc. Chem. Commun.* 789
137 Kyerematen, G. and Sandberg, F. (1986) *Acta Pharm. Sueca* **23**, 101
138 Sticher, O. *et al.* (1979) *Planta Med.* **35**, 253
139 Bettini, V. *et al.* (1984) *Fitoterapia* **55** (6), 323
140 Bettini, V. *et al.* (1985) *Fitoterapia* **56** (1), 3
141 Karatodorof, K. and Kalarova, R. (1977) *Izn, Durzh Inst. Kontrol Lek Svedstva* **10**, 103–9 (via BIOSIS)
142 Mix, D. B. *et al.* (1982) *J. Nat. Prod.* **45** (6), 657
143 Che, C-T. *et al.* (1984) *J. Nat. Prod.* **47** (2), 331
144 Mose, J. R. (1966) *Arzneim. Forsch.* **16**, 118
145 Henrickson, C. U. (1970) *Z. Immunitaetsforsch.* **5**, 425
146 Tympner, K. D. (1981) *Z. Angew. Phytother.* **5**, 181
147 Wagner, H. in "Economic and Medicinal Plant Research Vol. 1". Pub. Academic Press. (1985) UK
148 Strauch, R. and Hiller, K. (1974) *Pharmazie* **10/11**, 656
149 Mengs, M. (1982) *Z. Angew. Phytother.* **5**, 187
150 Rao, P. R. S. P. and Rao, E. V. (1977) *Curr. Sci.* **48** (18), 640
151 Gonnet, J-F. (1981) *Biochem. Syst. Ecol.* **9** (4), 299
152 Lavie, D. *et al.* (1964) *Phytochem.* **3**, 52
153 Rawson, M. D. (1966) *Lancet* **1**, 1121
154 Konopa, J. *et al.* in "Advances in Antimicrobial and Antineoplastic Chemotherapy Vol. 2", Ed. M. Semonsky, Pub. Avicenna Press (1972) Prague

155 Habs, M. *et al.* (1984) *J. Cancer Res. Clin. Oncol.* **108** (1), 154
156 Belkin, M. *et al.* (1952) *J. Nat. Cancer Inst.* **13**, 742
157 Kupchan, S. M. *et al.* (1965) *Science* **150**, 1827
158 Wolters, B. (1965) *Planta Med.* **13**, 189
159 Willuhn, G. and Kothe, U. (1983) *Arch. Pharm.* **316** (8), 678
160 Henning, W. (1981) *Lebens. Unters. Forsch.* **173**, 180
161 Senchute, G. V. and Boruch, I. F. (1976) *Rastit. Resur.* **12** (1), 113
162 Lietti, A. *et al.* (1976) *Arzneim. Forsch.* **26** (5), 829
163 Jarboe, C. H. *et al.* (1967) *J. Med. Chem.* **10**, 448
164 Jarboe, C. H. *et al.* (1969) *J. Org. Chem.* **34**, 4202
165 Jarboe, C. H. (1966) *Nature* **212**, 837
166 Ojewole, J. A. O. (1983) *Fitoterapia* **5**, 203
167 Glombitza, K. W. and Lentz, G. (1981) *Tetrahedron* **37** (22), 3861
168 Glombitza, K. W. *et al.* (1977) *Planta Med.* **32** (1), 33
169 Criado, M. T. *et al.* (1983) *I.R.C.S. Med. Sci.* **11** (3), 286
170 Quang-Liem, P. and Laur, M. H. (1976) *Biochimie* **58** (11/12), 1367
171 Quang-Liem, P. and Laur, M. H. (1974) *Biochimie* **56** (6/7), 925
172 Curro, F. *et al.* (1976) *Arch. Med. Interna.* **28** (1), 19
173 Phillips, D. J. H. (1979) *Environ. Pollut.* **18** (1), 31
174 "The Alkaloids. Vol. XVII" Ed. R. H. F. Manske, and R. Rodrigo. Pub. Academic Press (1979)
175 Elliott, J. Q. Pat. US 4515779 (1985) USA
176 Collins, K. R. Pat. EP 25649 (1981) Europe
177 Ladanyi, P. Pat. CH 638973 (1983) Switzerland
178 Maiti, M. *et al.* Febs Lett **142**, 280
179 "A Handbook of Medicinal Herbs", J. A. Duke, Pub. CRC Press (1985)
180 Krick, W. *et al.* (1983) *Z. Naturforsch. Sect. C Biosci.* **38** (9/10), 689
181 Bambhole, V. D. and Jiddewar, G. G. (1985) *Sach. Ayurveda* **37** (9), 557
182 Nawwar, M. A. M. and Buddrus, J. (1981) *Phytochem.* **20**, 2446
183 "An Atlas of Medicinal Plants of Middle America", J. F. Morton. Pub. Charles C. Thomas (1981) USA
184 Urzúa, A. and Acuna, P. (1983) *Fitoterapia* **4**, 175
185 Bombardelli, E. *et al.* (1976) *Fitoterapia* **47**, 3
186 Kreitmar, H. (1952) *Pharmazie* **7**, 507
187 Levy-Appert-Collins, M. C. and Levy, J. (1977) *J. Pharm. Belg.* **32**, 13
188 Herz, W. *et al.* (1977) *J. Org. Chem.* **42** (13), 2264
189 Bohlmann, F. *et al.* (1977) *Phytochem.* **16**, 1973
190 Vollmar, A. *et al.* (1986) *Phytochem.* **25**, 377
191 Wagner, H. (1972) *Phytochem.* **11**, 1504
192 Benoit, P. S. *et al.* (1976) *Lloydia* **39**, 160
193 Luthy, J. *et al.* (1984) *Pharm. Acta. Helv.* **59** (9/10), 242
194 Fell, K. R. and Peck, J. M. (1968) *Planta Med.* **4**, 411
195 Khodshaev, B. U. *et al.* (1984) *Khim. Prir. Soedin* **6**, 802
196 Kato, Y. (1946) *Folia Pharmacol. Jap.* **42**, 37 (via CA 47: 1843)
197 Inouye, H. *et al.* (1974) *Planta Med.* **25**, 285

198 Wink, M. *et al.* (1981) *Planta Med.* **43** (4), 342
199 Murakoshi, I. *et al.* (1986) *Phytochem.* **25** (2), 521
200 Viscardi, P. *et al.* (1984) *Pharmazie* **39** (11), 781
201 Brum-Bousquet, M. *et al.* (1981) *Planta Med.* **43** (4), 367
202 Brum-Bousquet, M. and Delaveau, P. (1981) *Plant. Med. Phytother.* **15** (4), 201
203 Kurihara, T. and Kikuchi, M. (1980) *Yakugaku Zasshi* **100** (10), 1054
204 Young, N. *et al.* (1984) *Biochem. J.* **222** (1), 41
205 Aquino, R. *et al.* (1985) *J. Nat. Prod.* **48** (3), 502
206 Ireland, C. R. *et al.* (1981) *Phytochem.* **20**, 1569
207 Aquino, R. *et al.* (1985) *J. Nat. Prod.* **48** (5), 811
208 Konopa, J. *et al.* (1974) *Arzneim. Forsch.* **24** (10), 1554
209 Panossian, A. G. *et al.* (1983) *Planta Med.* **47** (1), 17
210 Vartanian, G. S. *et al.* (1984) *Byull. Eksp. Biol. Med.* **97** (3), 295
211 Suganda, A. G. *et al.* (1983) *J. Nat. Prod.* **46** (5), 626
212 Didry, N. and Pinkas, M. (1982) *Plant. Med. Phytother.* **16** (4), 249
213 Kaiser, R. *et al.* (1975) *J. Agric. Food Chem.* **23**, 943
214 Battersby, A. R. *et al.* (1967) *J. Chem. Soc. Chem. Commun.* 1277
215 Ciaceri, G. (1972) *Fitoterapia* **43**, 134
216 Phillipson, J. D. and Anderson, L. A. (1984) *Pharm. J.* **233**, 80 and 111
217 Swaitek, L. *et al.* (1986) *Planta Med.* **6**, 60P
218 'Naturally Occurring Quinones", R. H. Thomson. 2nd Ed. Pub. Academic Press (1971)
219 Rauwald, H-W. and Just, H-D. (1981) *Planta Med.* **42**, 244
220 Wagner, H. *et al.* (1978) *Planta Med.* **33**, 53
221 Van Os, F. H. L. (1976) *Pharmacology* **14** (Suppl. 1), 7, 18
222 Pailer, M. and Haslinger, E. (1972) *Monatsh. Chem.* **103**, 1399 (via [5])
223 Jeremic, D. *et al.* (1985) *Tetrahedron* **41** (2), 357
224 Hegnauer, R. and Kooiman, P. (1978) *Planta Med.* **33** (1), 13
225 Sourgens, H. *et al.* (1982) *Planta Med.* **45**, 78
226 Gumbinger, H. G. *et al.* (1981) *Contraception* **23** (6), 661
227 Karimov, L. *et al.* (1975) *Khim. Prir. Soedin* **11**, 433
228 Delorme, P. *et al.* (1977) *Plant. Med. Phytother.* **11**, 5
229 Yamanouchi, S. *et al.* (1976) *Yakugaku Zasshi* **96** (12), 1492
230 Ichihara, A. *et al.* (1978) *Tetrahedron Letters* **33**, 305
231 Ichihara, A. *et al.* (1968) *Tetrahedron* **44**, 3961
232 Schulte, K. *et al.* (1967) *Arzneim. Forsch.* **17**, 829
233 Naya, K. *et al.* (1972) *Chem. Lett.* **3**, 235
234 Yamada, Y. *et al.* (1975) *Phytochem.* **14**, 582
235 Takeda, H. and Kiriyami, S. (1979) *J. Nutr.* **109** (3), 388
236 Dombradi, G. (1970) *Chemotherapy* **15**, 250
237 Morita, K. *et al.* (1984) *Mutat. Res.* **129** (1), 25
238 Tsujita, J. *et al.* (1979) *Nutr. Rep. Int.* **20** (5), 635
239 Bryson, P. D. *et al.* (1978) *J. Am. Med. Ass.* **239** (20), 2157
240 Nonaka, G. I. *et al.* (1982) *J. Chem. Soc. Perkin Trans.* **10** (4), 1067
241 Tanaka, T. *et al.* (1984) *Chem. Pharm. Bull* **32** (1), 117
242 Tanaka, T. *et al.* (1983) *Phytochem.* **22** (11), 2575

243 Nonaka, G. I. *et al.* (1984) *Chem. Pharm. Bull.* **32** (2), 483
244 Tanake, T. *et al.* (1985) *J. Chem. Res (S)* **6**, 176
245 Kosuga, T. *et al.* (1984) *Chem. Pharm. Bull.* **32** (11), 448
246 Kosuga, T. *et al.* (1981) *Yakugaku Zasshi* **101** (6), 501
247 Sunstar Inc. (1980) Pat. JP 80/120509 Japan
248 Martin, R. *et al.* (1985) *Planta Med.* **51** (3), 198
249 Ben'ko, G. N. (1983) *Rastit. Resur.* **19** (4), 516
250 Morozova, S. S. *et al.* (1981) *Rastit. Resur.* **17** (1), 101
251 Bombardelli, E. *et al.* (1972) *Fitoterapia* **43**, 3
252 Vanhoutte, P. M. (1986) Ch. 23 in "Advances in Medicinal Phytochemistry", Ed. D. Barton and W. D. Ollis. Pub. John Wiley
253 Mauz, Ch. *et al.* (1985) *Pharm. Acta Helv.* **60**, 4
254 Novotný, L. *et al.* (1961) *Tet. Lett.* **20**, 697
255 Gonçalves de Lima, O. *et al.* (1972) via CA 81:86157
256 Seshadri, T. F. (1972) *Phytochem.* **11**, 881
257 Lowry, J. B. (1973) *Nature* **241**, 61
258 Baruah, R. N. *et al.* (1985) *Phytochem.* **24** (1), 2641
259 Keller, K. *et al.* (1985) *Planta Med.* **51** (1), 6
260 Rohr, M. and Naegeli, P. (1979) *Phytochem.* **18** (2), 279 and 328
261 Rohr, M. *et al.* (1979) *Phytochem.* **18** (2), 279
262 Iguchi, M. *et al.* (1973) *Tet. Lett.* **29**, 2759
263 Seiber, J. N. *et al.* (1982) *Phytochem.* **21** (9), 2343
264 Takaoka, D. *et al.* (1975) *Nippon Kagaku Kaishi* **12**, 2192
265 Stone, J. E. and Blundell, M. J. (1951) *Anal. Chem.* **23**, 771
266 El Feraly, M. *et al.* (1980) *J. Nat. Prod.* **43**, 407
267 Hopf, H. and Kandler, O. (1977) *Phytochem.* **16**, 1715
268 Debelmas, A. M. and Rochat, J. (1967) *Plant. Med. Phytother.* **1**, 23
269 Harries, N. *et al.* (1978) *J. Clin. Pharm.* **2**, 171
270 Haginiwa, H. *et al.* (1963) *Yakagaku Zasshi* **83**, 623 (via [5])
271 Popinigis, I. *et al.* (1980) *Trib. Farm.* **48** (1/2), 24
272 Cam, J. (1973) *Bol. Soc. Quim. Peru* **39** (4), 204
273 Herz, W. *et al.* (1972) *Phytochem.* **11**, 3061
274 Evans, F. J. *et al.* (1975) *J. Pharm. Pharmacol.* **27**, 91P
275 Fairbairn, J. W. *et al.* (1977) *J. Pharm. Sci.* **66**, 1300
276 Fairbairn, J. W. and Simic, S. (1964) *J. Pharm. Pharmacol.* **16**, 450
277 Laurens, A. and Paris, R. R. (1976) *Plant. Med. Phytother.* **11**, 16
278 Ogunlana, E. O. and Ramstad, E. (1975) *Planta Med.* **27**, 354
279 Sullivan, J. T. *et al.* (1982) *Planta Med.* **44**, 175
280 Giono, P. *et al.* (1971) *Journées Medicales Dakar* (via [33])
281 Senayake, U. M. *et al.* (1978) *J. Agric. Food Chem.* **20**, 822
282 Nohara, T. *et al.* (1982) *Phytochem.* **21** (8), 2130
283 Nohara, T. *et al.* (1985) *Phytochem.* **24** (8), 1849
284 Hikino, H. "Economic and Medicinal Plant Research", Vol I. Pub. Academic Press (1985) UK
285 Otsuka, H. *et al.* (1982) *Yakugaku Zasshi* **102**, 162
286 Morimoto, S. *et al.* (1982) Abstr. 28th Ann. Meeting Japan Pharm. Soc. p555 (via 285)

287 Harada, M. and Yamazaki, R. (1981) Abstr. 64th Meeting Kanto Branch Japan Pharmacol. Soc. p27

288 Harada, M. and Hirayama, Y. (1979) *ibid* 60th Meeting p34

289 Tahara, K. *et al.* (1986) 6th Int. Conf. Prostaglandins and Related Compounds, Florence, Italy. June 3rd–6th. Pub. Fondzione Giovanni Lorenzini

290 Nagai, H. *et al.* (1982) *Jpn. J. Pharmacol.* **32** (5), 813

291 Sham, J. S. K. *et al.* (1984) *Planta Med.* **2**, 177

292 Merlini, L. *et al.* (1967) *Tetrahedron* **23**, 3129

293 Sakan, T. *et al.* (1967) *Tetrahedron* **23**, 4635

294 Sastry, S. D. *et al.* (1972) *Phytochem.* **11**, 453

295 Tagawa, M. and Murai, F. (1983) *Planta Med.* **47**, 109

296 Young, L. A. *et al.* in "Recreational Drugs", Pub. Berkeley Publishing Co. (1977) USA (via [298])

297 Margolis, J. S. in "Complete Book of Recreational Drugs", Pub. Cliff House Books 1978. USA. (via [298])

298 Sherry, C. J. *et al.* (1981) *Quart. J. Crude Drug Res.* **19** (1), 31

299 Harvey, J. W. *et al.* (1978) *Lloydia* **41**, 367

300 Hatch, R. C. (1972) *Amer. J. Vet. Res.* **33**, 143

301 Masada, Y. *et al.* (1971) *J. Food Sci.* **36**, 858

302 Camara, B. and Moneger, R. (1978) *Phytochem.* **17**, 91

303 Gal, I. E. (1967) *Pharmazie* **22**, 120

304 Monsereenusorn, Y. *et al.* (1982) *Crit. Rev. Toxicol* **10**, 321

305 Polonsky, J. (1960) *Bull. Soc. Chim. France* 1845

306 Polonsky, J. (1973) *Fortschr. Chem. Org. Natur.* **30**, 101

307 "The Alkaloids. Vol XVII." Eds. R. H. F. Manske and R. Rodrigo. Pub: Academic Press 1979

308 Bjeldanes, L. F. and Kim, I. (1977) *J. Org. Chem.* **42**, 2333

309 Fehr, D. (1979) *Pharmazie* **34**, 658

310 Yu, R. S. and You, S. Q. (1984) *Acta Pharm. Sinica* **19** (8), 566

311 Garg, S. K. *et al.* (1979) *Phytochem.* **18**, 1580 and 1764

312 Garg, S. K. *et al.* (1980) *Planta Med.* **38**, 363

313 Harborne, J. B. in "The Biology and Chemistry of the Umbelliferae", Ed. V. N. Heywood. Pub. Academic Press (1971)

314 Lewis, D. A. *et al.* (1985) *Int. J. Crude Drug Res.* **28** (1), 27

315 Sluis, W. G. van der *et al.* (1980) *Planta Med.* **39**, 268

316 Neshta, N. M. *et al.* (1983) *Khim. Prir. Soed.* **1**, 106

317 Bishay, D. W. *et al.* (1978) *Planta Med.* **33**, 422

318 D'Agostino, M. *et al.* (1985) *Boll. Soc. Ital. Biol. Sper.* **61** (2), 165

319 Lacroix, R. *et al.* (1973) *Tunisie Med.* **51**, 327 (via [5])

320 Damiani, P. *et al.* (1983) *Fitoterapia* **54**, 213

321 Holub, M. and Samek, Z. (1977) *Collect. Czech. Chem. Commun.* **42**, 1053

322 Herisset, A. *et al.* (1971) *Plant. Med. Phytother.* **5** (3), 234

323 Herisset, A. *et al.* (1974) *Plant. Med. Phytother.* **8** (4), 306 and 287

324 Isaac, O. (1979) *Planta Med.* **35** (2), 3

325 Gasic, O. *et al.* (1983) *Fitoterapia* **2**, 51

326 Redaelli, C. *et al.* (1981) *Plant Med.* **42**, 288
327 "Plant Flavonoids in Biology and Medicine". Pub. Alan R. Liss Inc. (1986)
328 Redaelli, C. *et al.* (1981) *J. Chrom.* **209**, 110
329 Jakovlev, V. *et al.* (1983) *Planta Med.* **49** (2), 67
330 Jakovlev, V. *et al.* (1979) *Planta Med.* **35** (2), 3
331 Isaac, O. (1979) *Planta Med.* **35** (2), 118
332 Szelenyi, I. *et al.* (1979) *Planta Med.* **35** (3), 218
333 Achterrath-Tuckerman, U. *et al.* (1980) *Planta Med.* **39** (1), 38
334 Vilagines, P. *et al.* (1985) *C.R. Acad. Sci. (III)* **301** (6), 289
335 Habersang, S. (1979) *Planta Med.* **37** (2), 115
336 Lefort, D. *et al.* (1969) *Planta Med.* **17**, 261
337 Sleumer (1947) *Pharm. Ztg.* **83**, 165
338 Tsotsoriya, G. *et al.* (1977) *Kromatogr. Met. Farm.* 172 (via CA 90:51421)
339 "The Medicinal and Poisonous Plants of Southern and Eastern Africa", Watt, J. M. and Breyer-Brandwijk, M. G. 2nd Ed. Pub. Livingstone (1962)
340 Wagner, H. in "The Biology and Chemistry of the Compositae", Eds V. N. Heywood *et al.* Pub. Academic Press (1977)
341 Kawabata, S. and Deki, M. (1977) *Kanzei Chuo. Bunsek.* **17**, 63 (via [5])
342 Proliac, A. and Blanc, M. (1976) *Helv. Chem. Acta* **58**, 2503
343 Balbaa, S. *et al.* (1973) *Planta Med.* **24**, 133
344 Benoit, P. S. *et al.* (1976) *Lloydia* **39**, 160
345 Dalal, S. R. *et al.* (1953) *J. Ind. Chem. Soc.* **30**, 455
346 Ghosal, S. *et al.* (1973) *J. Pharm. Sci.* **62**, 926
347 Goyal, H. *et al.* (1981) *J. Res. Ayur. Siddha.* **2** (3), 286
348 Sharma, P. V. (1982) *Indian J. Pharm. Sci.* **44** (2), 36
349 Hikano, H. *et al.* (1984) *Shoyakugku Zasshi* **38**, 359
350 Komatsu, M. *et al.* (1971) *Jpn. Kokai* **71** (27), 558 (via [5])
351 Buchalter, L. (1971) *J. Pharm. Sci.* **60**, 144
352 Isogai, A. *et al.* (1977) *Agric. Biol. Chem.* **41**, 1779
353 Allured, S. E. (1975) *Cosmet. Perf.* **90** (4), 69
354 Atanasova Shopova, A. S. and Rusinov, K. S. (1970) *Izv. Inst. Fiziol. Bulg. Akad. Sci.* **13**, 89 (via [5])
355 Corrigan, D. *et al.* (1978) *Phytochem.* **17**, 1131
356 Burnett, A. R. and Thomsom, R. H. (1968) *J. Clin. Soc.* (6), 854
357 Bhan, M. K. *et al.* (1976) *Ind. J. Chem.* **14**, 475
358 Buckova *et al.* (1970) *Acta Fac. Pharm. Univ. Comeniana* **19**, 7
359 Delas, R. *et al.* (1947) 66th Cong. French Ass. Prog. Sci. Sect. Pharmacol *Toulouse Med.* **49**, 57
360 Berkowitz, W. F. *et al.* (1982) *J. Org. Chem.* **47**, 824
361 Narayanan, C. S. and Matthew, A. G. (1985) *Ind. Perf.* **29** (1/2), 15
362 Leete, E. in "The Alkaloids Vol. 1", Ed. S. W. Pelletier. Pub. John Wiley (1983)
363 Blumenkopf, T. A. and Heathcock, C. H. *ibid* Vol. 5 (1985)

364 Homstedt, B. *et al.* (1977) *Phytochem.* **16**, 1753
365 Aynilian, G. *et al.* (1974) *J. Pharm. Sci.* **63**, 1938
366 Novak, M. and Salemink, C. (1987) *Planta Med.* **53** (1), 113
367 Connolly, J. D. *et al.* (1972) *J. Chem. Soc. (P)* 1145
368 Ferguson, G. *et al.* (1973) *J. Chem. Soc. Chem. Comm.* 281
369 Oga, S. *et al.* (1981) *Planta Med.* **42** (3), 310
370 Radics, L. *et al.* (1975) *Tet. Lett.* **48**, 4287
371 Suntry Ltd (1984) Pat. JP 84/20298 Japan
372 Shibata, M. (1977) *J. Chem. Soc. Jpn.* **97**, 911
373 Jarry, H. *et al.* (1985) *Planta Med.* **4**, 316
374 Genazzani, E. *et al.* (1962) *Nature* **194**, 544
375 Shibata, M. *et al.* (1980) *Yakugaku Zasshi* **100**, 1143
376 Flom, M. S. *et al.* (1967) *J. Pharm. Sci.* **56**, 1515
377 Strigina, L. I. *et al.* (1975) *Phytochem.* **15**, 1583
378 Strigina, L. I. *et al.* (1976) *Khim. Prir. Soedin.* **5**, 619
379 Di Carlo, F. I. *et al.* (1964) *J. Reticuloendothelial. Soc.* **1**, 224
380 Santavy, F. (1957) *Pharm. Zentralhalle* **96**, 307
381 Fell, K. R. and Ramsden, D. (1967) *Lloydia* **30**, 123
382 Bhat, S. V. *et al.* (1977) *Tet. Lett.* **19**, 1669
383 De Sousa, N. J. *et al.* (1983) *Med. Res. Rev.* **3**, 201
384 Metzger, H. and Lindner, E. (1981) *Arzneim. Forsch.* **31**, 1248
385 Zinkel, D. F. (1975) *Chemtech.* **5** (4), 235
386 "Plant Drug Analysis", Ed. H. Wagner *et al.* Pub. Springer-Verlag (1984)
387 Didry, N. *et al.* (1982) *Ann. Pharm. Fr.* **40** (1), 75
388 Engalycheva, E. I. *et al.* (1982) *Farmatsiya* **31** (2), 37
389 Hirono, I. *et al.* (1979) *J. Natl. Canc. Inst.* **63** (2), 469
390 Röder, E. *et al.* (1981) *Plant Med.* **43**, 99
391 Hirono, I. *et al.* (1976) *Gann* **67** (1), 125
392 Kraus, C. *et al.* (1985) *Planta Med.* **51** (2), 89
393 Bhandari, P. and Gray, A. I. (1985) *J. Pharm. Pharmacol.* **37**, 50P
394 Furuya, T. and Araki, K. (1968) *Chem. Pharm. Bull.* **16**, 2512
395 Culvenor, C. J. J. *et al.* (1980) *Experientia* **36**, 377
396 Branchlij *et al.* (1982) *Experientia* **38**, 1085
397 Monograph in The Irish Pharmacy Journal, May 1984, 171
398 Roitman, J. N. (1981) *Lancet* i, 944
399 Gray, A. I. *et al.* (1983) *J. Pharm. Pharmacol.* **35**, 13P
400 Gracza, L. *et al.* (1985) *Arch. Pharm.* **312** (12), 1090
401 Kozhina, I. S. *et al.* (1970) *Rastit. Resur.* **6**, 345
402 Franz, G. (1969) *Planta Med.* **17**, 217
403 Mascolo, N. *et al.* (1987) *Phytother. Res.* **1** (1), 28
404 Stamford, I. F. and Tavares, I. A. (1983) *J. Pharm. Pharmacol.* **35**, 816
405 Schoental, R. *et al.* (1970) *Cancer Res.* **30**, 2127
406 Weston, C. F. M. *et al.* (1987) *Brit. Med. J.* **295**, 183
407 Taylor, A. and Taylor, N. C. (1963) *Proc. Soc. Exp. Biol. Med.* **114**, 772
408 White, R. D. *et al.* (1983) *Toxicol Lett.* **15**, 25

409 Hayashi, K. *et al.* (1980) *Chem. Pharm. Bull.* **28**, 1954
410 Hayashi, K. *et al.* (1981) *Chem. Pharm. Bull.* **29**, 2725
411 Takase, M. *et al.* (1982) *Chem. Pharm. Bull.* **30**, 2429
412 Delle Monache, G. *et al.* (1971) *Tet. Lett.* **8**, 659
413 Ferrari, M. *et al.* (1971) *Phytochem.* **10**, 905
414 Ram, A. S. and Devi, H. M. (1983) *Indian J. Bot.* **6** (1), 21
415 Gijbels, M. J. M. *et al.* (1982) *Fitoterapia* **53** (1/2), 17
416 Bandyukova, V. and Khalmatov, K. (1967) *Khim. Prir. Soedin.* **3**, 57
417 "Guide des Plantes Medicinales". P. Schauenberg and F. Paris Pub. Delachaux et Niestle (1969) Switzerland
418 Hahn, S. J. (1973) *K'at'ollick Taehak Uihak. Nonmunj.* **25**, 127 (via [5])
419 Stipanovic, R. D. *et al.* (1975) *Phytochem.* **14**, 1077
420 Dorsett, P. H. *et al.* (1975) *J. Pharm. Sci.* **64**, 1073
421 Farkas, L. in "Pharmacognosy and Phytochemistry 1st Int. Cong. Munich 1971". Pub. Springer-Verlag (1971)
422 Nat. Coord. Gp. Male Fert. (1978) *Chin. Med. J.* **4**, 417 (via [48])
423 Dai, R. X. *et al.* (1978) *Acta Biol. Exp. Sinica* **11**, 27 (via [48])
424 Liu, Z. Q. *et al.* (1981) in "Recent Advances in Fertility Regulation. Beijing 1980", Eds. C. C. Fen *et al.* Pub. S. A. Atar, Geneva
425 Qian, S. Z. *et al.* (1980) *Chin. Med. J.* **93**, 477
426 Hamasaki, Y. and Tae, H. H. (1985) *Biochim. Biophys. Acta* **843** (1), 37
427 Vilain, B. *et al.* (1986) 6th Int. Conf. Prostaglandins and Related Compounds. Florence, Italy. June 3rd–6th. Pub. Fondzione Giovanni Lorenzini
428 Paslawska, S. and Piekos, R. (1976) *Planta Med.* **30**, 216
429 Hejtmanek, M. and Dadak, V. (1959) *Ceskoslov. Mykol.* **13**, 183 (via [5])
430 Racz-Kotilla, E. and Mozes, E. (1971) *Rev. Med.* **17**, 82 (via [5])
431 Kiesewetter, R. and Muller, M. (1958) *Pharmazie* **13**, 777
432 Bell, E. A. and Jansen, D. H. (1971) *Nature* **229**, 136
433 Ghosal, S. *et al.* (1971) *Planta Med.* **24**, 434
434 Grecu, V. L. and Cucu, V. (1975) *Planta Med.* **25**, 247
435 Karl, C. *et al.* (1981) *Planta Med.* **41**, 96
436 Middleton, E. and Drzewiecki, G. (1984) *Biochem. Pharmacol.* **33**, 3333
437 Busse, W. W. *et al.* (1984) *J. All. Clin. Immunol.* **73**, 801
438 Borisov, M. I. (1974) *Khim. Prir. Soedin.* **10**, 82
439 Hecker, E. (1968) *Cancer Res.* **28**, 2338
440 Evans, F. J. and Taylor, S. E. (1983) *Prog. Chem. Org. Nat. Prod.* **44**, 1
441 Berenblum, I. and Shubik, P. (1947) *Brit. J. Cancer* **1**, 379
442 Nishizuka, Y. (1984) *Nature* **308**, 693
443 "Naturally Occurring Phorbol Esters", Ed. F. J. Evans. Pub. CRC Press (1986)
444 Ohta, Y. *et al.* (1966) *Tet. Lett.* **52**, 6365

445 Ikeda, R. M. (1962) *J. Food Sci.* **27**, 455
446 Batterbee, J. E. *et al.* (1969) *J. Chem. Soc. (C)*, 2470
447 Prabhu, B. R. and Mulchandani, N. B. (1985) *Phytochem.* **24** (2), 329
448 Akhtardziev, K. *et al.* (1984) *Farmatsiya* **34** (3), 1
449 Mladenov, I. V. (1982) *C.R. Acad. Bulg. Sci.* **35** (8), 1165
450 Shcheptoin, B. M. *et al.* (1984) *Vrach Delo* **6**, 18
451 Varo, P. T. and Heinz, D. E. (1970) *J. Agric. Food. Chem.* **18**, 234 & 239
452 Harborne, J. B. and Williams, C. E. (1972) *Phytochem.* **11**, 1741
453 Davidyants, E. S. *et al.* (1984) *Khim. Prir. Soedin.* **5**, 666
454 Dominguez, X. A. and Hinojosa, M. (1976) *Planta Med.* **30**, 68
455 Auterhoff, H. and Häufel, H. P. (1968) *Arch. Pharm.* **301**, 537
456 Jin, J. (1966) *Lloydia* **29** (3), 250
457 Rauwald, H-W. and Huang, D-T. (1985) *Phytochem.* **24** (7), 1557
458 Hansel, R. *et al.* (1980) *Phytochem.* **19**, 857
459 Kotobuki Seiyaku, K. K. (1981) Pat. JP 81/10117 Japan
460 Baba, K. *et al.* (1981) *Yakugaku Zasshi* **101** (6), 538
461 Appleton, R. A. and Enzell, C. R. (1971) *Phytochem.* **10**, 447
462 Karlsson, K. *et al.* (1972) *Acta Chem. Scand.* **26**, 1383
463 Wahlberg, I. *et al.* (1972) *Acta Chem. Scand.* **26**, 1383
464 Lichti, H. and Von Wartburg, A. (1964) *Tet. Lett.* **15**, 835
465 Tunmann, P. and Stierstorfer, N. *Tet. Lett.* **15**, 1697
466 Sticher, O. (1977) *Deutsche Apoth. Ztg.* **32**, 1279
467 Haag-Berrurier, M. *et al.* (1978) *Plant. Med. Phytother.* **12** (3), 197
468 Erdos, A. *et al.* (1978) *Planta Med.* **34**, 97
469 Eichler, O. and Koch, C. (1970) *Arzneim. Forsch.* **20** (1), 107
470 Circosta, C. *et al.* (1984) *J. Ethnopharmacol.* **11**, 259
471 Abramowitz, M. (1979) *Med. Lett.* **21**, 30
472 Dranik, L. I. (1970) *Khim. Prir. Soed.* **6**, 268
473 Kosawa, M. *et al.* (1976) *Chem. Pharm. Bull.* **24**, 220
474 Gijbels, M. J. *et al.* (1983) *Sci. Pharm.* **51**, 414
475 Harborne, J. B. (1969) *Phytochem.* **8**, 1729
476 Pagnani, F. and Ciarallo, G. (1974) *Boll. Chim. Farm.* **113** (1), 30
477 Petkov, V. and Markovska, V. (1981) *Plant. Med. Phytother.* **15** (3), 172
478 Harborne, J. B. (1969) *Phytochem.* **8**, 1449
479 Ulubelen, A. *et al.* (1971) *Lloydia* **34** (2), 258
480 Becker, H. (1982) *Deutsche Apoth. Ztg.* **122** (45), 2320
481 Jacobson, M. (1967) *J. Org. Chem.* **32**, 1646
482 Bohlmann, F. and Hoffman, H. (1983) *Phytochem.* **22** (5), 1173
483 Wagner, H. *et al.* (1984) *Arzneim. Forsch.* **34**, 659
484 Schulte, K. E. *et al.* (1967) *Arzneim. Forsch.* **17**, 825
485 Bauer, R. *et al.* (1987) *Phytochem.* **26** (4), 1198
486 Von Röder, E. *et al.* (1984) *Deutsche Apoth. Ztg.* **124** (45), 2316
487 Bauer, R. *et al.* (1985) *Helv. Chim. Acta* **68**, 2355
488 Bauer, R. *et al.* (1986) Abstr. Conf. Phytochem. Soc. Eur., 3-5th Sept. Lausanne 1986

489 May, G. and Willuhn, G. (1978) *Arneim. Forsch.* **28**, 1
490 Wacker, A. and Hilbig, W. (1978) *Planta Med.* **33**, 89
491 Harnischfeger, G. and Stolze, H. (1980) *Notabene Medici* **10**, 484
492 Vomel, Th. (1985) *Arzneim. Forsch.* **35** II (9), 1437
493 Mose, J. R. (1983) *Med. Welt* **34**, 51
494 Stimpel, M. *et al.* (1984) *Infect. Immunol.* **46** (3), 845
495 Samochowie, C. E. *et al.* (1979) *Wiad. Parazyt.* **25** (1) 77
496 Lawrie, W. *et al.* (1964) *Phytochem.* **3**, 267
497 Richter, W. and Willuhn, G. (1977) *Pharm. Ztg.* **122**, 1567
498 Richter, W. and Willuhn, G. (1974) *Deutsche Apoth. Ztg.* **114**, 947
499 Inoue, T. and Sato, K. (1975) *Phytochem.* **14**, 1871
500 Paulo, E. (1976) *Folia Biol.* **24** (2), 213
501 Kerimov, S. S. and Chishov, O. S. (1974) *Khim. Prir. Soed.* **10**, 254
502 Khvorost, P. P. and Komissarenko, N. F. (1976) *Khim. Prir. Soed.* **6**, 820
503 Vishnakova, S. A. *et al.* (1977) *Rastit. Resur.* **13**, 428
504 Keisawetter, R. and Muller, M. (1958) *Pharmazie* **13**, 777
505 Prakash, A. O. (1981) *Planta Med.* **41**, 258
506 Bhargava, S. K. and Dixit, V. P. (1985) *Plant. Med. Phytother.* **19** (1), 29
507 Hiller, K. in "Les Ombellifers: Contributions Pluridisciplinaires a la Systematique." Perpignan 18–21 May 1977. Pub. CNRS (1978)
508 Hiller, K. in "The Biology and Chemistry of the Umbelliferae". Ed. V. N. Heywood Pub. Academic Press (1971)
509 Erdelmeier, C. A. J. and Sticher, O. (1985) *Planta Med.* **51** (5), 407
510 Lisciani, R. *et al.* (1984) *J. Ethnopharmacol* **12** (3), 263
511 Ikeda, R. M. *et al.* (1962) *J. Food. Sci.* **27**, 455
512 Boukef, K. *et al.* (1976) *Plant. Med. Phytother.* **10**, 24, 30, 119
513 Blanc, P. and De Saqui-Sannes, G. (1972) *Plant. Med. Phytother.* **6** (2), 106
514 Atallah, A. and Nicholas, H. (1972) *Phytochem.* **11**, 1860
515 El-Naggar, L. *et al.* (1978) *Lloydia* **41**, 73
516 Baslas, B. K. and Agarwal, R. (1980) *Curr. Sci.* **49**, 311
517 Evans, F. J. and Kinghorn, A. D. (1977) *Bot. J. Linn. Soc.* **74**, 23
518 F. J. Evans in "Naturally Occurring Phorbol Esters". Ed. F. J. Evans Pub. CRC Press (1986)
519 Williamson, E. M. *et al.* (1980) *J. Pharm. Pharmacol.* **32**, 373
520 Williamson, E. M. *et al.* (1981) *Biochem. Pharmacol.* **30** (18), 2691
521 Williamson, E. M. and Evans, F. J. (1981) *Acta. Pharmacol. et Toxicol.* **48**, 47
522 Wright, S. and Burton, J. L. (1982) *Lancet* ii, 1120
523 Midwinter, R. E. *et al.* (1982) *Lancet* i, 339
524 Pye, J. K. *et al.* (1985) *Lancet* ii, 373
525 Horrobin, D. F. (1983) *J. Reprod. Med.* **28** (7), 465
526 Haslett, C. *et al.* (1983) *Int. J. Obesity* **7** (6), 549
527 Ten Hoor, F. (1980) *Nutr. Metab.* **24** (Suppl. 1), 162
528 Seaman, G. V. F. *et al.* (1979) *Lancet* i, 1139

529 Harkiss, K. J. and Timmins, P. (1973) *Planta. Med.* **23**, 342
530 Salama, O. and Sticher, O. (1983) *Planta Med.* **47**, 90
531 Betts, T. J. (1968) *J. Pharm. Pharmacol.* **20**, 61S
532 Karlsen, J. *et al.* (1969) *Planta Med.* **17**, 281
533 Rothbacher, H. and Kraus, A. (1970) *Pharmazie* **25**, 566
534 Albert-Puleo, M. (1980) *J. Ethnopharmacol.* **2**, 337
535 Kunzemann, J. and Hermann, K. (1977) *Z. Lebens. Unters Forsch.* **164**, 194
536 El-Khrisy, E. A. M. *et al.* (1980) *Fitoterapia* **51**, 273
537 Stahl, E. (1980) *Deutsche Apoth. Ztg.* **45**, 2324
538 Forster, H. B. *et al.* (1980) *Planta Med.* **40** (4), 309
539 Gershbein, L. L. (1977) *Food Cosmet. Toxicol.* **15** (3), 173
540 Bohlmann, F. and Zdero, C. (1982) *Phytochem.* **21** (10), 2543
541 Govindachari, T. R. *et al.* (1964) *Tetrahedron* **21** (6), 1509
542 Romo de Viva, A. and Jiminez, H. (1965) *Tetrahedron* **21** (7), 1742
543 Hylands, D. M. and Hylands, P. (1986) Abstr. Phytochem. Soc. Eur. Meeting, Lausanne 3–5th Sept 1986 P17
544 Berry, M. I. (1984) *Pharm. J.* **232**, 611
545 Johnson, E. S. *et al.* (1985) *Brit. Med. J.* **291**, 569
546 Collier, H. O. J. *et al.* (1980) *Lancet* ii, 922
547 Makheja, A. N. and Bailey, J. M. (1981) *Lancet* ii, 1054
548 Heptinstall, S. *et al.* (1985) *Lancet* i, 1071
549 Buck, A. C. *et al.* (1986) 6th Int. Conf. Prostaglandins and Related Compounds. Florence, Italy. June 3rd–6th. Pub. Fondzione Giovanni Lorenzi
550 Siewek, F. *et al.* (1985) *Z. Naturforsch.* **40** (1/2), 8
551 Swann, K. and Melville, C. (1972) *J. Pharm. Pharmacol.* **24**, 170P
552 Weinges, K. and Von der Eltz, H. (1978) *Justus Leibigs Ann. Chem.* 1968
553 Jerznanowska, Z. and Pijewska, L. (1954) *Acta Polon. Pharm.* **11**, 1 (via CA 48:11000)
554 Pethes, E. *et al.* (1973) *Herba Hung.* **12**, 101
555 Grancia, D. *et al.* (1985) *Ceskoslov. Farm.* **34** (6), 209
556 Lassère, B. *et al.* (1983) *Naturwissensch.* **70**, 95
557 Toth, L. *et al.* (1980) *Pharmazie* **35**, 334
558 Girardon, P. *et al.* (1985) *Planta Med.* **51** (6), 533
559 Hardman, R. *et al.* (1980) *Phytochem.* **19**, 698
560 Bohmann, M. B. *et al.* (1974) *Phytochem.* **13**, 1513
561 Sood, A. R. *et al.* (1976) *Phytochem.* **15**, 351
562 Adamska, M. and Lutomski, J. (1971) *Planta Med.* **20**, 224
563 Ribes, G. *et al.* (1986) *Proc. Soc. Exp. Biol. Med.* **183**, 159
564 Ribes, G. *et al.* (1986) *Ann. Nutr. Metab.* **28**, 37
565 Ribes, G. *et al.* (1986) *Phytother. Res.* **1** (1), 40
566 Abdo, M. S. and Al-Khafawi, A. A. (1969) *Planta Med.* **17**, 14
567 Al-Meshal, I. A. *et al.* (1985) *Fitoterapia* **56** (4), 232
568 Cohn, J. N. (1974) *J. Am. Med. Ass.* **229**, 1911
569 Thomas, R. *et al.* (1974) *J. Pharm. Sci.* **63**, 1649

570 Itokawa, H. *et al.* (1987) *Planta Med.* **53** (1), 32
571 Mitsui, S. *et al.* (1976) *Chem. Pharm. Bull.* **24**, 2377
572 Wichtl, M. (1963) *Planta Med.* **11**, 53
573 Thomas, A. G. *et al. Tetrahedron* **32**, 2261
574 Burrell, J. W. K. *et al.* (1976) *Tet. Lett.* **30**, 2837
575 Naef, F. *et al. Helv. Chim. Acta* **58**, 1016
576 Jessenne, M. G. *et al.* (1974) *Plant. Med. Phytother.* **8**, 241
577 Malteru, K. E. and Faegri, A. (1982) *Acta Pharm. Sueca.* **19**, 43
578 Lu, G. B. *et al.* (1984) *Yao Hsueh Husueh Pao* **19** (8) 636 (via Medline)
579 Augusti, K. T. and Mathew, P. T. (1974) *Experientia* **30**, 468
580 Whitaker, J. R. (1976) *Adv. Food. Res.* **22**, 73
581 Block, E. *et al.* (1984) *J. Am. Chem. Soc.* **106**, 8295
582 Apitz-Castro, R. *et al.* (1983) *Thromb. Res.* **32**, 155
583 Kabelik, J. (1970) *Pharmazie* **25**, 266
584 Jain, R. C. and Vyas, C. R. (1974) *Brit. Med. J.* **2**, 730
585 Brahmachari, M. D. and Augusti, K. T. (1962) *J. Pharm. Pharmacol.* **14**, 254 and 617
586 Augusti, K. T. and Benaim, M. E. (1974) *Clin. Chim. Acta* **60**, 121
587 Chaudhuri, B. N. *et al.* (1984) *Biomed. Biochim. Acta* **41** (7), 1045
588 Schoetan, A. *et al.* (1984) *Experientia* **40** (3), 261
589 Wenkert, E. *et al.* (1971) *Experientia* **28**, 377
590 Jensen, S. R. *et al.* (1987) *Phytochem.* **26** (6), 1725
591 Inouye, H. *et al.* (1968) *Tet. Lett.* 4429
592 Inouye, H. *et al.* (1970) *Chem. Pharm. Bull.* **18**, 1856
593 Bricout, J. (1974) *Phytochem.* **13**, 2819
594 Lewis, J. R. and Gupta, P. (1971) *J. Chem. Soc. Chem. Comm.* **4**, 629
595 Atkinson, J. E. *et al.* (1969) *Tetrahedron* **25**, 1507
596 Rulko, F. (1976) *Pr. Nauk. Akad. Med. Wroclawin* **8**, 3 (via [5])
597 Sadritdinov, F. (1971) *Farmakol. Alkaloidov Serdechnykh Glikozidov* 146 (via [5])
598 Swietek, L. and Dombrowicz, E. (1984) *Farm. Pol.* **40** (12), 729
599 Fikenscher, L. H. and Hegnauer, R. *Plant. Med. Phytother.* **3** (3), 183
600 Reinbold, A. M. and Popa, P. D. (1974) *Khim. Prir. Soedin.* 589
601 Rodriguez, M-C. *et al.* (1984) *Phytochem.* **23** (7), 1467
602 Sticher, O. and Lahloub, M. F. (1982) *Planta Med.* **30**, 124
603 Rovesti, P. (1957) *Ind. Perf.* **12**, 334
604 Narasimhan, S. and Govinarajan, V. S. (1978) *J. Food. Tech.* **13**, 31
605 Hikino, H. in "Economic and Medicinal Plant Research Vol. 1", Pub. Academic Press (1985) UK
606 Suekawa, M. *et al.* (1984) *J. Pharmacobio.-Dyn* **7** (11), 836
607 Mowrey, D. B. and Clayson, D. E. (1982) *Lancet* **ii**, 655
608 Kasahara, Y. and Hikino, H. (1983) *Shoyakugaku Zasshi* **37**, 73
609 Abdurada, M. *et al.* (1982) *Proc. Symp. Wakan-Yaku* **15**, 162
610 Kikuchi, F. *et al.* (1982) *Chem. Pharm. Bull.* **30**, 754
611 Sugaya, A. *et al.* (1975) *Shoyakugaku Zasshi* **29**, 160
612 Gujral, S. *et al.* (1978) *Nutr. Rep. Int.* **17**, 183
613 Doskotch, R. W. and Vanevenhoven, P. W. (1967) *Lloydia* **30**, 141

614 Braquet, P. and Godfroid, J. J. (1986) *Trends Pharm. Sci.* **7**, 397
615 Nunez, D. *et al.* (1986) 6th Int. Conf. Prostaglandins and Related Compounds, Florence, Italy. June 3rd–6th. Pub. Fondzione Giovanni Lorenzini
616 Touvay, C. *et al.* (1986) *ibid.*
617 Publisi, L. (1986) *ibid.*
618 Peter, H. *et al.* (1966) *Arzneim. Forsch.* **16**, 719
619 Schafflor, K. and Reeh, P. W. (1985) *Arzneim. Forsch.* **35** II (8), 1283
620 Braquet, P. *et al.* (1985) *Lancet* **i**, 1501
621 Chung, K. F. *et al.* (1987) *Lancet* **i**, 248
622 Reuse-Bourgain, M. (1986). 6th Int. Conf. Prostaglandins and Related Compounds. Florence, Italy. June 3rd–6th. Pub. Fondzione Giovanni Lorenzini
623 Hellegouarch, A. *et al.* (1985) *Gen. Pharmacol.* **16** (2), 129
624 Gessner, B. *et al.* (1985) *Arzneim. Forsch.* **35** II, (9), 1459
625 Becker, L. and Skipworth, G. (1975) *J. Am. Med. Ass.* **231**, 1162
626 Phillipson, J. D. and Anderson, L. A. (1984) *Pharm. J.* **232**, 161
627 Shoji, J. in "Advances in Chinese Medicinal Materials Research", Ed. H. M. Chang *et al.* Pub. World Scientific Pub. Co. (1985) Singapore and USA
628 Konno, C. *et al.* (1984) *Planta Med.* **50** (5), 434
629 Takahashi, M. and Yoshikura, M. (1966) *Yakugaku Zasshi* **86**, 1051 and 1053
630 Kitigawa, I. (1983) *Yakugaku Zasshi* **103**, 612
631 Hansen, L. and Boll, P. M. (1986) *Phytochem.* **25** (2), 285
632 Singh, V. K. *et al.* (1984) *Planta Med.* **50**, 462
633 Singh, V. K. *et al.* (1983) *Planta Med.* **47**, 234
634 Hiai, S. in "Advances in Chinese Medicinal Materials Research", Ed. H. M. Chang *et al.* Pub. World Scientific Pub. Co. (1985) Singapore and USA
635 Matsuda, H. *et al.* (1986) *Chem. Pharm. Bull.* **34** (3), 1153
636 Fulder, S. J. (1981) *Am. J. Chin. Med.* **9**, 112
637 Salto, H. and Lee, Y. U. (1978) *Proc. 3rd Int. Ginseng Symp.* 109
638 Avakian, E. V. *et al.* (1984) *Planta Med.* **50**, 151
639 Baldwin, C. A. *et al.* (1986) *Pharm. J.* **237**, 583
640 Bader, G. *et al.* (1987) *Pharmazie* **42** (2), 140
641 Goswami, A. *et al.* (1984) *Phytochem.* **23** (4), 837
642 Metzer, J. *et al.* (1984) *Pharmazie* **39** (12), 869
643 Lassere, B. *et al.* (1983) *Naturwissenschaft* **70**, 95
644 Gleye, J. *et al.* (1974) *Phytochem.* **13**, 675
645 Haginiwa, J. and Harada, M. (1962) *Yakugaku Zasshi* **82**, 726
646 Preininger, V. in "The Alkaloids Vol. XV", Ed. R. H. F. Manske Pub. Academic Press (1975)
647 Timmermann, B. *et al.* (1985) *Phytochem.* **24** (5), 1031
648 Barberan, F. A. T. (1986) *Fitoterapia* **57** (2), 67
649 Camps, F. *et al.* (1985) *An. Quim. 81* C (1), 74
650 Bull, L. B. *et al.* in "The Pyrrolizidine Alkaloids", Pub. Wiley (1968) NY

651 Qualls, C. W. and Segall, H. J. (1978) *J. Chrom.* **15**, 202
652 Toppel, G. and Hartmann, T. (1986) *Planta Med.* **6**, 25P
653 Van Dooren, Bos, R. *et al.* (1981) *Planta Med.* **42**, 385
654 Mansour, R. M. A. and Saleh, N. A. M. (1981) *Phytochem.* **20**, 1180
655 King, F. E. and Wilson, J. G. (1964) *J. Chem. Soc.* 4011
656 Majuinder, P. L. and Bhattacharya, M. (1974) *Chem. Ind.* 77
657 Katochvil, J. F. *et al.* (1971) *Phytochem* **10**, 2529
658 Schrecker, A. W. (1957) *J. Am. Chem. Soc.* **79**, 3823
659 Wagner, H. and Grevel, J. (1982) *Planta Med.* **45**, 98
660 Ficarra, P. *et al.* (1984) *Farm. Ed. Prat.* **39** (5) 148
661 Ficarra, P. *et al.* (1984) *Farm. Ed. Prat.* **39** (10) 342
662 Ammon, H. P. T. and Handel, M. (1981) *Planta Med.* **43**, 105, 209 and 313
663 Iwamoto, M. *et al.* (1981) *Planta Med.* **42** (1), 1
664 Rewerski, W. *et al.* (1971) Arzneim. Forsch. **21**, 886
665 Beretz, A. *et al.* (1980) *Planta Med.* **39** (3), 241
666 Horhammer, L. *et al.* (1965) *Tet. Lett.* 1707
667 Bachelard, H. S. and Trikojus, V. M. (1963) *Austral. J. Biol. Sci.* **16**, 147
668 Ockendon, J. G. and Buczki, S. T. (1979) *Trans. Br. Mycol. Soc.* **72**, 156
669 Kupchan, S. M. *et al.* (1961) *Lloydia* **24** (1), 17
670 Sandberg, F. and Thorsen, R. (1962) *Lloydia* **25** (3) 201
671 Winkler, C. and Wichtle, M. (1985) *Pharm. Acta Helv.* **60** (9/10), 234
672 Karrer, W. (1950) *Helv. Chim. Acta* **33**, 433
673 Roberts, M. F. (1975) *Phytochem.* **14**, 2395
674 Roberts, M. F. (1980) *Planta Med.* **39**, 216
675 Hendriks, H. *et al.* (1983) *Pharm. Weekblad* **5**, 281
676 Woerdenbag, H. J. *et al.* (1987) *Phytother. Res.* **2** (2), 76
677 Pederson, E. (1975) *Phytochem.* **14**, 2086
678 Vollmar, A. *et al.* (1986) *Phytochem.* **25** (2), 377
679 Karawya, M. S. *et al.* (1969) *Lloydia* **32**, 76
680 Mahmood, Z. F. *et al.* (1983) *Fitoterapia* **4**, 153
681 Bardwaj, D. K. *et al.* (1978) *Phytochem.* **17**, 1440
682 Vanhaelen, M. and Vanhaelen-Fastre, R. (1975) *Phytochem.* **14**, 2709
683 Vanhaelen-Fastre, R. and Vanhaelen, M. (1976) *Planta Med.* **29**, 179
684 Farnsworth, N. R. *et al.* (1975) *J. Pharm. Sci.* **64** (4), 535
685 Hartley, R. D. (1968) *Phytochem.* **7**, 1641
686 Hartley, R. D. and Fawcett, C. H. (1968) *Phytochem.* **7**, 1395
687 Moir, M. *et al.* (1980) *Phytochem.* **19** (10), 2201
688 Kumai, A. and Okamoto, R. (1984) *Toxicol. Lett.* **21** (2), 203
689 Bravo, L. *et al.* (1974) *Boll. Chim. Farm.* 306
690 Hansel, R. *et al.* (1982) *Planta Med.* **45** (4), 224
691 Wohlfart, R. (1983) *Deutsche Apoth. Ztg.* **123**, 1637
692 Schmalreck, A. F. *et al.* (1975) *Can. J. Microbiol.* **21**, 205
693 Caujolle, F. *et al.* (1969) *Agressologie* **10**, 405 (via [5])
694 Nicholas, H. J. (1964) *J. Pharm. Sci.* **53**, 895

695 Busby, M. C. *et al.* (1983) *Proc. R. IR. Acad. Sect. B* **83**, 1
696 Henderson, M. S. and McCrindle, R. (1969) *J. Chem. Soc. Chem. Comm.* **15**, 2014
697 Popa, D. P. *et al.* (1968) *Khim. Prir. Soed.* **4** (6), 345
698 Popa, D. P. and Salei, L. A. (1973) *Rastit. Resur.* **9** (3), 384
699 Popa, D. P. *et al.* (1974) *Rastit. Resur.* **10** (3), 365
700 Karryev, M. O. *et al.* (1976) *Izv. Akad. Nauk. Turkm. Ser. Biol.* **3**, 86
701 Pandler, W. W. and Wagner, S. (1963) *Chem. Ind.* **42**, 1693
702 Brieskorn, C. H. and Feilner, K. (1968) *Phytochem.* **7**, 485
703 Bartarelli, I. M. (1966) *Boll. Chim. Farm.* **105**, 787
704 Cahen, R. (1970) *C R Soc. Biol.* **164**, 1467
705 Savona, G. *et al.* (1976) *J. Chem. Soc. (P)* **1**, 1607
706 Savona, G. *et al.* (1977) *J. Chem. Soc. (P)* **1**, 322
707 Konoshima, T. and Lee, K-H. (1986) *J. Nat. Prod.* **49** (4), 650
708 Vogel, G. in "Pharmacognosy and Phytochemistry", Ed. H. Wagner and L. Horhammer. Pub. Springer-Verlag (1971)
709 Preziosi, P. and Manca, P. (1965) *Arzneim. Forsch.* **15**, 404
710 Rao, G. S. *et al.* (1974) *J. Pharm. Sci.* **63**, 471
711 Proserpio, G. *et al.* (1980) *Fitoterapia* **2**, 113
712 Evans, W. C. and Somanabandu, A. (1977) *Phytochem.* **16**, 1859
713 Phillipson, J. D. and Melville, C. (1960) *J. Pharm. Pharmacol.* **12**, 506
715 Pohl, R. W. (1955) *Am. Fern J.* **45**, 95
716 Gibelli, C. (1931) *Arch. Int. Pharmacodyn.* **41**, 419
717 Bate-Smith, E. C. (1978) *Phytochem.* **17**, 267
718 Der Mardirossian, A. *et al.* (1976) *J. Toxicol. Environ. Health* **1**, 939
719 Dutta, T. and Basu, U. P. (1968) *Ind. J. Exp. Biol.* **6** (3), 181
720 Boiteau, P. *et al.* (1949) *Compt. Rend. Acad. Sci.* **228**, 1165
721 Dutta, T. and Basu, U. P. (1967) *Ind. J. Chem.* **5**, 586
722 Rao, P. S. and Seshadri, T. R. (1969) *Curr. Sci.* **38**, 77
723 Asakawa, Y. *et al.* (1982) *Phytochem.* **21** (10), 2590
724 Allegra, G. *et al.* (1981) *Clin. Terap.* **99**, 507
725 Bossé, J-P. *et al.* (1979) *Ann. Plastic Surg.* **3** (1), 13
726 Vecchaio, A. D. *et al.* (1984) *Farm. Ed. Prat.* **39** (10), 355
727 Di Carlo, F. I. *et al.* (1964) *J. Reticuloendothelial Soc.* **1** 224
728 Morisset, R. *et al.* (1987) *Phytother. Res.* **1** (3), in press
729 Joulain, D. (1976) *Riv. Ital. Ess. Prof. Piante Off. Ar. Sap. Cosm.* **48**, 479
730 Opdyke, D. L. J. (1978) *Food Cosmet. Toxicol.* **16** (Suppl. 1), 787
731 Huoven, K. *et al.* (1985) *Acta Pharm. Fenn.* **99**, 94
732 Kisakurek, M. V. *et al.* in "The Alkaloids. Vol. 1", Ed. S. W. Pelletier, Pub. John Wiley (1983)
733 "Marihuana", G. C. Nahas, Pub. Springer-Verlag (1976)
734 Turner, C. E. *et al.* (1980) *J. Nat. Prod.* **43**, 169
735 Yamaudi, T. (1975) *Phytochem.* **14**, 2189
736 Fairbairn, J. W. *et al. J. Pharm. Pharmacol.* **28**, 130
737 Segelman, A. *et al.* (1977) *J. Pharm. Sci.* **66**, 1358

738 Paris, R. R. *et al.* (1976) *Plant. Med. Phytother.* 10, 144
739 Kettenes-Van den Bosch, J. J. and Salemink, C. A. (1978) *Recl. Trav. Chim. Pays-Bas* 97, 221
740 Gill, E. W. *et al.* (1970) *Nature* 228, 135
741 Burstein, S. and Ozman, K. (1982) *Biochem. Pharmacol.* 34, 2019
742 Fairbairn, J. W. and Pickens, J. T. (1981) *Br. J. Pharmacol.* 72, 401
743 Barrett, M. L. *et al.* (1985) *Biochem. Pharmacol.* 34, 2019
744 Evans, A. T. *et al.* (1985) *J. Pharm. Pharmacol.*
745 Evans, A. T. *et al.* (1987) *FEBS* 211, 119
746 Evans, A. T. *et al.* (1987) *Biochem. Pharmacol.* 36, 2035
747 Formukong, E. *et al.* (1986) *J. Pharm. Pharmacol.*
748 Berrens, L. and Young, E. (1963) *Int. Arch. All. Appl. Immunol.* 22, 51
749 "The Alkaloids XXV. Chemistry and Pharmacology", Ed. A. Brossi, Pub. Academic Press (1985)
750 Stancioff, D. J. and Renn, D. W. (1975) *A. C. S. Symp. Ser.* 15, 282
751 Thomson, A. W. and Horne, C. H. W. (1976) *Br. J. Exp. Pathol.* 57, 455
752 Tscherche, R. in "Pharmacognosy and Phytochemistry", Ed. H. Wagner and L. Horhammer, Pub. Springer-Verlag (1971)
753 Hostettmann, K. in "Advances in Medicinal Plant Research", Ed. A. J. Vlietinck and R. A. Domisse, Pub. Verlagsgesellschaft (1985)
754 Balansard, G. *et al.* (1980) *Planta Med.* 39, 234
755 Julien, J. *et al.* (1985) *Planta Med.* (3), 205
756 Mahran, G. H. *et al.* (1975) *Planta Med.* 29, 127
757 Hill, K. in "The Alkaloids. Vol. 1", Ed. S. W. Pelletier, Pub. John Wiley (1983)
758 Craveiro, A. A. *et al.* (1979) *J. Nat. Prod.* 42, 169
759 Singh, S. and Stacey, B. E. (1973) *Phytochem.* 12, 1701
760 Wagner, H. (1973) in "Chemistry in Biochemical Classification", Nobel Symposium (1973)
761 Pietta, P. and Zio, C. (1983) *J. Chrom.* 260, 497
762 Schwartz, J. S. P. *et al.* (1964) *Tetrahedron* 20, 1317
763 Stamm, O. A. *et al.* (1958) *Helv. Chim. Acta* 41, 2006
764 Heller, W. and Tamm, C. (1975) *Helv. Chim. Acta.* 58, 974
765 Nordal, A. *et al.* (1966) *Acta Chem. Scand.* 20, 1431
766 Aurousseau, M. *et al.* (1965) *Ann. Pharm. Franc.* 23, 251 (via 5)
767 Linde, H. (1983) *Arch. Pharm.* 316 (11), 971
768 Nair, A. G. R. and Subramanian, S. (1962) *J. Sci. Ind. Res. India* 21B, 437
769 Jain, S. R. and Sharma, S. N. (1967) *Planta Med.* 15 (4), 439
770 Mukherjee, S. K. *et al.* (1963) *Ind. Med. Gaz.* 3, 97
771 Shrothi, D. S. *et al.* (1963) *Ind. J. Med. Res.* 51, 464
772 Desai, V. B. and Sirsi, M. (1966) *Ind. J. Pharmac.* 28, 340
773 Dupaigne, P. (1974) *Plantes Med. Phytother.* 8, 104
774 Desai, V. B. and Rupawala, E. N. (1966) *Ind. J. Pharm.* 29, 235
775 Karawya, M. S. *et al.* (1981) *Fitoterapia* 4, 175
776 Inoue, O. *et al.* (1978) *J. Chem. Res.* 144

777 Yagi, A. *et al.* (1978) *Chem. Pharm. Bull.* **26**, 1798
778 Okamura, N. *et al.* (1981) *Chem. Pharm. Bull.* **29**, 676 and 3507
779 Shibata, S. *et al.* (1970) *Phytochem.* **9**, 677
780 Ikram, M. *et al.* (1981) *J. Nat. Prod.* **44**, 91
781 Woo, W. S. *et al.* (1979) *Phytochem.* **18**, 353
782 Cyong, J. *et al.* (1979) *Proc. Symp. Wakan-Yaku* **12**, 1
783 Cyong, J. and Hanabusa, K. (1980) *Phytochem.* **19**, 2747
784 Cyong, J. and Takahashi, M. (1982) *Chem. Pharm. Bull.* **30**, 1081
785 Ahn, Y. S. *et al.* (1982) *Korean J. Pharmacol.* **18** (1), 17
786 Freidrich, H. and Engelshowe, R. (1978) *Planta Med.* **33**, 251
787 Thomas, A. F. (1972) *Helv. Chim. Acta* **56**, 1800
788 De Pascuale Teresa, J. (1977) *An. Quim.* **73** (3), 463 (via 5)
789 Thomas, A. F. (1972) *Helv. Chim. Acta* **55**, 2429
790 Lounasmaa, M. *et al.* (1975) *Planta Med.* **28**, 16
791 Widen, C-J. and Puri, H. S. (1980) *Planta Med.* **40**, 284
792 Hansel, R. and Beiersdorff, H. U. (1955) *Arzneim. Forsch.* **9**, 581
793 Smith, R. M. (1979) *Tetrahedron* **35** (3), 437
794 Seshadri, T. R. (1972) *Phytochem.* **11**, 881
795 Maurya, R. *et al.* (1984) *J. Nat. Prod.* **47**, 179
796 Maurya, R. *et al.* (1985) *J. Nat. Prod.* **48**, 313
797 Mathé, I. *et al.* (1982) *Planta Med.* **45**, 158
798 Raynaud, J. and Mnajed, H. (1972) *C. R. Acad. Sci. Paris* **274**, 1746
799 Freudenberg, K. and Weinges, K. (1959) *Tet. Lett.* **17**, 19
800 Pelletier, S. W. *et al.* in "The Alkaloids Vol. 2", Pub. John Wiley (1984)
801 Hogg, J. W. *et al.* (1974) *Phytochem.* **13**, 868
802 Tori, K. *et al.* (1976) *Tet. Lett.* **5**, 387
803 Tada, H. *et al.* (1976) *Chem. Pharm. Bull.* **24**, 667
804 Novak, M. (1985) *Phytochem.* **24** (4) 585
805 Ter Heide, R. *et al.* (1970) *J. Chrom.* **50**, 127
806 Herisset, A. *et al.* (1971) *Plant. Med. Phytother.* **5**, 305
807 Mukherjee, B. D. and Trenkle, R. W. (1973) *J. Agric. Food Chem.* **21**, 298
808 Timiner, R. *et al.* (1975) *J. Agric. Food Chem.* **23**, 53
809 Kaiser, R. and Lamparsky, D. (1977) *Tet. Lett.* **7**, 665
810 Ianova, L. G. *et al.* (1977) *Khim. Prir. Soedi.* **1**, 111
811 Becchi, M. and Carrier, M. (1980) *Planta Med.* **38** (3), 267
812 Giner, R. *et al.* (1986) *Planta Med.* **6**, 83P
813 Paris, R. (1977) *Plant. Med. Phytother.* **11** (Suppl.), 129
814 Paris, R. and Delaveau, P. (1977) *Plant. Med. Phytother.* **11** (Suppl.), 198
815 Ruban, G. *et al.* (1978) *Acta Crystalogr. Sect. B* **34** (4), 1163 (via BIOSIS)
816 Rees, S. and Harborne, J. (1984) *Bot. J. Linn. Soc.* **89** (4), 313
817 Marquardt, P. *et al.* (1976) *Planta Med.* **30**, 68
818 Huang, Z-J. *et al.* (1982) *J. Pharma. Sci.* **71** (2), 270
819 Röder, E. *et al.* (1983) *Planta Med.* **49**, 57

820 Zalkow, L. H. *et al.* (1979) *J. Chem. Soc. Perkin Trans.* 1, 1542
821 Laufke, R. (1958) *Planta Med.* 6, 237
822 Tschesche, R. *et al.* (1959) *Naturwissensch.* 46, 109
823 Bleier, W. *et al.* (1965) *Pharm. Acta Helv.* 40, 554
824 Tschesche, R. in "Pharmacognosy and Phytochemistry", Ed. H. Wagner and L. Horhammer, Pub. Springer-Verlag (1971)
825 Kopp, B. and Kubelka, W. (1982) *Planta Med.* 45, 87
826 Slater, C. A. (1961) *J. Sci. Agric. Food* 12, 732
827 Stanley, W. L. and Jurd, L. (1971) *J. Agric. Food Chem.* 19, 1106
828 Tatum, J. H. and Berry, R. E. (1977) *Phytochem.* 16, 109
829 Breitweiser, K. (1943) *Pharmazie Ind.* 10, 76
830 Killacky, J. *et al.* (1976) *Planta Med.* 30, 310
831 Van Hulle, C. (1970) *Pharmazie* 25, 620
832 Bhardwaj, D. K. *et al.* (1977) *Phytochem.* 16, 401
833 Bhardwaj, D. K. *et al.* (1977) *Phytochem.* 15, 352
834 Bhardwaj, D. K. and Singh, R. (1977) *Curr. Sci.* 46, 753
835 Saitoh, T. *et al.* (1976) *Chem. Pharm. Bull.* 24, 752
836 Saitoh, T. *et al.* (1976) *Chem. Pharm. Bull.* 24, 1242
837 Saitoh, T. *et al.* (1978) *Chem. Pharm. Bull.* 26, 752
838 Saitoh, T. *et al.* (1976) *Chem. Pharm. Bull.* 24, 991
839 Kinoshita, T. *et al.* (1978) *Chem. Pharm. Bull.* 26, 141
840 Kinoshita, T. *et al.* (1978) *Chem. Pharm. Bull.* 26, 135
841 Tanaka, S. *et al.* (1987) *Planta Med.* 53 (1), 5
842 Segal, R. *et al.* (1985) *J. Pharm. Sci.* 74 (1), 79
843 Amagaya, S. *et al. J. Pharmacobiodyn.* 7 (12), 923
844 Kiso, Y. *et al.* (1984) *Planta Med.* 50, 298
845 Hayashi, Y. *et al.* (1979) *Yakuri to Chiryo* 7, 3861
846 Epstein, M. T. *et al.* (1977) *Brit. Med. J.* 19, 488
847 Neilsen, I. and Pedersen, R. S. (1984) *Lancet* 1, 8389
848 Rees, W. D. W. *et al.* (1979) *Scand. J. Gastroenterol.* 14, 605
849 Bardhan, K. D. *et al.* (1978) *Gut* 19, 779
850 Watanabe, Y. and Watanabe, K. (1980) *Proc. Symp. Wakan-Yaku* 13, 16
851 Yagura, T. *et al.* (1978) *Proc. Symp. Wakan-Yaku* 11, 79
852 Kumagai, A. and Takata, M. (1978) *Proc. Symp. Wakan-Yaku* 11, 73
853 Karawya, M. S. *et al.* (1971) *J. Ass. Off. Ann. Chem.* 54 (6), 1423
854 Gross, D. (1971) *Forts. Chem. Org. Nat.* 29, 1
855 Ayer, W. A. and Habgood, T. E. in "The Alkaloids Vol. XI", Ed. R. H. F. Manske, Pub. Academic Press (1968)
856 Gijbels, M. J. *et al.* (1982) *Planta Med.* 44, 207
857 Gijbels, M. J. *et al.* (1981) *Chromatographia* 14 (8), 451
858 Lawrence, B. M. (1980) *Perf. Flav.* 5, 29
859 Albulescu, D. *et al.* (1975) *Farmacia* 23, 159
860 Fischer, F. C. and Svendson, A. B. (1976) *Phytochem.* 15, 1079
861 Yu, S. R. and You, S. Q. (1984) *Yao Hsueh Hsueh Pao* 19 (8), 566
862 Keeler, R. F. (1975) *Lloydia* 38, 56
863 Morton, J. F. (1975) *Morris Arbor. Bull.* 26, 24 (via [5])

864 Nowacki, E. *et al.* (1976) *Biochem. Physiol. Pflanz.* **169**, 183

865 Gestetner, B. (1974) *Phytochem.* **10**, 2221

866 Berrang, B. (1974) *Phytochem.* **13**, 2253

867 Tapper, B. A. *et al.* (1975) *J. Sci. Food. Agric.* **26**, 277

868 Larher, F. *et al.* (1983) *Plant Sci. Lett.* **29** (2/3), 315

869 Malinow, M. R. *et al.* (1977) *Steroids* **29**, 105

870 Catalano, S. *et al.* (1976) *Phytochem.* **15**, 22

871 "The Encyclopaedia of Herbs and Herbalism", Ed. M. Stuart, Pub. Orbis (1979)

872 Sanford, K. J. and Heinz, D. E. (1971) *Pharm. Acta Helv.* **59** (9/10), 242

873 Forrest, T. P. *et al.* (1973) *Naturwissenschaft.* **60**, 257

874 Forrest, J. E. and Heacock, R. A. (1972) *Lloydia* **35**, 440

875 Baldry, J. *et al.* (1976) *Int. Flav. Food. Add.* **7**, 28

876 Trim, A. R. and Hill, R. (1952) *Biochem. J.* **50**, 310

877 Nung, V. N. *et al.* (1971) *Plant. Med. Phytother.* **5**, 177

878 Imperato, F. (1982) *Phytochem.* **21** (8), 2158

879 Jain, S. R. and Sharma, S. N. (1967) *Planta Med.* (4), 439

880 Twaij, H. A. A. *et al.* (1985) *Indian J. Pharmacol.* **17** (1), 73

883 Widen, C. J. (1971) *Helv. Chim. Acta* **54**, 2824

884 Calderwood, J. M. *et al. J. Pharm. Pharmacol.* **21**, 55 S

885 Bottari, F. *et al.* (1972) *Phytochem.* **11**, 2519

886 Puri, H. S. *et al.* (1978) *Planta Med.* **33**, 177

887 Dewick, P. *et al.* (1982) *Phytochem.* **20**, 2277

888 Hartwell, J. L. and Detly, W. E. (1950) *J. Am. Chem. Soc.* **72**, 246

889 Stoll, A. *et al.* (1954) *J. Am. Chem. Soc.* **76**, 5004 and 6431

890 Stoll, A. *et al.* (1955) *J. Am. Chem. Soc.* **77**, 1710

891 Wartburg, A. *et al.* (1957) *Helv. Chim. Acta* **40**, 1331

892 Chatterjee, R. (1952) *Econ. Bot.* **6**, 342

894 Auterhoff, H. and May, O. (1958) *Planta Med.* **6**, 240

894 Jardine, I. in "Anticancer Agents Based on Natural Product Models", Ed. Cassady, J. M. and Douros, J. D., Pub. Academic Press (1980)

895 Kasprzyk, Z. and Pyrek, J. (1968) *Phytochem.* **7**, 1631

896 Kasprzyk, Z. and Wilkomyrski, B. (1973) *Phytochem.* **13**, 2299

897 Pyrek, J. (1977) *Roczniki Chemii* **51**, 1141, 2331 and 2493

898 Wilkomirski, B. (1985) *Phytochem.* **24** (12), 3067

899 Vecherko, L. P. *et al.* (1975) *Khim. Prir. Soed.* **11** (3), 366

900 Samochowiec, E. *et al.* (1979) *Wiad. Parazytol.* **25** (1), 77

901 Lossner, G. (1968) *Planta Med.* **16**, 54

902 Herrmann, K. (1962) *Lebens. Unters. Forsch.* **116**, 224

903 Tomoda, M. *et al.* (1980) *Chem. Pharm. Bull.* **28**, 824

904 Kochich, P. *et al.* (1983) *Sov. J. Bioorg. Chem.* **9** (2), 121

905 Tomoda, M. *et al.* (1987) *Planta Med.* **53** (1), 8

906 Blaschek, W. and Franz, G. (1986) *Planta Med.* **6**, 76P

907 Kardosova, A. *et al.* (1983) *Coll. Czech. Commun.* **45**, 2082

908 Gudej, J. (1981) *Acta Pol. Pharm.* **38**, 385

909 Schimmer, O. *et al.* (1980) *Planta Med.* **40** (1), 68

910 Gijbels, M. J. M. *et al.* (1985) *Fitoterapia* **61** (1), 17
911 Baruah, R. N. *et al.* (1985) *Planta Med.* (6), 531
912 Hausen, B. M. *et al.* (1984) *Planta Med.* (3), 229
913 Masterova, I. *et al.* (1987) *Phytochem.* **26** (6), 1844
914 Nagy, E. *et al.* (1984) *Z. Naturforsch.* **39B** (12), 1813
915 Lindeman, A. *et al.* (1982) *Lebens. Wiss. und Tachnol.* **15** (5), 286
916 Barnaulov, O. D. *et al.* (1977) *Rastit. Resur.* **13** (4), 661
917 Thieme, H. (1965) *Pharmazie* **20**, 113
918 Genig, A. Y. *et al.* (1977) *Mater, S'ezola Farm. B. SSR* **3**, 162
919 Haslam, E. *et al.* (1985) in *Ann. Proc. Phytochem. Soc. Eur.* **25**, 252
920 Barnaulov, O. D. and Denisenko, P. (1980) *Farmakol. Toksicol.* **43** (6), 700
921 Barnaulov, O. D. (1978) *Rastit. Resur.* **14** (4), 573
922 Kasarnovski, L. S. (1962) *Tr. Khar'kovsk Farmats. Inst.* **2**, 23
923 Abou-Donia, A. H. A. (1976) Ph.D Thesis, Faculty of Pharmacy, University of Alexandria, Egypt.
924 Plouvier, V. (1963) *Compt. Rend.* **257**, 4061
925 Hong, N. D. *et al.* (1983) *Korean J. Pharmacog.* **14** (2), 51
926 "The Alkaloids", D. R. Dalton, Pub. Marcel Dekker Inc. (1979)
927 Kapadia, G. J. and Fayez, M. B. (1970) *J. Pharm. Sci.* **59**, 1699
928 Stout, G. H. *et al.* (1970) *J. Am. Chem. Soc.* **92**, 1070
929 Nyborg, J. and La Cour, T. (1975) *Nature* **257**, 824
930 Schildknecht, H. *et al.* (1970) *Chem. Ztg* **94**, 347
931 Kupchan, S. M. and Baxter, R. L. (1974) *Science* **187**, 652
932 Pelter, A. and Hansel. R. (1968) *Tet. Lett.* **19**, 2911
933 Wagner, H. *et al.* (1971) *Tet. Lett.* **22**, 1985
934 Neu, R. (1960) *Arch. Pharm.* **293**, 269
935 Desplaces, A. *et al.* (1975) *Arzneim.-Forsch.* **25**, 89
936 Tuchweber, B. *et al.* (1973) *J. Med.* **4**, 327
937 Vogel, G. *et al.* (1984) *Toxicol. Appl. Pharmacol.* **51**, 265
938 Hruby, K. *et al.* (1983) *Hum. Toxicol.* **2** (2), 183
939 Poser, G. (1971) *Arzneim.-Forsch.* **21**, 1209
940 Benda, I. and Zenz, W. (1973) *Wien. Med. Wschr.* **123**, 512
941 Devault, R. L. and Rosenbrook, W. (1973) *J. Antibiotic.* **26**, 532
942 Qiu, S. J. *et al.* (1981) *Chin. J. Cardiol.* **9**, 61
943 Franz, H. *et al.* (1981) *Biochem. J.* **195**, 481
944 Luther, P. *et al.* (1980) *Int. J. Biochem.* **11**, 429
945 Olsnes, S. *et al.* (1982) *J. Biol. Chem.* **257**, 1371
946 Woynarvski, J. M. *et al.* (1980) *Hoppe-Seyglers Z. Physiol. Chem.* **361** (10), 1525 and 1535
947 Becker, H. and Exner, J. (1980) *Z. Pflanzenphysiol.* **97**
948 Muller, J. (1962) *Ger. Offen.* DE 1, 130, 112
949 Bloksma, N. *et al.* (1982) *Planta Med.* **46**, 221
950 Kwaja, T. A. *et al.* (1980) *Experientia* **36**, 599
951 Wagner, H. *et al.* (1986) *Planta Med.* (2), 102
952 Franz, H. (1985) *Pharmazie* **40** (2), 97
953 Samuellson, G. *et al.* (1981) *Acta Pharm. Sueca* **18**, 179

954 Rentea, R. *et al.* (1981) *Lab. Invest.* **44** (1), 43
955 Stirpe, F. *et al.* (1982) *J. Biol. Chem.* **257** (22), 13271
956 Salzer, G. and Muller, H. (1978) *Prax. Klin. Pneumol.* **32** (11), 721
957 Salzer, G. and Havelec, L. (1978) *Onkologie* **1** (6), 264
958 Hassauer, W. *et al.* (1979) *Onkologie* **2** (1), 28
959 Schilling, G. *et al.* (1975) *Leibigs Ann. Chem.* **230**
960 Malakov, P. *et al.* (1985) *Phytochem.* **24** (10), 2341
961 Kartnig, T. *et al.* (1985) *J. Nat. Prod.* **48** (3), 494
962 Reuter, G. and Diehl, H. J. (1970) *Pharmazie,* **25**, 586
963 Tschesche, R. *et al.* (1980) *Phytochem.* **19**, 2783
964 Chang, C. F. and Li, C. Z. (1986) *Chung, I. Chieh Ho Tsa Chih* **6** (1), 39
965 Peng, Y. (1983) *Bull. Chin. Mat. Med.* **8**, 41
966 Xia, X. X. (1983) *J. Trad. Chin. Med.* **3**, 185
967 Duquenois, P. (1965) *Mem. Soc. Bot. Fr.* 41
968 Bate-Smith, E. C. *et al. Phytochem.* **7**, 1165
969 Guerin, J. C. and Reveillere, H. P. (1985) *Ann. Farm. Fr.* **43** (1), 77
970 Nano, G. M. *et al.* (1976) *Planta Med.* **30**, 211
971 Jork, H. and Juel, S. (1979) *Arch. Pharm.* **312**, 540
972 Juel, S. *et al.* (1976) *Arch. Pharm.* **309**, 458
973 Hoffmann, B. and Herrmann, K. (1982) *Z. Lebens. Unters. Forsch.* **174** (3), 211
974 Stefanovic, M. *et al.* (1982) *Glas. Khem. Drush. Beogr.* **47** (3), 7
975 Kaul, V. K. *et al.* (1976) *Ind. J. Pharm.* **38** (1), 21
976 Deshpande, V. H. (1968) *Tet. Lett.* 1715
977 Nomura, T. *et al.* (1983) *Planta Med.* **47**, 151
978 Kimura, Y. *et al.* (1986) *J. Nat. Prod.* **94** (4), 639
979 Swiatek, L. *et al.* (1982) *Planta Med.* **30**, 153, 12P
980 Maurer, B. and Greider, A. (1977) *Helv. Chim. Acta* **60**, 1155
981 Srivastava, K. C. and Rastogi, S. C. (1969) *Planta Med.* **17**, 189
982 Gaind, K. N. and Saini, T. S. (1968) *Ind. J. Pharm.* **30**, 233
983 Pernet, R. (1972) *Lloydia* **35**, 280
984 Brieskorn, C. H. (1983) *Phytochem.* **22** (5), 1207
985 Brieskorn, C. H. (1983) *Phytochem.* **22** (1), 187
986 Brieskorn, C. H. (1980) *Tet. Lett.* **21** (6), 1511
987 Brieskorn, C. H. and Noble, P. (1983) *Phytochem.* **22** (5) 1207
988 Mincione, E. and Iavarone, C. (1972) *Chim. Ind.* **54**, 424 and 525
989 Bajaj, A. C. and Dev, S. (1982) *Tetrahedron* **38** (19), 2949
990 Mester, L. *et al.* (1979) *Planta Med.* **37** (4), 367
991 Kodama, M. *et al.* (1975) *Tet. Lett.* **35**, 3065
992 Ruecker, G. (1972) *Arch. Pharm.* **305** (7), 486
993 Malhotra, S. C. and Ahuja, M. M. S. (1971) *Ind. J. Med. Res.* **59** (10), 1621
994 Srivastava, M. *et al.* (1984)*J. Biosci.* **6** (3), 277
995 Arora, R. B. *et al.* (1972) *Ind. J. Med. Res.* **60** (6), 929
996 Tripathi, S. N. *et al.* (1975) *Ind. J. Exp. Biol.* **13** (1), 15
997 Joseph, M. I. *et al.* (1987) *Pharmazie* **42** (2), 142

998 Hughes, R. E. *et al.* (1980) *J. Sci. Food Agric.* **31**, 1279
999 Anonymous (1982) *Vet. Hum. Toxicol.* **24**, 247
1000 Willaman, J. J. and Schubert, B. G. (1961) *Tech. Bull.* **1234**, USDA. Washington DC (via [183])
1001 Sanford, K. J. and Heinz, D. E. (1971) *Phytochem.* **10**, 1245
1002 Gottleib, O. R. (1979) *J. Ethnopharmacol.* **1**, 309
1003 Sarath-Kumara, S. J. *et al.* (1985) *J. Sci. Food. Agric.* **36** (2), 93
1004 Rasheed, A. *et al.* (1984) *Planta Med.* **50** (2), 222
1005 Forrest, J. E. *et al.* (1974) *J. Chem. Soc. Perkin Trans.* 1 (2), 205
1006 Isogai, A. *et al.* (1973) *Agric. Biol. Chem.* **37**, 198 and 1479
1007 Misra, V. *et al.* (1978) *Ind. J. Med. Res.* **67**, 482
1008 Bennett, A. *et al.* New Eng. J. Med. **290**, 110
1009 Shafkan, I. *et al.* (1977) *New Eng. J. Med.* **296**, 694
1010 Pecevski, J. *et al.* (1980) *Toxicol. Lett.* **7**, 739
1011 Miller, E. C. *et al.* (1983) *Cancer Res.* **43**, 1124
1012 Kim, *et al.* (1978) *Biochim. Biophys. Acta* **537**, 22
1013 Effertz, B. *et al.* (1979) *Z. Pflanzenphysiol.* **92**, 319
1014 Tschersche, R. in "Pharmacognosy and Phytochemistry", Ed. H. Wagner and L. Horhammer, Pub. Springer-Verlag (1971)
1015 Anand, C. L. (1971) *Nature* **233**, 496
1016 Connor, J. *et al.* (1975) *J. Pharm. Pharmacol.* **27**, 92
1017 Gabrinowicz, J. W. (1974) *Med. J. Aust.* **ii**, 306
1018 Augusti, K. T. (1976) *Curr. Sci.* **45**, 863
1019 Spare, C. G. and Virtanen, A. I. (1963) *Acta Chem. Scand.* **17**, 641
1020 Maugh, T. H. (1979) *Science* **204**, 293
1021 Dorsch, W. *et al.* (1984) *Eur. J. Pharmacol.* **107** (1), 17
1022 Dorsch, W. *et al.* (1986). 6th Int. Conf. Prostaglandins and Related Compounds. Florence, Italy. June 3rd–6th. Pub. Fondzione Giovanni Lorenzini.
1023 Liakopoulou-Kyriakides, M. *et al.* (1985) *Phytochem.* **24** (3), 600 and (7), 1593
1024 Lund, E. D. and Bryan, W. L. (1977) *J. Food Sci.* **42**, 385
1025 Shaw, P. E. and Coleman, R. L. (1971) *J. Agric. Food Chem.* **19**, 1276
1026 Natarajan, S. *et al.* (1976) *Econ. Bot.* **30**, 38
1027 Wilson, W. and Shaw, P. E. (1977) *J. Agric. Food Chem.* **25**, 211
1028 Tatum, J. H. and Berry, R. E. (1977) *Phytochem.* **16**, 1091
1029 Tsukida, K. *et al.* (1973) *Phytochem.* **12**, 2318
1030 Morita, N. *et al.* (1973) *Chem. Pharm. Bull.* **21**, 600
1031 El Moghazy, A. M. *et al.* (1980) *Fitoterapia* **5**, 237
1032 Baltassat, F. *et al.* (1985) *Plant Med. Phytother.* **18** (4), 194
1033 Guha, *et al.* (1979) *J. Nat. Prod.* **42**, 1
1034 MacLeod, A. J. *et al.* (1985) *Phytochem.* **24** (11), 2623
1035 Ashraf, M. *et al.* (1980) *Pak. J. Sci. Ind. Res.* **23** (3/4), 128
1036 Chaudhary, S. K. *et al.* (1986) *Planta Med.* (6), 462
1037 Innocenti, G. *et al.* (1976) *Planta Med.* **29**, 165
1038 Bennati, E. and Fedeli, E. (1968) *Boll. Chim. Farm.* **107**, 716
1039 Bennati, E. (1968) *Boll. Chim. Farm.* **110**, 664

References

1040 Lutomski, J. and Malek, B. (1975) *Planta Med.* **27**, 381
1041 Loehdefink, J. and Kating, H. (1974) *Planta Med.* **25**, 101
1042 Poethke, W. *et al.* (1970) *Planta Med.* **18**, 303
1043 Schilcher, H. (1968) *Z. Naturforsch.* **23B**, 1393
1044 Proliac, A. and Raynaud, J. (1986) *Pharmazie* **41** (9), 673
1045 Aoyagi, N. *et al.* (1974) *Chem. Pharm. Bull.* **22**, 1008
1046 Lutomski, J. and Wrocinski, T. (1960) *Buil. Inst. Ros. Lec.* **6**, 176
1047 Budzianowski, J. *et al.* (1985) *J. Nat. Prod.* **48** (2), 336
1048 Geraci, D. *et al.* (1978) *Immunochem.* **15**, 491
1049 Atal, C. K. *et al.* (1975) *Lloydia* **38**, 256
1050 Richard, M. L. *et al.* (1976) *J. Food Sci.* **36**, 584
1051 Raina, M. L. *et al.* (1976) *Planta Med.* **30**, 198
1052 Traxter, J. T. (1971) *J. Agric. Food Chem.* **19**, 1135
1053 Clark and Menary (1981) *Econ. Bot.* **35**, 59
1054 Hefendehl, F. W. and Murray, M. J. (1973) *Planta Med.* **23**, 101
1055 Kantarev, N. and Peicev, P. (1977) *Folia Med.* **19** (1), 41
1056 Kaul, J. L. and Trojanek (1966) *Lloydia* **29**, 25
1057 Janot, M-M. *et al.* (1962) *Bull. Soc. Chim. Fr.* 1079
1058 Gosset-Garnier, J. *et al.* (1965) *Bull. Soc. Chim. Fr.* 676
1059 Hesse, M. "Indolalkaloide in Tabellen", Pub. Springer-Verlag (1964 and 1968)
1060 Rudski, E. and Grzywaz, Z. (1977) *Dermatologia* **155** (2), 115
1061 Texier, O. *et al.* (1984) *Phytochem.* **23** (12), 2903
1062 Pourrat, H. and Pourrat, A. (1966) *Bull. Soc. Chim. Fr.* 2410
1063 Pourrat, H. *et al.* (1979) *Ann. Pharm. Fr.* **37**, 441
1064 Pourrat, H. *et al.* (1982) *Ann. Pharm. Fr.* **40**, 373
1065 Kolesnik, *et al.* (1963) *Chem. Abs.* **59**, 7856
1066 Banerji, R. *et al.* (1981) *Indian Drugs* **19**, 121
1067 Amoros, M. *et al.* (1979) *Plant. Med. Phytother.* **13**, 122
1068 Amoros, M. and Girre, R. L. (1977) *Phytochem.* **26** (3), 787
1069 Yamada, Y. *et al.* (1978) *Phytochem.* **17**, 1798
1070 Roschin, V. I. *et al.* (1985) *Khim. Prir. Soedin.* **1**, 122
1071 Zinkel, D. F. *et al.* (1972) *Phytochem.* **11**, 425 and 3387
1072 Walewska, E. and Thieme, H. (1969) *Pharmazie* **24**, 423
1073 Bolkart, K. H. *et al.* (1968) *Naturwissenschaften* **55**, 445
1074 Foder, G. B. and Colasenko, B. in "Alkaloids Vol. 3", Ed. S. W. Pelletier, Pub. John Wiley (1985)
1075 Lebedov-Kosov, V. I. (1980) *Rastit. Resur.* **16**, 403
1076 Oshio, H. and Inoye, H. (1982) *Planta Med.* **44**, 204
1077 Endo, T. *et al.* (1981) *Chem. Pharm. Bull.* **29**, 1000
1078 Maksyutina, N. P. (1972) *Farm. Z. H.* **27** (1), 59 (via Biol. Abs. 54:68742)
1079 Pailer, V. M. *et al.* (1969) *Planta Med.* **17** (2), 139
1080 Petricic, J. (1966) *Arch. Pharm. Ber. Dtsch. Pharm. Ges.* **299** (12), 1007
1081 Pagani, F. (1975) *Boll. Chim. Farm.* **114** (8), 450
1082 Costello, C. H. and Butler, C. L. (1950) *J. Am. Pharm. Ass. Sci. Ed.* **39**, 233

1083 Gross, M. *et al.* (1975) *Phytochem.* **14**, 2263
1084 Corbett, M. and Billets, S. (1975) *J. Pharm. Sci.* **64**, 1715
1085 Baer, H. in "Toxic Plants", Ed. A. D. Kinghorn, Pub. Columbia Press (1979)
1086 Wagner, H. *et al.* (1986) Abstr. Phytochem. Soc. Eur. Conf. Lausanne Switzerland 3rd–5th Sept. 1986
1087 Sick, W. W. and Shin, K. H. (1976) *Yakhak Hoe Chi.* **20** (3), 149
1088 Shin, K. H. *et al.* (1979) *Soul Taehakkyo Saengyak Opjukjip* **18**, 90
1089 Sick, W. W. *et al.* (1976) *Soul Taehakkyo Saengyak Opjukjip* **15**, 103
1090 McPherson, A. in "Toxic Plants", Ed. A. D. Kinghorn, Pub. Columbia Press (1979)
1091 Tomlinson, J. A. *et al.* (1974) *J. Gen. Virol.* **22**, 225
1092 Aron, G. M. and Irvin, J. D. (1980) *Antimicrob. Agents Chem.* **17**, 1032
1093 Ussberg, M. A. *et al.* (1977) *Ann. N.Y. Acad. Sci.* **284**, 431
1094 Woo, W. S. and Kang, S. S. (1978) Chem. Abs. 88:4750z
1095 Lewis, W. H. (1979) *J. Am. Med. Ass.* **242** (25), 2759
1096 Jizba, J. *et al.* (1971) *Tett. Let.* **18**, 1329
1097 Constantinescu, E. *et al.* (1966) *Pharmazie* **21**, 121
1098 Tanake, T. *et al.* (1986) *Chem. Pharm. Bull.* **34** (2), 656
1099 Thieme, H. and Benecke, R. (1969) *Pharmazie* **24**, 567
1100 El-Masry, S. *et al.* (1981) *Planta Med.* **41**, 61
1101 Fairbairn, J. W. and Williamson, E. M. (1978) *Phytochem.* **17**, 2087
1102 Fish, F. *et al.* (1975) *Lloydia* **38**, 268
1103 Fish, F. and Waterman, P. G. (1973) *J. Pharm. Pharmac.* **25S**, 115
1104 Thieme, H. and Winkler, H. J. (1971) *Pharmazie* **7**, 434
1105 Miller, J. N. in "Industrial Gums", Ed. R. L. Whistler, Pub. Academic Press (1973)
1106 Cordell, G. A. in "The Alkaloids Vol. XVI", Ed. R. H. F. Manske, Pub. Academic Press (1977)
1107 Oshio, H. and Inouye, H. (1982) *Planta Med.* **44**, 204
1108 Popov, S. (1978) *IUPAC Int. Symp. Chem. Nat. Prod.* **11** (2), 61 (via CA 92:59170)
1109 Ershoff, B. H. (1976) *J. Food Sci.* **41**, 949
1110 Khorana, M. L. *et al.* (1958) *Ind. J. Pharm.* **20**, 3
1111 Tomoda, M. *et al.* (1987) *Planta Med.* **53** (1), 8
1112 Gasco, A. *et al.* (1974) *Tet. Lett.* **38**, 3431
1113 Pourrat, A. *et al.* (1980) *J. Pharm. Belg.* **35** (4) 277
1114 Evans, F. J. and Schmidt, R. J. (1980) *Planta Med.* **38**, 289
1115 Tewary, J. P. and Srivasta, M. C. (1968) *J. Pharm. Sci.* **57**, 328
1116 Schabort, J. C. (1978) *Phytochem.* **17**, 1062
1117 Wagner, H. *et al.* (1980) *Planta Med.* **38**, 204
1118 Kupchan, S. M. and Streelman, D. R. (1976) *J. Org. Chem.* **41**, 3481
1119 Murae, T. *et al.* (1973) *Tetrahedron* **29**, 1515
1120 Murae, T. *et al.* (1975) *Chem. Pharm. Bull.* **23** (9), 2191
1121 Wagner, H. *et al.* (1979) *Planta Med.* **36**, 113
1122 Ohmoto, T. and Koike, K. (1983) *Chem. Pharm. Bull.* **31**, 3198

1123 Geissmann, T. (1964) *Ann. Rev. Pharmacol.* **4**, 305
1124 O'Neill, M. *et al.* (1987) *Abs. Brit. Soc. Parasit.* Meeting March 1987
1125 Bray, D. H. *et al.* (1987) *Phytother. Res.* **1** (1), 22
1126 Lyon, R. L. *et al.* (1973) *J. Pharm. Sci.* **62**, 218
1127 Adolf, A. and Hecker, E. (1980) *Tet. Lett.* **21**, 2887
1128 Segall, H. J. and Krick, T. P. (1979) *Toxicol. Lett.* **4**, 193
1129 Bradbury, R. B. and Culvenor, C. C. J. (1954) *Aust. J. Chem.* **7**, 378
1130 Schoental, R. (1968) *Cancer Res.* **28**, 2237
1131 Marczal, G. (1963) *Herba Hung.* **2**, 343
1132 Henning, W. (1981) *Lebens. Unters. Forsch.* **173**, 1
1133 Bamford, D. S. *et al.* (1970) *Br. J. Pharmacol.* **40** (1), 161P
1134 Beckett, A. *et al.* (1954) *J. Pharm. Pharmacol.* **6**, 785
1135 Burn, J. H. and Withell, E. R. (1941) *Lancet* **2**, 1
1136 Guggolz, J. *et al.* (1961) *Agric. Food Chem.* **9** (4), 331
1137 Kattaev, N. S. *et al.* (1972) *Khim. Prir. Soed.* **6**, 806
1138 Dewick, P. (1977) *Phytochem.* **16**, 93
1139 Sachse, J. (1974) *J. Chrom.* **96** (1), 123
1140 Yoshihara, T. *et al.* (1977) *Agric. Biol. Chem.* **41** (9), 1679
1141 Lagarias, J. C. *et al.* (1979) *J. Nat. Prod.* **42**, 220 and 663
1142 Hilp, K. *et al.* (1975) *Arch. Pharm.* **308**, 429
1143 Fujise, Y. *et al.* (1965) *Chem. Pharm. Bull.* **13**, 93
1144 Dedio, I. and Kozlowski, J. (1977) *Acta Pol. Pharm.* **34**, 97
1145 Horejsi, V. and Kocourek, J. (1978) *Biochim. Biophys. Acta* **538**
1146 Koster, J. *et al.* (1983) Planta Med. **48**, 131
1147 Kartnig, T. *et al.* (1985) *Pharm. Acta Helv.* **60** (9/10), 253
1148 Scholz, R. and Rumpler, H. (1986) *Planta Med.* (6), 58P
1149 Williams, V. *et al.* (1983) *Phytochem.* **22**, 569
1150 Zwaving, J. H. (1972) *Planta Med.* **21**, 254
1151 Zwaving, J. H. (1974) *Pharm. Weekbl.* **109**, 1169
1152 Oshio, H. *et al.* (1974) *Chem. Pharm. Bull.* **22**, 823
1153 Van Os, F. H. L. (1976) *Pharmacol.* **14** (Suppl. 1), 7
1154 Tsuboi, *et al.* (1977) *Chem. Pharm. Bull.* **25**, 2708
1155 Kashiwada, Y. *et al.* (1984) *Chem. Pharm. Bull.* **32** (9), 3461
1156 Nonaka, G. *et al.* (1977) *Chem. Pharm. Bull.* **25**, 2300
1157 Freidrich, H. and Holhe, J. (1966) *Arch. Pharm.* **299**, 857
1158 Fairbairn, J. W. (1976) *Pharmacol.* **14** (Suppl. 1), 48
1159 Koedan, A. and Gijbels, M. J. M. (1978) *Z. Naturforsch.* **33C**, 144
1160 Litvinenko, V. I. *et al.* (1970) *Planta Med.* **18**, 243
1161 Brieskorn, C. H. and Michel, H. (1968) *Tet. Lett.* **30**, 3447
1162 Houlihan, C. M. *et al.* (1985) *J. Am. Oil. Chem. Soc.* **62** (1), 96
1163 Brieskorn, C. H. and Domling, H. J. (1969) *Z. Lebens. Unters. Forsch.* **14**, 10
1164 Brieskorn, C. H. and Zweyrohn, G. (1970) *Pharmazie* **25**, 488
1165 Tattje, D. H. E. (1970) *Pharm. Weekbl.* **105**, 1241
1166 Novak, I. *et al.* (1965) *Pharmazie* **20**, 738
1168 Varga, E. *et al.* (1976) *Fitoterapia* **47**, 107
1169 Rozsa, Z. *et al.* (1980) *Planta Med.* **39**, 218

1170 Novak, I. *et al.* (1967) *Planta Med.* **15**, 132
1171 Reisch, J. *et al.* (1976) *Phytochem.* **15**, 240
1172 Grundon, M. F. in "The Alkaloids Vol. 11", Pub. Royal Soc. Chem. (1981)
1173 Reisch, J. *et al.* (1967) *Pharmazie* **22**, 220 and (1970) **25**, 435
1174 Van Duuren, B. L. *et al.* (1971) *J. Natl. Cancer Inst.* **46**, 1039
1175 Robbins, R. C. (1967) *J. Atheroscler. Res.* **7**, 3
1176 Krolikowska, M. and Wolbis, M. (1979) *Acta Pol. Pharm.* **36**, 469
1177 Zoz *et al.* (1976) *Rastit. Resur.* **12** (3), 411 (via CA 85:174257)
1178 Tamas, M. *et al.* (1981) *Clujul. Med.* **54** (1), 73 (via CA 96:149036)
1179 Franck, H. P. (1975) *Deutch. Apoth. Ztg.* **115**, 1206
1180 "The Chemistry of Lignans", Ed. C. B. S. Rao, Pub. Andhra University Press (1978) Andhra Pradesh, India
1181 Caldes, G. *et al.* (1981) *J. Gen. Appl. Microbiol.* **27**, 157
1182 Xu, S. X. (1986) *Chung Yao Tung Pao* **11** (2), 42 (via Datastar)
1183 Dhingra, V. K. *et al.* (1975) *Ind. J. Chem.* **13**, 339
1184 Duquenois, P. (1972) *Bull. Soc. Pharm. Strasbourg* **15**, 149
1185 Brieskorn, C. H. and Bichele, W. (1971) *Deutsch Apoth. Ztg.* **111**, 141
1186 Murko, D. *et al.* (1974) *Planta Med.* **25**, 295
1187 Francke, W. (1982) *Econ. Bot.* **36** (2), 163
1188 Adams, D. R. *et al.* (1975) *Phytochem.* **14**, 1459
1189 Patnikar, S. K. and Naik, C. G. (1975) *Tet. Lett.* **15**, 1293
1190 Demole, D. R. *et al.* (1976) *Helv. Chim. Acta* **59**, 737
1191 Elmunajied, D. T. *et al.* (1965) *Phytochem.* **4** (4), 587
1192 Tschesche, R. *et al.* (1969) *Chem. Ber.* **102**, 1253
1193 Thurmon, F. M. (1942) *New Eng. J. Med.* **227** (4), 128
1194 Sethi, M. L. *et al.* (1976) *Phytochem.* **15**, 1773
1195 Segelman, A. B. *et al.* (1976) *J. Am. Med. Ass.* **236**, 477
1196 Chowdhury, B. K. *et al.* (1976) *Phytochem.* **15**, 1803
1197 Borchet, P. *et al.* (1973) *Cancer Res.* **33**, 575
1198 Hartwell, J. L. *et al.* (1953) *J. Chem. Soc.* **75**, 235
1199 Haensel, R. *et al.* (1964) *Planta Med.* **12**, 169
1200 Wagner, H. and Flachsbarth, H. (1981) Planta Med. **41**, 244
1201 Wagner, H. *et al.* (1984) *Arzneim. Forsch.* **34**, 659
1202 Kimura, Y. *et al.* (1985) *Planta Med.* **51**, 132
1203 Kimura, Y. *et al.* (1984) *Planta Med.* **50**, 290
1204 Kubo, M. *et al.* (1984) *Chem. Pharm. Bull.* **32** (7), 2724
1205 Takido, M. *et al.* (1979) Yakugaku Zasshi **99** (4), 443–444
1206 Nicollier, G. F. *et al.* (1981) *J. Agric. Food Chem.* **29**, 1179
1207 Yagmai, M. S. and Benson, G. G. (1979) *J. Nat. Prod.* **42** (2), 229
1208 Kimura, Y. *et al.* (1987) *Phytother. Res.* **1** (1), 48
1209 Kojima, H. *et al.* (1987) *Phytochem.* **26** (4), 1107
1210 Shibata, S. in "Progress in Phytochemistry Vol. 6", Ed. Reinhold *et al.*, Pub. Pergamon Press (1980)
1211 Shoji, J. *et al.* (1971) *Yakugaku Zasshi* **91**, 198
1212 Sakuma, S. *et al.* (1975) *Abs. 95th Ann. Meet. Pharm. Soc. Japan* **2**, 247
1213 Corner, J. J. *et al.* (1962) *Phytochem.* **1**, 73

1214 Fairbairn, J. W. (1964) *Lloydia* **27**, 79

1215 Fairbairn, J. W. and Shrestha, A. B. (1967) *Lloydia* **30**, 67

1216 Lemli, J. and Cuveele, J. (1975) *Phytochem.* **14**, 1397P

1217 Christ, B. *et al.* (1978) *Arzneim. Forsch.* **28**, 225

1218 Lemli, J. *et al.* (1981) *Planta Med.* **43**, 11

1219 Martinod, P. *et al. Politecnica* **4** (1), 34 (via CA 92:37745)

1220 Kuroda, K. and Tagaki, K. (1968) *Nature* **220**, 707

1221 Kuroda, K. and Kaku, T. (1969) *Life Sci.* **8** (1), 151

1222 Hill, R. K. in "The Alkaloids Vol. 2", Ed. S. W. Pelletier, Pub. John Wiley (1984)

1223 Kuroda, K. and Tagaki, K. (1969) *Arch. Int. Pharmacodyn* **178** (2), 382 and 392

1224 Kuroda, K. *et al.* (1976) *Cancer Res.* **36**, 1900

1225 Ghosh, P. *et al.* (1977) *Lloydia* **40** (4), 636

1226 Polonsky, J. *et al.* (1978) *Experientia* **34** (9), 1122

1227 Plowman, T. (1969) *Econ. Bot.* **23**, 2

1228 Barnes, C. S. and Loder, J. W. (1962) *Aust. J. Chem.* **15**, 322

1229 Asakawa, Y. and Takemoto, T. (1979) *Experientia* **35**, 1429

1230 Kifakh, S. Y. and Blinova, K. F. (1984) *Khim. Prir. Soed.* **5**, 658

1231 Furuta, T. *et al.* (1986) *Phytochem.* **25** (2), 517

1232 Higuchi, R. *et al.* (1987) *Phytochem.* **26** (1), 229

1233 Labriola, R. A. and Denlofeu, V. (1969) *Experientia* **25**, 124

1234 Lallouette, P. *et al.* (1967) *C.R.A.S. Paris D* **265**, 582

1235 Topping, D. L. *et al.* (1980) *Proc. Nutr. Soc. Aust.* **5**, 195

1236 Janeczko, Z. (1980) *Acta Polon. Pharm.* **37**, 559

1237 Tamano, M. and Koketsu, J. (1982) *Agric. Biol. Chem.* **46**, 1913

1238 Vostrowsky, O. *et al.* (1984) *Z. Lebens. Unters. Forsch.* **179**, 125

1239 Hurabielle, H. *et al.* (1982) *Planta Med.* **45**, 55

1240 Hëfer, O. and Nikiforov, A. (1982) *J. Nat. Prod.* **45** (4), 455

1241 Nieschultz, O. and Schmersahl, P. (1968) *Arzneim. Forsch.* **18** (10), 1330

1242 Murray, M. J. *et al.* (1972) *Crop Sci.* **12**, 723

1243 Subramanian, S. S. and Nair, A. G. R. (1972) *Phytochem.* **11**, 452

1244 Afifi-Yazar, F. and Sticher, O. (1980) *Helv. Chim. Acta* **63**, 1905

1245 Sticher, O. *et al.* (1982) *Planta Med.* **45**, 159

1246 Wojcik, E. (1981) *Acta Polon. Pharm.* **38**, 621

1247 Karawya, M. S. *et al.* (1973) *Planta Med.* **23**, 213

1248 Garcia-Casado, P. *et al.* (1977) *Pharm. Acta Helv.* **52**, 218

1249 British Pharmaceutical Codex 11th Ed. Pub. Pharmaceutical Society Press (1979) UK

1250 Vega, F. A. (1976) *An. Rev. Acad. Farm.* **42** (1), 81

1251 Hakim, F. S. and Evans, F. J. (1976) *Pharm. Acta Helv.* **52**, 117

1252 Mathic, C. and Ourrison, G. (1964) *Phytochem.* **3**, 115, 133, 377, 379

1253 Holzl, J. and Ostrowski, E. (1986) *Planta Med.* **6**, 62P

1254 Freytag, W. E. (1984) *Deutsch. Apoth. Ztg.* **124** (46), 2383

1255 Kitanov, G. *et al.* (1984) *Khim. Prir. Soed.* **2**, 269

1256 Suzuki, O. *et al.* (1984) *Planta Med.* **3**, 272

1257 Muldner, H. and Zoller, M. (1984) *Arneim. Forsch.* **34** II (8), 918

1258 Huneck, S. (1968) *Tetrahedron* **19**, 479

1259 Ayuga, C. *et al.* (1985) *An. R. Acad. Farm* **51** (2), 321

1260 Vichnanova, S. A. *et al.* (1973) *Planta Med.* (Suppl.), 185

1261 Croft, S. *et al.* (1985) *Ann. Trop. Med. Parasitol.* **79** (6), 651

1262 Wagner, H. *et al.* (1986) Abstr. Phytochem. Soc. Eur. Lausanne 3–5th Sept. 1986 43P

1263 Lewis, Y. S. *et al.* (1960) *Food Sci.* **9**, 405 and (1961) **10**, 49

1264 Lee, P. L. *et al.* (1975) *J. Agric. Food Chem.* **23**, 1195

1265 Holopainen, M. (1968) *Planta Med.* (6), 20P

1266 Schearer, W. R. (1984) *J. Nat. Prod.* **47** (6), 964

1267 Ognyanov, I. and Tochorova, M. (1983) *Planta Med.* **48**, 181

1268 Nano, G. M. *et al.* (1983) *Fitoterapia* (4), 135

1269 Banthorpe, D. V. *et al.* (1973) Planta Med. **23**, 64

1270 Von Rudloff (1961) *Can. J. Chem.* **39**, 1200

1271 Beuscher, N. and Kopanski, L. (1986) *Planta Med.* (6), 111P

1272 Vomel, T. (1985) *Arzneim. Forsch.* **35** II (9), 1437

1273 Miguel, J. D. (1976) *J. Agric. Food Chem.* **24**, 833

1274 Svendsen, A. B. and Karlsen, J. (1966) *Planta Med.* **14**, 376

1275 Montes, G. M. *et al.* (1981) *An. Real Acad. Farm.* **47** (3), 285

1276 Van den Broucke, C. O. *et al.* (1983) *Pharm. Weekbl.* **5** (1), 9

1277 Harkiss, K. J. and Linley, P. (1979) *Planta Med.* **35**, 61

1278 Sullivan, G. (1968) *J. Agric. Food Chem.* **30** (3), 609

1279 Lund, K. and Rimpler, H. (1985) *Deutsche Apoth. Ztg.* **125** (3), 105

1280 Anderson, D. M. W. and Bridgeman, M. M. E. (1985) *Phytochem.* **24** (10), 2301

1281 Fang, S. *et al.* (1982), *You Ji Hua Xue* **2**, 26

1282 Whistler, R. L. *et al.* (1976) *Adv. Carbohydr. Chem. Biochem.* **32**, 235

1283 Osswald, H. (1968) *Arzneim. Forsch.* **18**, 1495

1284 Polonski, J. (1985) *Prog. Chem. Org. Nat. Prod.* **47**, 221

1285 Casinovi, C. G. *et al.* (1964) *Tet. Lett.* 3991

1286 Varga, E. *et al.* (1980) *Planta Med.* **40**, 33

1287 Ohmoto, T. *et al.* (1981) *Chem. Pharm. Bull.* **29**, 390

1288. Ravindranath, V. and Satyanarayana, M. N. (1980) *Phytochem.* **19**, 2031

1289 Krishnamurthy, N. *et al.* (1976) *Trop. Sci.* **18**, 37

1290 Srimal, R. C. and Dhawan, C. N. (1973) *J. Pharm. Pharmacol.* **25**, 447

1291 Nagarajan, K. and Arya, V. P. (1982) *J. Sci. Ind. Res.* **41**, 232

1292 Wagner, H. *et al.* (1986) 6th Int. Conf. Prostaglandins and Related Compounds. Florence, Italy. June 3rd–6th. Pub. Fondzione Giovanni Lorenzini.

1293 Kiso, Y. *et al.* (1983) *Planta Med.* **49**, 185

1294 Garg, S. K. (1974) *Planta Med.* **26**, 225

1295 Basu, A. B. (1971) *Ind. J. Pharm.* **33**, 131

1296 Dhar, M. L. *et al.* (1968) *Ind. J. Exp. Biol.* **6**, 232

1297 Marker, R. E. *et al.* (1940) *J. Chem. Soc.* **60**, 2620

1298 Costello, C. H. and Lynn, E. V. (1950) *J. Am. Pharm. Ass.* **39**, 117

1299 Jahodar, L. *et al.* (1978) *Pharmazie* 33 (8), 536
1300 Jahodar, L. *et al.* (1981) *Pharmazie* 36 (2), 294
1301 Denford, K. E. (1973) *Experientia* 29, 939
1302 Jahodar, L. *et al.* (1985) *Cesk. Farm.* 34 (5), 174
1303 Frohne, D. (1970) *Planta Med.* 18, 1
1304 Hendriks, H. *et al.* (1981) *Planta Med.* 42 (1), 62
1305 Hazelhoff, B. *et al.* (1979) *Pharm. Weekbl. Sci. Ed.* 1, 71
1306 Hansel, V. R. and Schultz, J. (1982) *Deutsch. Apoth. Ztg.* 122 (5), 215
1307 Hendricks, H. and Bruins, A. B. (1980) *J. Chrom.* 190, 321
1308 Hendricks, R. *et al.* (1977) *Phytochem.* 16, 1853
1309 Bos, R. *et al.* (1983) *Phytochem.* 22 (6), 1505
1310 Thies, P. W. and Funke, S. (1966) *Tet. Lett.* 11, 1155
1311 Van Meer, J. H. and Labadine, R. P. (1981) *J. Chrom.* 205 (1), 206
1312 Popov, S. *et al.* (1974) *Phytochem.* 13, 2815
1313 Funke, E. D. and Friedrich, H. (1975) *Planta Med.* 28, 215
1314 Torssell, K. and Wahlberg, K. (1966) *Tet. Lett.* 4, 445
1315 Gross, D. *et al.* (1971) *Arch. Pharm.* 304, 19
1316 Bounthanh, C. *et al.* (1981) *Planta Med.* 41, 21
1317 Becker, H. *et al.* (1983) *Planta Med.* 49 (1), 64
1318 Eickstedt, K. W. von (1969) *Arzneim. Forsch.* 19, 995
1319 Veith, J. *et al.* (1986) *Planta Med.* (3), 179
1320 Hendriks, H. *et al.* (1985) *Planta Med.* (3), 28
1321 Reidel, E. *et al.* (1982) *Planta Med.* 46, 219
1322 Braun, R. *et al.* (1982) *Deutsche Apoth. Ztg.* 122, 1109
1323 Bounthanh, C. *et al.* (1983) *Planta Med.* 49, 138
1324 Braun, R. *et al.* (1984) *Planta Med.* 1
1325 Leathwood, P. D. and Chauffard, F. (1983) *J. Psychiatr. Res.* 17 (2), 115
1326 Leathwood, P. D. *et al.* (1982) *Pharmacol. Biochem. Behav.* 17, 65
1327 McIlroy, R. J. in "The Plant Glycosides", Pub. Arnold (1951) London
1328 Farnsworth, N. R. (1968) *Lloydia* 246
1329 Nahrstedt, A. *et al.* (1981) *Planta Med.* 42 (4), 313
1330 King, L. A. *et al.* (1985) *Hum. Toxicol.* 4 (4), 355
1331 Papanov, G. Y. and Malakov, P. Y. (1981) *Z. Naturforsch. (B)* 36, 112
1332 Su, K. L. *et al.* (1983) *Lloydia* 36, 72 and 80
1333 Odinstsova, N. V. (1960) *Farmakol. i Toxicol.* 23, 132 (via CA 54:25303)
1334 Gupta, K. R. and Niranjan, G. S. (1982) *Planta Med.* 46, 240
1335 Markham, K. R. *et al.* (1970) *Phytochem.* 9, 2359
1336 Beuscher, N. and Kopanski, L. (1985) *Planta Med.* 51, 381
1337 Jana, M. and Raynaud, J. (1971) *Plant. Med. Phytother.* 5, 301
1338 Kawai, M. and Matsuura, T. (1970) *Tetrahedron* 26, 1743
1339 Yamaguchi, H. *et al.* (1974) *Yakugaku Zasshi* 94, 1115
1340 Freidrich, H. and Kruger, N. (1974) *Planta Med.* 26, 327
1341 Bernard, P. *et al. J. Pharm. Belg.* 26, 661
1342 Messerschmidt, W. (1967) *Arch. Pharm.* 300, 550
1343 Messerschmidt, W. (1968) *Arzneim. Forsch.* 18, 1618

1344 Freidrich, H. and Kruger, N. (1974) *Planta Med.* **25**, 138
1345 Sticher, O. *et al.* (1971) *Deutsche Apoth. Ztg.* **111**, 1795
1346 Marco, J. L. *et al. Phytochem.* **21** (10), 2567
1347 Bruno, M. *et al.* (1985) *Phytochem.* **24** (11), 2597
1348 Tschesche, R. and Struckmeyer, K. (1976) *Chem. Ber.* **109**, 2901
1349 Gupta, G. S. and Behari, M. (1972) *J. Ind. Chem. Soc.* **49**, 317
1350 Bertelli, D. J. and Crabtree, J. H. (1968) *Tetrahedron* **24**, 2079
1351 Vostrowski, O. *et al.* (1981) *Z. Naturforsch. (C)* **36** (5/6), 369
1352 Zakirov, S. K. *et al.* (1976) *Khim. Prir. Soedin.* **4**, 548
1353 Akhmedov, I. S. *et al.* (1970) *Khim. Prir. Soedin.* **6**, 691
1354 Beauhaire, J. and Fourrey, J-L. (1982) *J. Chem. Soc. Perk. Trans.* 861
1355 Schneider, Von G. and Mielke, B. (1979) *Deutsche Apoth. Ztg.* **119** (25), 977
1356 Beauhaire, J. *et al.* (1981) *Tet. Lett.* **22** (24), 2269
1357 Kasymov, S. Z. *et al.* (1979) *Khim. Prir. Soed.* **5**, 658
1358 Greger, H. (1978) *Phytochem.* **17**, 806
1359 Hoffman, B. and Herrmann, K. (1982) *Z. Lebens. Unters. Forsch.* **174** (3), 211
1360 Swiatek, L. and Dombrowicz, E. (1984) *Farm. Pol.* **40** (12), 729
1361 Dermanovic, S. *et al.* (1976) *Glas, Hem. Drus.* **41**, 287 (via CA 87:98796h)
1362 Baumann, I. C. *et al.* (1975) *Z. Allg. Med.* **51** (17), 784
1363 Del Castillo, J. *et al.* (1975) *Nature* **253**, 365
1364 Kinloch, J. D. (1971) *Practitioner* **206**, 44
1365 Stahl, E. and Gerard, D. (1983) *Z. Lebens. Unters. Forsch.* **176** (1), 1
1366 Miller, F. M. and Chow, L. M. (1954) *J. Am. Chem. Soc.* **76**, 1353
1367 Verzár-Petri, G. *et al.* (1979) *Herba Hung.* **18** (2), 83
1368 Falk, A. J. *et al.* (1974) *Lloydia* **37**, 598
1369 Chandler, R. F. *et al.* (1982) *Econ. Bot.* **36** (2), 203
1370 Cuong, B. N. *et al.* (1979) *Phytochem.* **18**, 331
1371 Smolenski, S. J. *et al.* (1967) *Lloydia* **30**, 144
1372 Falk, A. J. *et al.* (1975) *J. Pharm. Sci.* **64**, 1838
1373 Midiwo, J. O. and Runkunga, G. M. (1985) *Phytochem.* **24** (6), 1390
1374 Fairbairn, J. W. and El Muhtadi, F. J. (1972) *Phytochem.* **11**, 263
1375 Mujumdar, R. B. *et al.* (1972) *Ind. J. Chem.* **10**, 677
1376 Vohora and Kumar (1971) *Planta Med.* **20**, 100
1377 Clark, J. T. *et al. Science* **225**, 847
1378 Buffum, J. (1982) *J. Psychoactive Drugs* **17**, 131
1379 Shiobara, Y. *et al.* (1985) *Phytochem.* **24** (11), 2629
1380 Hikino, H. *et al.* (1970) *Chem. Pharm. Bull.* **18**, 752
1381 Matthes, H. W. D. *et al.* (1980) *Phytochem.* **19**, 2643

Index of Botanical Synonyms, Local Names and Related Species

Index of Botanical Names

Index of Plant Names